FOURTH EDITION

EVALUATING THE
HEALTHCARE
SYSTEM

FOURTH EDITION

EVALUATING THE

HEALTHCARE

SYSTEM

Effectiveness, Efficiency, and Equity

Charles E. Begley | David R. Lairson | Robert O. Morgan

Paul J. Rowan | Rajesh Balkrishnan, contributing author

HAP

AUPHA

Health Administration Press, Chicago, Illinois

Association of University Programs in Health Administration,
Arlington, Virginia

Your board, staff, or clients may also benefit from this book's insight. For more information on quantity discounts, contact the Health Administration Press Marketing Manager at (312) 424–9470.

Library of Congress Cataloging-in-Publication Data

Begley, Charles E., 1947-
  Evaluating the healthcare system : effectiveness, efficiency, and equity / authored by Charles E. Begley, David Lairson, and Robert O. Morgan. — Fourth edition.
    pages cm
  ISBN 978-1-56793-523-3 (alk. paper)
  1. Medical care—United States—Evaluation. 2. Medical care—Research—United States. 3. Medical policy—United States—Evaluation. I. Lairson, David, 1948- II. Morgan, Robert O. III. Title.
  RA399.A3E95 2013
  362.1072—dc23
                                2012041896

The paper used in this publication meets the minimum requirements of American National Standard for Information Sciences—Permanence of Paper for Printed Library Materials, ANSI Z39.48-1984. ♾™

Acquisitions editor: Carrie McDonald; Project manager: Jennifer Seibert; Cover designer: Scott Miller; Layout: PerfecType

Found an error or a typo? We want to know! Please e-mail it to hapbooks@ache.org, and put "Book Error" in the subject line.

For photocopying and copyright information, please contact Copyright Clearance Center at www.copyright.com or at (978) 750–8400.

Health Administration Press
A division of the Foundation of the American
    College of Healthcare Executives
One North Franklin Street, Suite 1700
Chicago, IL 60606–3529
(312) 424–2800

Association of University Programs
    in Health Administration
2000 North 14th Street
Suite 780
Arlington, VA 22201
(703) 894–0940

BRIEF CONTENTS

DETAILED CONTENTS

PREFACE

This book defines the three broad perspectives of health services research—effectiveness, efficiency, and equity—and illustrates their application in the evaluation of health services, systems, and policies. The nature and scope of health services research are described in the context of a model of health that recognizes healthcare, behavioral, and environmental determinants. The continuum of personal and community-based health services addressed by health services research is defined, as are the different levels of analysis. A brief history of health services delivery, research, and policy in the United States is presented along with an international overview.

The text presents the conceptual frameworks, definitions, and methods of each perspective and follows up with discussions of current policies and programs addressing each perspective and their performance. The book ends by relating health services research to the principal aims of policy analysis; the case study in Chapter 9 applies and integrates the three perspectives of health services research in the evaluation of a recent policy change concerning disparities in breast cancer screening and early diagnosis.

This book lends itself to any program that trains students how to assess the effectiveness, efficiency, or equity of health services and formulate and evaluate policies designed to improve health services delivery. The primary audiences for the book are practicing professionals and graduate students in public health, health administration, and the healthcare professions as well as federal, state, and local policymakers and program planners charged with the design and conduct of policy-relevant health services research. Professionals and students in medical sociology, the behavioral sciences, and public administration interested in conducting applied or policy-oriented health and health services research will also find the book of considerable interest. We developed and applied the perspective presented in the book in a course we have offered to masters and doctoral students in public health since 1986.

Revisions to this edition draw on a growing body of research on the social, economic, behavioral, and health services determinants of clinical and population health and explore the distinct and complementary roles of personal health services, community-based public health services, and public policy in improving the health of individuals and communities. Chapter 1 provides an updated, integrative framework of the contributions of health services research to describing and evaluating the performance of health services and systems with respect to the objectives of effectiveness, efficiency, and equity. Many areas in the book have been updated and refined, including discussion on the evolving nature and focus of health services research, the three perspectives of health services research and their relationship to other methods of inquiry, the levels of health services research analysis, the objectives and practices of policy analysis, and the international perspective on health services research and policy. The historical summary of health services research and delivery in the United States also has been updated to include discussion on the Patient Protection and Affordable Care Act (ACA).

As in previous editions, Chapters 2, 4, and 6 introduce the objectives, concepts, and methods of effectiveness, efficiency, and equity research, respectively, while Chapters 3, 5, and 7 review the policy strategies that have emerged to accomplish these objectives and the criteria and evidence used to measure their success. The effectiveness chapters (2 and 3) introduce and apply a conceptual framework that integrates methods for assessing the effectiveness of medical and nonmedical interventions from the population and clinical perspectives. The Donabedian structure/process/outcome model is retained as the prevailing analysis model, but additional models are reviewed, including the Glasgow RE-AIM model, and interrelationships among these models are reviewed. A new focus emphasizes the strengths and weaknesses of published effectiveness analyses, noting the nature of the sampled population, the nature of the data analyzed, and the wide range of effectiveness study designs. As in the previous edition, Chapter 3 reviews ways in which policy and program efforts might be effective for sustaining and improving health and ways that policy efforts can be evaluated using population-wide indicators as benchmarks for outcomes.

The efficiency discussion (Chapters 4 and 5) examines the concepts of production and allocation efficiency and major findings regarding the performance of the US and other countries' healthcare systems with respect to these objectives. Updated material on the cost, financing, and level of efficiency of the US healthcare system relative to other major industrial countries is included. Findings from the Oregon policy experiment, which used a lottery system to assign eligibility for enrollment in a limited number of Medicaid slots, highlight recent research on the benefits of insurance coverage for low-income individuals. The chapter discusses aspects of the ACA that address cost control and the efficiency of healthcare delivery, provides updated information on historical changes to the structure of the health services system in the United States, and explains how failure to address efficiency and equity concerns led to the development of the ACA in 2009. The ACA is contrasted with Enthoven's model for a universal health insurance system based on managed competition. Pay for performance, accountable care organizations, and medical homes are introduced as new payment and service delivery models designed to improve the efficiency and quality of the health services delivery system in the United States.

Chapters 6 and 7 introduce a conceptual framework grounded in emerging and expanded theoretical dimensions of deliberative, distributive, and social justice and use it to assess the progress of the US health services system in achieving equity along each of these dimensions. All of the material and references have been updated, and a discussion of the equity objectives of the ACA has been incorporated. The conceptual framework section has been revised to more prominently discuss the historical role of distributive justice as a paradigm for assessing equity in health services research. The study design section now includes a brief discussion of the role of nonrandomized data and designs and references methods that have been developed to address issues arising from their use. The organization discussion in the section on distributive justice has been updated to reflect infrastructure changes, and the financing discussion has been updated to reflect the coverage changes introduced by the ACA. The section on at-risk populations has been expanded to reflect recent literature on health equity disparities related to predisposing, enabling, and need-related characteristics. The section on realized access has been revised to emphasize the mutable factors shown to affect access and explain disparities (e.g., insurance, education).

Chapters 8 and 9 describe the interrelationships between the objectives, concepts, and methods of effectiveness, efficiency, and equity research and the objectives and principles of policy analysis in formulating and evaluating health policy. A new section in Chapter 8 discusses the stages of the policymaking process and the factors that influence it. Existing material on the roles that policy analysts can, do, and should play in the policymaking process has been updated, as has the section on the challenges and limitations of applying health services research in policy analysis. Chapter 9 presents a new case study illustrating the kinds of information and analyses involved in applying health services research in an evaluation of a policy change. The case is concerned with determining the outcomes of introducing Medicaid coverage for the National Breast and Cervical Cancer Early Detection Program. The major objectives and features of this government program are described, and its implementation in Texas is summarized. The chapter illustrates policy analysis by describing and evaluating key elements of the Medicaid change.

This book makes unique contributions to the field of health services research: It (1) presents and applies an integrative framework for defining health services research as a field of study involving the application of concepts and methods of effectiveness, efficiency, and equity in evaluating health policies and programs; (2) reviews and integrates the conceptual, methodological, and empirical contributions of health services research to addressing these issues; and (3) illustrates how the perspectives and methods of effectiveness, efficiency, and equity research can be used to anticipate and pose relevant questions to inform current and future health policy debates.

Charles E. Begley
David R. Lairson
Robert O. Morgan
Paul J. Rowan

ACKNOWLEDGMENTS

The authors gratefully acknowledge the thoughtful and constructive comments provided by the Health Administration Press reviewers. We want to extend a particular thank-you to our former colleague Lu Ann Aday for her major contribution to earlier editions of the text and for generously offering her time to edit early versions of this edition. We also want to acknowledge our former colleague and coauthor Carl H. Slater, MD, for his role in establishing the foundation for the effectiveness chapters in the first and second editions.

Special thanks go to Imelda Garcia, director, Texas Department of State Health Services, Bureau of Community Health, and her staff for supplying the Texas Breast and Cervical Cancer Services Program data for the case study.

We also gratefully acknowledge our graduate students Jinhai Huo, Tong Han Chung, and Bumyang Kim for contributing work to Chapters 4, 5, and 9 and especially Janki Panchal for locating and compiling sources for the entire manuscript and for identifying, learning, and effectively using software to manage the references.

We are grateful for the supportive environment at the University of Texas School of Public Health, which made it possible for us to write the book as a routine part of our faculty roles and responsibilities and to obtain the administrative support that we received for this project from our secretaries, Sherri Curry and Regina Fisher.

Finally, we owe a special debt to the students in our course on health services delivery and performance throughout the years who stimulated and challenged us to stay up to date on current policies and programs, revise and sharpen the ideas put forth in this book, and keep up with the changing field of health services research. All of us feel that our understanding of the concepts of effectiveness, efficiency, and equity has been broadened and deepened in the process of writing this edition. Our hope is that those who read it will be similarly rewarded.

INTRODUCTION TO HEALTH SERVICES RESEARCH AND POLICY ANALYSIS

Chapter Highlights

1. *Health services research (HSR)* produces evidence of the performance of personal and community-based health services and systems, and *policy analysis* applies this evidence to define policy problems and evaluate possible solutions.
2. HSR provides frameworks, criteria, measures, and methods for evaluating health services, systems, and policies from three major perspectives: effectiveness, efficiency, and equity.
3. *Effectiveness* examines the degree to which health services preserve or improve the health of patients and populations. *Efficiency* evaluates the relationship between health outcomes and the resources required to produce them. *Equity* concerns fair distribution of health and health services.

Introduction

The Institute of Medicine (IOM 1995) defines HSR as a basic and applied field that "examines the use, costs, quality, accessibility, delivery, organization, financing, and outcomes of health care services to increase knowledge and understanding of the structure, processes, and effects of health services for individuals and populations." Health policy analysis has been defined as "the process of assessing, and deciding among, alternatives based on their usefulness in satisfying one or more goals or values" (Munger 2000). Because the aims of HSR and policy analysis overlap, it is useful to examine how these two fields can be integrated in practice. This chapter introduces the fields of HSR and policy analysis and presents a framework for integration. The chapters that follow present HSR concepts and methods for assessing the effectiveness, efficiency, and equity of health services and systems. The final chapters of the book detail principles and practices for applying HSR in policy analysis and include a case study illustrating their application.

Overview of Health Services Research

Objectives and Focus

The IOM definition acknowledges that HSR contributes to basic and applied research and concerns the study of health services that affect the health of individuals and populations. In 2000, an Academy for Health Services Research and Health Policy committee clarified the role of HSR as "the multidisciplinary field of scientific investigation that studies how social factors, financing systems, organizational structures and processes, health technologies, and personal behaviors affect access to health services, the quality and cost of health services, and ultimately our health and well-being. Research may focus on individuals, families, organizations, institutions, communities, and populations" (Lohr and Steinwachs 2002). The population health focus was reinforced in 2002 when the National Information Center on Health Services Research and Health Care Technology noted that "the goal of HSR is to provide information that will eventually lead to improvements in the health of the citizenry" (NICHSR 2007).

In 2007, AcademyHealth, the organization formed to represent the field of HSR, conducted a series of activities focusing on the future HSR workforce. In an editorial summarizing the discussions, Colby and Baker (2009) noted the continuing "flexible and evolving foci and boundaries of the field driven by the push of intellectual progress as well as the pull of societal changes and policy events," predicting that future demand for HSR "will depend on its ability to continue to answer important questions that matter to both public and private decision makers." They reinforced the policy application of HSR, quoting a previous challenge to the field by John Eisenberg, former director of the Agency for Healthcare Research and Quality: "Put research to work to improve policies, clinical practice, and outcomes!"

These HSR definitions and foci highlight the following features of the field:

1. Its interdisciplinary contribution to the development and application of theories regarding the operation of an array of personal healthcare services and community-based health interventions and systems
2. Its focus on understanding the relationship between health services and other determinants of health
3. Its study of the influence of health services and other determinants of health on the health and well-being of individuals and populations
4. Its application to real-world policy and program questions and issues

A study may be classified as HSR if it concerns services delivered through the personal healthcare system, defined broadly as any transaction between a healthcare provider and a client for the purpose of promoting the health of the client. Health services may also fall within the domain of the public health system and involve community-based interventions aimed at promoting community health, such as immunization programs, sanitation and disease control, health education, and occupational health and safety programs. The breadth of services addressed by HSR is illustrated by the continuum presented in Exhibit 1.1. One end encompasses preventive services, largely devoted to primary prevention in the community. The center of the continuum is the personal healthcare system, largely identified by the delivery of outpatient and inpatient services to patients who are ill. The other end comprises health services that deliver long-term treatment and rehabilitation to disabled individuals and persons with chronic illness as well as palliative care for the terminally ill.

HSR is inherently interdisciplinary, drawing on theories and methods from numerous fields including biology, sociology, psychology, political science, epidemiology, demography, economics, law, ethics, and medicine, among others (Choi and Greenberg 1982; Ginzberg 1991; NICHSR 2007; Pittman 2010). The uniqueness of HSR among other fields of inquiry is shown in Exhibit 1.2, which compares the objectives of HSR and those of other fields of health-related research. Basic biomedical research, such as virology or cardiology, is primarily concerned with the development and testing of theories to explain biological phenomena and develop potential preventive and curative innovations, while clinical research aims to evaluate the efficacy of clinical interventions in patients and populations. Public health research conceptualizes and investigates the role of social and environmental factors in producing population health and the efficacy of community-based interventions on population health.

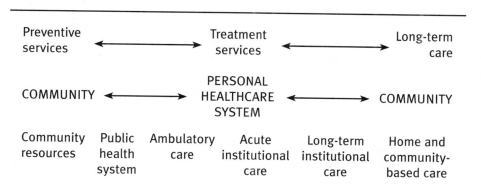

EXHIBIT 1.1
Continuum
of Healthcare
Services

Source: Aday (2001, Figure 5.1, 118). Copyright © 2001. This material is used by permission of John Wiley & Sons, Inc.

EXHIBIT 1.2

Comparison of Health Services Research Objectives and Those of Other Types of Health-Related Research

Biomedical Research	Clinical Research	HSR	Public Health Research
Research on cells, tissues, organs, organ systems, normal development, and disease processes	Patient-level research on prevention and treatment of illness; efficacy of interventions	Effectiveness, efficiency, and equity of personal and community-based health services and delivery systems	Community and environmental influences on health and illness; efficacy of population-based interventions

In some cases HSR draws on biomedical and clinical research to investigate challenges in the organization and delivery of health services. HSR also draws on other fields, such as economics, psychology, political science, and management science, for frameworks, methods, and evaluative criteria. Developments in economics, such as new methods of modeling consumer choice, or in psychology, such as new insight into health risk behavior, may contribute to health services researchers' understanding of the effectiveness of health services. HSR further draws on the public health field to understand the relationships among health services, community-based determinants of health, and challenges in the organization and delivery of community-based interventions aimed at influencing population health.

Health Services Research Perspectives

As discussed at the beginning of this chapter, HSR provides frameworks and methods for assessing health services and systems with respect to the objectives of effectiveness, efficiency, and equity. **Effectiveness** focuses on the intended and desired outcomes produced by health services and is measured by health preservation or improvement. Efficacy, a component of effectiveness, is limited to evaluating the degree of success an intervention (e.g., receiving a clinically recommended dose of a drug) delivers under ideal conditions. Effectiveness also concerns the outcomes realized under a range of practice conditions. These outcomes include not only health outcomes, such as disease symptoms, physical and mental functioning, mortality, and life expectancy, but also the impact of health outcomes on economic productivity, quality of life, and well-being.

The second major objective of HSR is to monitor and evaluate the **efficiency** of health services and delivery systems. When evaluating efficiency, analysts view health services delivery as either an outcome or an input. When health services delivery is viewed as an outcome, evaluation focuses on production efficiency (i.e., the combination of inputs required to produce services at the lowest costs); when health services delivery is viewed as an input, the focus is on allocative efficiency (i.e., the best combination of services) in the production of health. The allocative efficiency of health services delivery is judged in terms of *opportunity costs*—foregone health improvements that could have been achieved had the resources been invested in alternative health improvement efforts (e.g., investing in economic development versus personal health services in a poor country). Allocative efficiency depends on the cost and effectiveness of a given health service relative to the cost and effectiveness of other health-related service or non-service investments. Ultimately, maximization of health services performance requires both production efficiency (the minimum cost of producing a given set of services) and allocative efficiency (the optimal combination of service and non-service health investments).

Equity is concerned with distributional fairness in the delivery of health services and in health status among subgroups of a population. *Procedural equity* refers to the extent to which the structural and process features of health services delivery result in an equitable distribution of services for individuals and population subgroups with comparable needs and wants. *Substantive equity*, the ultimate test of the equity of health services delivery, is the extent to which disparities in health are minimized among individuals and subgroups of a population. The normative relevance of variations in the structure and process of services (procedural equity) ultimately can be judged by the contributions of these variations to reducing inequities in health (substantive equity) across individuals, groups, and populations.

The effectiveness, efficiency, and equity perspectives provide broad criteria for assessing the achievement of health services performance and policy objectives. The objectives of the three perspectives are often complementary. Improving the effectiveness of health services while holding resources constant increases efficiency; increased efficiency creates opportunities for improved effectiveness and equity. However, these objectives also may conflict. Maximizing effectiveness by allocating additional resources to improve health may compromise efficiency if the cost of the resources is high relative to their effectiveness. Maximizing effectiveness and efficiency by distributing resources to persons who would gain the most health may be deemed unfair in terms of procedural or substantive equity if the policy leads to an uneven distribution of health services or health status. In complex policy choices, such as choosing among alternative public and private strategies for financing health services, HSR facilitates maximally informed decisions by identifying and clarifying the objectives of those decisions and the trade-offs that must be made when objectives conflict.

Levels of Analysis

The effectiveness, efficiency, and equity perspectives of HSR offer specific criteria for evaluating health services and systems at clinical and population levels (Exhibit 1.3). At the **clinical level**, the focus is on personal health-care resources (technology, expertise, equipment, and facilities) and on organizations and systems that transform these resources into healthcare services and distribute them to individuals in a specific community or health system (Longest Jr. 2005). Outcomes are measured in terms of the health of individuals served by a single provider, an institution, a group of providers or institutions, or an entire healthcare system, and that information is used to assess the contribution of personal health services to improving or maintaining the health of service recipients. The clinical level also addresses the financing of health services. At this level, production efficiency is concerned with the combination of inputs required to produce services for individuals at the lowest costs and procedural equity assesses the fairness of health services delivery across individuals with comparable needs and wants.

At the **population level**, HSR assesses the design and contribution of personal and community efforts to improve population health. Population-level activities and services usually are conducted by public health agencies, but the personal healthcare system may overlap. For example, personal healthcare might be one component among other environmental, social,

EXHIBIT 1.3
Definitions of
Effectiveness,
Efficiency, and
Equity Criteria

| Criteria | Level of Analysis | |
	Clinical	Population
Effectiveness	*Clinical effectiveness:* Improving the health of individual patients through the delivery of healthcare services	*Population effectiveness:* Improving the health of populations through medical or nonmedical services
Efficiency	*Production efficiency:* Combining inputs to produce services at the lowest cost	*Production efficiency:* Combining inputs to produce services at the lowest cost *Allocative efficiency:* Combining health services and other health-related investments to produce maximum health given available resources
Equity	*Procedural equity:* Maximizing the fairness in the distribution of services across individuals *Substantive equity:* Minimizing the disparities in the distribution of health across individuals	*Procedural equity:* Maximizing the fairness in the distribution of services across groups *Substantive equity:* Minimizing the disparities in the distribution of health across groups

and biological interventions organized at the community level. Examples of public health activities include immunizations; sanitation; disease control; occupational health and safety; health education; epidemiology; and regulation of air, water, and food quality (NICHSR 2007). At this level, population effectiveness is concerned with how the mix of personal healthcare services and community-based social and environmental factors produces the greatest improvements in population health. Allocative efficiency at this level is concerned with identifying the mix of service and non-service investments in social and environmental interventions that produces the highest level of population health relative to the costs of production. Substantive equity at the population level is judged ultimately by the extent to which the health benefits of personal and community-based interventions are shared equitably across populations in the community.

Historical Perspective

Although HSR is a relatively young field of inquiry, its origins may be traced to the early 1900s in the United States. Selected historical contributions of HSR are highlighted in the following paragraphs to illustrate the evolving scope of the field and its role in the formulation of health policy. (For more detail, see Anderson 1991, Colby et al. 2008, Flook and Sanazaro 1973, IOM 1995, McCarthy and White 2000, and NICHSR 2007.)

The Flexner Report, based on a comprehensive study of medical schools in the United States and Canada, was published in 1910 (Flexner 1910). This report, requested in part by the American Medical Association (AMA) and sponsored in part by John D. Rockefeller's philanthropic education effort, the General Education Board, highlighted the great variation in physician training among 168 medical schools. Along with other events, publication of this report led to the closure of 20 percent of the medical schools reviewed (Hiatt and Stockton 2003), and the AMA gained influence over the standardization of medical education in the United States, including physician licensure requirements (Beck 2004). Thus, this systematic review of health services workforce characteristics and training affected private policy (through initiatives of the AMA) and instituted changes to public policy (through states' revision of physician licensure standards).

The Committee on the Costs of Medical Care, sponsored by several private foundations, was established in 1927. This prestigious 42-member committee played a major role in the design and conduct of research on the utilization and costs of personal healthcare services in the United States and on inequities of access that existed across income groups. The Committee published 28 reports, including a series of recommendations that affected and continue to affect how medical services are organized and delivered in the United States.

In 1935 and 1936, the Public Health Service, an agency of the US executive branch, conducted a national health survey and a census of hospitals. The purpose was to provide basic data on the health and health services needs of the population and on the financial structure of US hospitals. No such broad assessment of the profile of health services needs and resources had ever been attempted. An outgrowth of this early research was the development of the concept of service areas for hospitals and health centers.

In 1944, the American Hospital Association (AHA), a private beneficent organization, established its Commission on Hospital Services (AHA 2010). The commission provided the first complete inventory of the nation's hospitals. This inventory and the Public Health Service's hospital census identified a need for more general hospital beds, especially in rural areas. This finding prompted the passage of the federal government's Hill-Burton Act in 1946, which authorized a massive nationwide hospital survey and construction program.

The Commission on Chronic Illness, established in 1949 under the auspices of the AHA, AMA, American Public Health Association, and American Public Welfare Association, carried out a number of studies regarding long-term residential and community-based services and community prevalence and prevention of chronic illness. The AHA Commission on Financing, established in 1951, attempted to address many of the financing issues (i.e., factors affecting the cost, prepayment, and financing of services for non-wage-earning and low-income groups) that the 1944 AHA Commission on Hospital Services had not dealt with directly. The research carried out by these nationally representative, private beneficent organizations contributed to early deliberations concerning the appropriate role of the federal government in health services (e.g., the role of President Truman's Commission on the Health Needs of the Nation) and to the development of methods of survey research and statistical and economic analysis that provided the foundation for contemporary HSR.

The US Department of Health, Education, and Welfare was established in 1953, and the National Health Survey Act, which authorized the major data-gathering efforts of the National Center for Health Statistics, was passed in 1956. The research done under the auspices of these agencies documented the same inequities in health and health services among the poor, the disabled, and the elderly that the Committee on the Costs of Medical Care had identified 20 years earlier. Their findings provided empirical evidence of the need for Medicaid and Medicare. The establishment of these federal programs in 1965 initiated federally subsidized health services coverage for these groups.

The formalization of HSR at the federal level began with the creation of a National Institutes of Health study section on HSR in 1960, formed from the merger of Public Health Research and Hospital Facilities Research study sections. The lead federal agency supporting formal HSR activities, the National Center for Health Services Research and Development

(NCHSRD), was established in 1968. Over the following years, a number of other federal agencies (e.g., Veterans Administration, Health Care Financing Administration [now the Centers for Medicare & Medicaid Services (CMS)], National Institute of Mental Health, National Institute of Aging) and private foundations (e.g., Robert Wood Johnson Foundation, Commonwealth Fund, Kaiser Family Foundation, Pew Foundation) also assumed a greater role in the design and conduct of HSR activities.

The first national meeting of the Association for Health Services Research and the Foundation for Health Services Research was held in Chicago in June 1984. In 1989, NCHSRD received substantial funding for research on patient outcomes and medical effectiveness as a result of major outcomes research bills introduced by Congress, and the agency was subsequently renamed the Agency for Health Care Policy and Research (AHCPR) to reflect its policy-oriented focus. In 1999, AHCPR was reauthorized as the Agency for Healthcare Research and Quality, establishing it as the lead federal agency on the quality of HSR and the coordinator of HSR and all federal quality improvement efforts (AHRQ 2011).

In the mid-2000s, the term *comparative effectiveness research* came into prominence as health services researchers increasingly focused on contrasting the relative benefits of various medical treatments. Greater attention also was given to issues regarding the efficiency and equity of personal health services delivery posed by rising health services costs and gaps in insurance coverage. This rise has been characterized most commonly in terms of the effectiveness and efficiency implications of having an increasing portion of the US gross domestic product (GDP) claimed by health services but also in terms of the equity implications of rising health insurance premiums and consequent increases in the proportion of the population without health insurance.

By 2009, the promise of comparative effectiveness research as a policy strategy for more effective and efficient healthcare delivery was strong enough for the landmark American Recovery and Reinvestment Act to include more than a billion dollars of funding for this effort (Sox 2010). Following this significant economic stimulus legislation, Congress enacted the Patient Protection and Affordable Care Act (ACA) of 2010. The ACA includes a range of support for HSR, including grants for comparative effectiveness research; funding for the establishment of the Patient-Centered Outcomes Research Institute, Center for Medicare & Medicaid Innovation, and Independent Payment Advisory Board; and a significant role for HSR in the design, implementation, and evaluation of new coverage provisions and service delivery reforms.

Thus, recent years have seen unprecedented changes in HSR and increased appreciation of the role of the HSR perspectives (effectiveness, efficiency, and equity) in formulating and assessing health policy. This increased support suggests that the demand for HSR in the United States is likely to heighten significantly in coming years (Pittman 2010). Whether these developments will fulfill the promise on which they were promoted remains to be seen. They do, however, fully acknowledge the need for health services delivery that is effective, efficient, and equitable and the imperative to institute mechanisms for formally incorporating HSR into the policymaking process to ensure these aims are achieved.

Overview of Health Policy Analysis

The principal aims of health policy analysis are described as (1) the production of information relevant to understanding the importance and causes of policy problems and identifying and evaluating policy alternatives and (2) the translation of this information into reasonable arguments to guide governmental decision making (Bardach 2009; Dunn 2009; Munger 2000). The objectives of information gathering and the issues addressed in the field of health policy analysis overlap those of HSR: to document the origins, scope, and causes of quality, cost, and access problems in health services delivery that are of concern to policymakers (e.g., the proportion of the population or subgroups without health insurance, the components and causes of the rising cost of healthcare, the frequency of inappropriate care delivery and medical errors) and to estimate the probable consequences of alternative strategies for addressing such concerns (e.g., comparisons of various government programs or market-enhancing regulations designed to expand public and private coverage of health services or reduce waste in the delivery of healthcare services).

Information translation—increasingly demanded by policymakers (Colby and Baker 2009) and embraced by policy-oriented health services researchers—involves using existing empirical evidence and theory to develop reasonable characterizations of the nature, importance, and cause of a policy problem or to support a specific option among policy alternatives to achieve a given goal. The primary emphasis of this objective is normative and prescriptive: to provide a logical, evidence-based rationale for government action (e.g., the status quo regarding the mixture of public and private health insurance coverage versus a potential future state of greater public insurance) toward a desired goal (e.g., a maximal combination of effectiveness, efficiency, and equity of health services delivery), based on consideration of multiple criteria (e.g., cost versus quality versus access).

Health services researchers engaged in translation must become familiar with the complexities of the policymaking process and policy analysis. Although what constitutes a specific policy initiative from any branch of government (legislative, executive, or judicial) is usually fairly well specified, with objectives, rules, and responsibilities for implementation and outcomes, health policies that deal with a common condition or issue, taken together, may be fragmented, duplicative and, in some cases, conflicting. Thus, there is potential for conflict among policy objectives and tension between analysis and political influence in the policy process. The de facto influence of policy analysis in a given policy process varies depending on whether the process lends itself to rational problem solving or is driven by political consensus gathering. In a rational problem-solving process, policy evidence and reasoning tend to be highly valued in the debates that influence decisions. However, in a highly politicized, adversarial policy process, the primary constraint on action may be disagreement about the criteria to be used in selecting and judging policy rather than about the most effective strategy for achieving a mutual end.

Besides politics, a number of other factors may enhance or constrain the influence of policy analysis on policy decisions. Included among these factors are the attitudes, concerns, and opinions of the public and of special interest groups; these constituencies' ability to influence the decision-making process; the values of elected and nonelected officials; and the nature and content of competing items on the agenda (Longest Jr. 2005).

The primary research objectives of policy analysis contrast with those of other types of basic and applied scientific inquiry, including HSR (see Exhibit 1.4). Basic science and social science disciplines provide useful theories to explain biological or social phenomena (e.g., the economic theory of supply and demand to explain the operation of consumer and provider behavior in the medical services marketplace). These theories underlie the methods of HSR and the ways a policy analyst may describe and assess a policy problem or evaluate a policy proposal. Health program evaluation is concerned with assessing the effect of specific policies and programs (e.g., alternative health education, clinical screening strategies for cancer prevention) on a defined outcome of interest (e.g., survival, quality of life) and comparing the alternatives. A major activity of HSR has been evaluating the effect of community-based outreach, physician education, financial incentives, and other health services programs on preventive behavior and service use (Casale et al. 2007; Fisher et al. 2009; Grembowski 2001; Wennberg et al. 2007).

Bringing the benefits of HSR and policy analysis together in the policy process presents many challenges (Brownson et al. 2006; Gagnon, Turgeon, and Dallaire 2007). Although the interests of researchers and policy analysts may overlap, Brownson and colleagues (2006) describe the two factions as travelers in parallel universes who have differing perspectives, time frames, and incentives. Indeed, HSR has been criticized historically for not being sufficiently involved in the conduct of research that directly informs health policy decisions (Anderson 1991; Choi and Greenberg 1982; Flook and Sanazaro 1973; Ginzberg 1991; IOM 1995, 1991, 1979; Lavis et al. 2002; Tunis, Stryer, and Clancy 2003). However, compilations of HSR's contributions to health policy—its insight into both the causes of health system problems and the potential and actual consequences of major reforms—clearly indicate that the

EXHIBIT 1.4
Comparison of
Objectives of
Health Policy
Analysis and
Those of Other
Types of Inquiry

Type of Inquiry	Objective
Disciplinary research	To explain biological or social phenomena $X \longrightarrow Y$
Health services research	To describe and assess the performance of the healthcare system Structure Process Outcome $X \longrightarrow Y$
Health program evaluation	To evaluate the effect of health policies and programs $X_0 \longrightarrow Y_0$ $X_1 \longrightarrow Y_1$ $X_2 \longrightarrow Y_2$ $X_3 \longrightarrow Y_3$
Health policy analysis	To analyze and compare alternative (1) problem definitions and (2) health policy solutions (1) Problem analysis (2) Solution analysis X_1 vs. X_2 vs. $X_3 \longrightarrow X$ Y_1 vs. Y_2 vs. $Y_3 \longrightarrow Y$

lines between HSR and policy analysis are more aptly characterized as diffuse rather than distinct (Altman and Reinhardt 1996; Brown 1991; Colby et al. 2008; DeFriese, Ricketts III, and Stein 1989; Ginzberg 1991; Shi 1997; Shortell and Reinhardt 1992; White 1992). Organized efforts are being made to bring the fields closer together (Colby et al. 2008).

Integration of Health Services Research and Policy Analysis

A framework for integrating HSR and policy analysis is provided in Exhibit 1.5. This framework portrays the HSR focus on describing, analyzing, and evaluating the **structure**, **process**, and **outcomes** of health services

EXHIBIT 1.5
Framework for
Integrating
Health Services
Research and
Policy Analysis

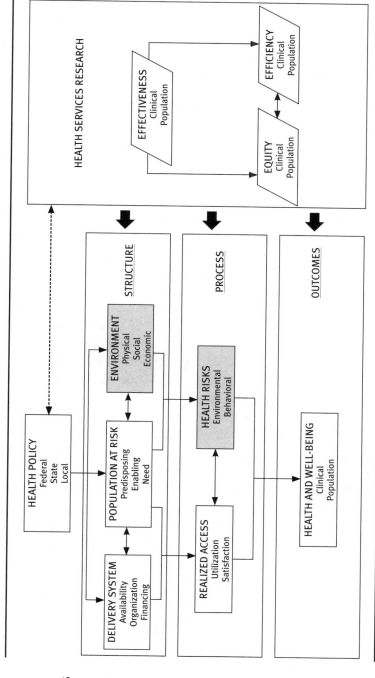

and systems while recognizing the influence of population characteristics and environmental factors on health. *Structure*, as defined by Donabedian (2003), refers to the availability, organization, and financing of health services and systems; the characteristics of the populations served by them; and the physical, social, and economic environments to which the populations are exposed. *Process* encompasses the transactions between patients and providers in the course of actual service delivery as well as the environmental and behavioral transactions exacerbating health risks. *Outcomes* are the consequences of health policies and services for the health and well-being of individuals and populations.

HSR provides basic descriptive data on the organization and delivery of health services, such as the number and distribution of providers, the percentage of the population that is uninsured, and the rates of service utilization. HSR also analyzes relationships among health services and other determinants of health (represented by the arrows in Exhibit 1.5) and the impact of the delivery system on the health and well-being of individuals and populations. The shaded boxes in Exhibit 1.5 represent the community-wide structural factors and environmental and behavioral risk factors that influence health, as described by Evans, Barer, and Marmor (1994) and extended by Roos and colleagues (1996) and Kindig (1997). Incorporation of environmental aspects and health risks acknowledges the important effect these factors have on health outcomes. For example, discriminatory housing practices may increase health disparities by increasing poor and ethnic/racial populations' exposure to environmental toxins. The provision of childcare centers in workplaces may increase infant health through breastfeeding. Income maintenance programs may reduce the stress of meeting survival needs and improve participants' diets. Pathways linking these factors to health and, in turn, affecting the demand for and use of health services are becoming increasingly recognized.

Information from both the clinical and population levels of HSR may be required to fully understand and interpret the effects of health policies. Commitments to developing medical technologies or procedures to optimize individual patient outcomes may fail to consider whether, given limited resources, they are the best investments for enhancing the health and well-being of the community as a whole (including service recipients and non-recipients). Treatments that have been demonstrated to be efficacious for individual patients may not be as effective when delivered across institutions or even within the same institution. System outcomes may be influenced by organizational and financial incentives that affect patterns of health services provision. Population outcome studies explore the health service and health status variations that may result from differential access to health services and from different styles of practice not detectable by outcomes research at the clinical level alone. A focus on the effects that personal lifestyles, behaviors (e.g., smoking), and attitudes (e.g., toward regular physical activity) have on individuals' health status may not fully reveal the array of social, structural, and environmental factors (e.g., poverty, lead paint, toxic waste) that may have consequences for the health of populations residing in a community.

Effectiveness is placed before efficiency and equity in the integrative framework (Exhibit 1.5) to indicate the central role it plays in assessing the efficiency of producing health benefits and the equitable distribution of these benefits and costs across groups. Evidence of the effectiveness of clinical or population-level interventions is needed to make informed judgments regarding the efficient allocation of resources and the types of services to which equitable access should be ensured.

This framework has been adapted and applied in a variety of policy contexts, such as evaluation of the availability of community child health services, the health and health services needs of homeless populations, and the effectiveness, efficiency, and equity of behavioral health services; comparative health systems analysis; and assessments of safety net programs (Aday et al. 1999; Aday and Awe 1997; Andersen 1995; Begley et al. 2002; Davidson et al. 2004; DuPlessis, Inkelas, and Halfon 1998; Gelberg, Andersen, and Leake 2000; Halfon and Hochstein 2002; IOM 2002b, 1993; Morgan et al. 2009). As reflected in Exhibit 1.5, effectiveness, efficiency, and equity research may lead to different conclusions regarding the best policy option. Optimally, analyses of competing health policy alternatives measure and evaluate each of these criteria and the trade-offs resulting from emphasizing some to the exclusion of others. The double-headed arrow between HSR and health policy indicates that health policy can directly influence the role and focus of HSR. There also is an increasing impetus, grounded in research on the fundamental social, economic, and environmental determinants of health, to expand HSR to better understand the role of non-service health determinants, such as education, employment, community development, and other social and economic determinants of health.

Chapters 2 through 7 describe the specific concepts and methods of HSR and present evidence for the effectiveness, efficiency, and equity perspectives of health services delivery and policy. Chapter 8 elaborates on the integration of HSR in policy analysis, and in Chapter 9 a case study of a policy change addressing health disparities illustrates how HSR can be applied to answer a specific policy question.

Overview of Health Services in the United States

As a foundation for the next chapters, the following discussion highlights the basic resource availability, organization, and financing characteristics of the US healthcare system, focusing in particular on the major issues and changes that have taken place over the past three decades in both personal and community health services.

Personal Health Services

Managed Care Systems

Managed care encompasses various forms of health maintenance organizations (HMOs), point-of-service plans (POSs), and preferred provider organizations (PPOs). HMOs guarantee delivery of a comprehensive prepaid benefit package to a voluntarily enrolled population through a system of care. POSs are HMOs that offer partial reimbursement for services an enrollee chooses to obtain outside the HMO network. PPOs contract to provide services at a discounted rate under conditions of utilization review that offer providers a wider network of enrolled populations—and enrolled populations a wider choice of providers—while restricting the scope or increasing the out-of-pocket costs of the benefits provided (Sultz and Young 2011).

HMO plans and enrollment have grown since the early 1970s. HMOs became vigorous competitors of traditional health insurance plans in several metropolitan areas, enrolling about 27 percent of covered workers by 2002 (Claxton et al. 2010). HMOs then began to lose ground to PPOs and nontraditional HMOs, which allow enrollees to select a non-HMO provider in exchange for a financial penalty. By 2009, HMO enrollment had declined to 20 percent of covered workers. In that same period, PPO enrollment grew from 52 percent to 60 percent of covered workers, reflecting consumer preference for a less restrictive form of managed care.

As growth in the commercial market slowed in the early to mid-1990s, managed care plans competed vigorously to enroll public beneficiaries. Seventeen percent of Medicare beneficiaries were enrolled in managed care plans in 1999. Strong growth was projected to continue, reaching one-third of beneficiaries by 2007 (Lamphere et al. 1997), but managed care enrollment share declined to 12 percent of the Medicare population by 2003 (CMS 2011b). With more generous payment, Medicare managed care enrollment rose to 18 percent in 2009. Managed care enrollment has remained strong in the Medicaid program, representing more than 70 percent (36.2 million) of Medicaid beneficiaries in 2009 (CMS 2011a).

Physician Organizations

Of the 740,867 physicians in patient care in 2008, 75.2 percent were in office-based practice, 14.6 percent were in training, and 10.3 percent were full-time hospital staff. Almost half of physicians in office-based practice were in primary care specialties (Smart 2010). Nearly all physician practices had one or more managed care contracts, and around one-third had contracts with capitation payment (Havlicek 1996; Wassenaar and Thran 2003).

The physician practice size has been growing. In 1965, about 90 percent of physicians were in solo or two-person practice. By 1996, that number had decreased to 41 percent, and by 2004, to 33 percent. The average number of physicians per medical practice was 20.4 in 2004, ranging from 7.8 in obstetrics/gynecology to 41.5 in radiology. About 25 percent of patient care physicians were in solo practice in 2007 and 2008 (Kane 2011).

Hospital Systems

The hospital industry also has undergone tremendous change. The past 40 years have seen rapid advancement in medical technology; the expansion of outpatient services; the growth of multihospital systems; the emergence of increased competition among hospitals and between hospitals and other providers; mergers and conversion of community not-for-profit hospitals to for-profit status; and a fundamental change in the Medicare payment system, which supplies about half of the hospital revenue in the United States. The shift, described in more detail later in this chapter, has been from a retrospective reimbursement system to a prospective payment system (PPS) based on diagnosis-related groups (DRGs) (CDC 2011c).

The number of community hospitals declined from 5,875 in 1975 to 5,010 in 2008; over the same period, total beds decreased from 942,000 to 808,000 (AHA 2010). The decline was accompanied by a shift toward investor-owned (for-profit) community hospitals and away from state and local government community hospitals. The former represented 13.2 percent of community hospitals in 1975 compared to 19.6 percent in 2008. However, not-for-profit community hospitals continue to represent the majority of hospitals and hospital beds (AHA 2010).

Another reaction to managed care and other cost containment strategies has been the development of strategic alliances between hospitals. Not-for-profit hospitals affiliated with other hospitals in their region during the 1990s to establish referral patterns, share services, and protect against the expansion of proprietary hospital chains (Luke, Begun, and Pointer 1989). In the proprietary sector, large hospital corporations have purchased hospitals in different markets and instituted centralized and standardized management practices to achieve greater efficiency and profits. Merger activity was especially strong in the mid-1990s, with 235 deals affecting 768 hospitals. Thereafter, merger activity decreased; only 52 transactions took place in 2009 (AHA 2009). This move to horizontal integration (coordination of similar services across providers) was followed by efforts to achieve vertical integration (coordination of different types of services, such as primary and specialty). Hospital systems and physician groups also formed organized systems of care in the 1990s (Shortell and Hull 1996). However, the trend toward vertical integration and tightly managed care failed to yield the anticipated efficiencies and was largely abandoned by hospitals, physician groups, and health plans across the nation by 2000 (Lesser et al. 2003; Robinson 2001).

The reacceleration of healthcare cost growth and the passage of the ACA have reinvigorated the search for more integrated and efficient healthcare delivery models, including accountable care organizations (ACOs) and patient-centered medical homes. These models, while more flexible for patients and providers, embody aspects of managed care, including care coordination, use of electronic medical records, a focus on primary care, and payment incentives for greater efficiency and quality. CMS and the ACA support development of these organizations, which are reviewed in Chapter 5.

Payment Arrangements

Until the 1980s, physicians in the United States controlled their means of payment and the amount they could charge through fee-for-service (FFS) reimbursement. Physician incomes were high relative to those of other professionals, and healthcare delivery practices were both inefficient and inequitable. The FFS system, which is difficult to understand and complex to administer, was the predominant form of payment. Under this system, overpayments for procedural care at the expense of visits and consultations have been well documented, as have wide variations in fees for identical services (Simon and Born 1996).

A new physician payment system under Medicare, the resource-based relative value scale (RBRVS), was developed in the early 1980s in response to these problems (Physician Payment Review Commission 1991). The relative value was the sum of physician work, practice expense, and malpractice costs, adjusted for geographic cost differences and converted to dollars using a conversion factor. The aim was to develop a physician payment system that would (1) rationalize FFS payments under Medicare, (2) reduce the rate of growth of physician expenditures, (3) protect Medicare enrollees' access to care, and (4) support quality care (Epstein and Blumenthal 1993).

The implementation of Medicare's PPS in 1984 was the cornerstone for a corresponding movement to contain hospital costs. Under PPS, hospitals are paid a prospectively determined amount per discharge rather than on a retrospective, reasonable-cost basis. Payment varies by DRG category and is updated annually to reflect changes in average reported charges among US hospitals (McClellan 1997). The Deficit Reduction Act of 2005 modified the DRG system to reduce payment for certain cases with hospital-acquired infections that could have been averted had care been provided according to evidence-based guidelines (CMS 2011c). In 2008, CMS expanded the payment system from 538 DRGs to 745 Medicare Severity DRGs (MS-DRGs) to better account for severity of illness. This change shifted payment toward hospitals with more severe cases (CMS 2010a). Hospital payment has been sharply affected by the growth in managed care and competition in the private sector since the 1990s. As a result, hospitals are increasingly engaging in cost cutting, participating in mergers, forging closer relations with physicians and other providers, assuming insurance functions, and contracting directly with employers. New payment initiatives, including pay for performance and bundled-payment experiments within the context of ACOs, are the latest healthcare reforms designed to restrain cost growth and yield greater value for money in healthcare.

Availability and Utilization

In the 1960s, the physician shortage in the United States appeared to be worsening. In response, federal and state governments greatly expanded investment in medical schools, thereby increasing the number of medical school graduates. These trends, along with the growth in managed care organizations, raised subsequent concerns in the 1980s and 1990s about a burgeoning physician surplus (NCHS 2011, 1997; Politzer et al. 1996; Reinhardt 1991; Weiner 1994).

Later reports suggested that there was no surplus of physicians in the United States (Salsberg and Forte 2002). The medical market has continued to absorb the growing number of physicians in both primary and specialty care. Demand kept pace with the increasing supply of physicians in the 1990s, driven by the aging population, the increasing complexity and intensity of treatments, physicians' reduced work hours, and the backlash against managed care (Staiger, Auerbach, and Buerhaus 2010). The policy to increase the number of primary care physicians in the 1990s failed to address the payment gap between primary care and specialists, and growth in the number of primary care practitioners has been slow relative to the growing demand for primary care, which, given the ACA's increased focus on the primary care–based medical home, is likely to further intensify (Bodenheimer and Pham 2010; Colwill, Cultice, and Kruse 2008). A critical shortage of hospital nurses and nursing school faculty also exists in many regions of the United States, particularly rural areas. These problems are worsening due to retirement (more nurses are exiting practice than entering) and the aging patient population (Buerhaus 2008).

HSR has documented substantial variations by geography in the levels of healthcare resources, rates of administering various medical diagnostic procedures, and rates of performing surgical operations. The association of these variations with health outcomes is a major focus of current research. The following paragraphs focus on evidence of this variation. Descriptive information on widely used indicators of the utilization of and satisfaction with healthcare is highlighted in Chapter 7.

Glover (1938) is credited with first reporting the phenomenon of variation in the rates of surgical procedures performed, specifically tonsillectomy rates in England. Since then, a host of studies have reported variation in the delivery rates of common surgical procedures, including within

US states (Lewis 1969; Wennberg and Gittelsohn 1973), within a Canadian province (Roos 1984), within countries (McPherson et al. 1981; Wennberg, Bunker, and Barnes 1980), and between countries (Bunker 1970; McPherson et al. 1982, 1981; Vayda 1973; Wennberg, Bunker, and Barnes 1980). All of these studies found that the rates varied as much as sixfold from one geographic area of a state/province to another and as much as threefold between countries. Variation also has been found in the rates of diagnostic and medical procedures administered in the United States (Chassin et al. 1986; Wennberg 1990). Using data from 16 university hospital or large community hospital market areas, Wennberg (1990) found that the ratios of high to low in the number of procedures per person varied from 2.0 for inguinal hernia repair to 3.6 for coronary artery bypass graft surgery to 19.4 for carotid endarterectomy. More recently, researchers have found that regions that practice the most intensive and costly form of care may achieve worse patient outcomes than those achieved by regions characterized by more conservative use of resources (Skinner and Staiger 2009; Skinner, Staiger, and Fisher 2010, 2006).

Studies have also demonstrated variation in breast cancer screening and treatment. For example, Sabatino and colleagues (2008) found that only 38 percent of uninsured women had undergone a mammogram within the previous two years versus 74 percent of insured women and that this disparity had not changed since 1993. Researchers continue to disentangle factors related to worse breast cancer outcomes for African-American women, including access to screening and care, disease characteristics, and cultural differences (Banerjee et al. 2007).

The ACA intends to change the organization and delivery of services in the US healthcare system by increasing regulation of health insurers, expanding government coverage programs, subsidizing the purchase of health insurance, developing health insurance exchanges for competing health plans, and experimenting with new payment and organization models to reduce variation in medical practice and control costs. These changes are designed to increase access to insurance and the demand for healthcare services while improving the performance of healthcare providers and systems. The net impact of these changes on the effectiveness, efficiency, and equity of US healthcare remains to be assessed by health services researchers. Their findings will help the United States tailor policy to keep moving toward the goal of achieving affordable healthcare for all citizens.

Expenditures and Financing

National healthcare expenditures for the complex and highly technological US medical care enterprise were $2.6 trillion in 2010, compared to $27.3 billion in 1960. During the same period, healthcare expenditures grew from $147 to $8,402 per capita and from 5.2 percent to 17.9 percent of GDP (CMS 2011c; Martin et al. 2011). Driven mainly by an increase in outpatient hospital services, spending on hospitals began increasing rapidly in 1997 and reached 12 percent growth in 2001 (Strunk, Ginsburg, and Gabel 2002). While hospital expenditures have continued growing, recent shifts in the distribution of spending for services mainly have been toward nursing home and home care. Hospital expenditures remain the largest share of total spending, followed by expenditures for physician services. Although the absolute levels of expenditures increased, the share for drugs declined from about 10 percent in 1960 to near 4 percent in 1982 and then rose again to 10 percent in early 2000 due to new drug development and more aggressive medical treatment guidelines (CMS 2011c; Martin et al. 2011; Thorpe 2005).

The growth of personal healthcare expenditures (i.e., spending for the direct provision of care to individuals) increased sharply after the passage of Medicare and Medicaid in 1965 and continued to trend upward in the 1970s, a period of high general inflation. Growth decreased initially in the 1980s in response to cost containment measures and the decline of general inflation. However, average annual cost increases between 9 and 10 percent continued during the late 1980s and early 1990s. Growth slowed again in the mid-1990s but reaccelerated in early 2000, only to slow yet again after 2003 and after the 2008 financial crisis (CMS 2011c). While healthcare cost growth has since slowed, it still exceeds the growth in income; as a result, an increasing percentage of income is being spent on healthcare. The major factors affecting the growth of personal health expenditures have been economy-wide inflation, medical price inflation in excess of general inflation, and the use and intensity of services per capita during periods of economic growth and decline (Martin et al. 2011).

Government and private insurers have expanded their roles in financing healthcare services in the United States. Government programs covered about 44 percent of the cost in 2009, almost double the proportion covered in 1960 (CMS 2011c). Around 14 percent of personal health expenditures were paid out of pocket in 2009, compared to 56 percent in 1960. Private insurance (primarily Blue Cross and Blue Shield plans), employer self-insurance, independent plans, and commercial insurance company plans covered 34 percent of the cost in 2009, compared to 21 percent in 1960. Despite the growth of government and private insurance, 50.7 million persons were uninsured in 2009, and an equal or greater number did not have adequate insurance coverage (DeNavas-Walt, Proctor, and Smith 2010; NCHS 2011). (Additional evidence on the uninsured is presented in Chapter 7.)

Changes in financing are under way in the US personal health services system. One of the primary objectives of the ACA is to expand health insurance coverage by requiring most individuals to obtain coverage, expanding Medicaid to low-income adults, providing premium assistance for the purchase of private insurance, using tax credits and penalties to encourage employers to offer coverage, and increasing regulation of the benefits of private coverage. A number of ACA coverage provisions are already in effect for the population under age 65, such as elimination of lifetime coverage limits and prohibition against canceling the coverage of policyholders who become sick, limits on insurance companies' administrative costs and profits, prohibition against denying coverage for children with preexisting medical conditions, and permission for adults aged 19 to 25 who cannot obtain health insurance through an employer to stay covered by their parents' health plan. Although these provisions are significant, the provisions with the largest potential impact on coverage do not take effect until 2014 and are expected to be fully implemented by 2019–2020. In 2014, all US citizens and legal immigrants will be required to have health insurance coverage or pay a tax penalty. The Medicaid expansions and health insurance exchanges will also be implemented in 2014.

Public Health

CMS estimated that expenditures for US public health activities by all levels of government were about 3 percent of total national health expenditures, or $64.1 billion, in 2007 (NCHS 2011). A 2008 survey of local public health agencies (LPHAs) conducted by the National Association of County and City Health Officials (NACCHO 2009) documented that the majority (60 percent) of local public health agencies were county based. The most common programs and services provided included adult and child immunizations, communicable disease surveillance, tuberculosis screening and treatment, food service establishment inspection, environmental health surveillance, food safety education, tobacco use prevention, and school / daycare center inspection.

The occupations LPHAs usually employed included public health nurses, environmental scientists, and administrative/clerical staff. In 2008, the average LPHA staff size in full-time equivalents (FTEs) was 58, with a median of 15 FTEs. Median annual LPHA expenditures were $1.12 million. The largest proportion of LPHA budgets came from local sources (25 percent), followed by state sources (20 percent). Funding streams varied by metropolitan and nonmetropolitan area location and the size of the population served. Local public health officials consistently indicated that workforce and partnerships with their local communities were their agencies' greatest strengths, while funding was consistently mentioned as their biggest challenge (NACCHO 2009).

Health departments face major additional challenges today. The September 11, 2001, terrorist attacks placed greater expectations and burdens on local and state health departments to expand their emergency response systems. With increased funding from the Centers for Disease Control and Prevention, the majority of health departments have hired additional staff, participated in tabletop emergency drills and exercises, and trained staff on emergency preparedness. A growing body of research on the social determinants of health has also broadened the public health mandate to develop intersectoral programs and policies to address them. These and other challenges are compelling health departments to reconsider their mission and ways to accomplish it. Fifty-eight percent of local public health departments reported supporting community efforts to address health disparities in 2008 (NACCHO 2009).

A series of IOM reports have assessed the strengths and limitations of the US public health system and suggested fruitful new directions for better achieving US public health policy objectives (IOM 2003, 2002a, 1988). The 1988 IOM report presented a vision for the future of public health in terms of the core public health functions of policy assessment, development, and assurance and ten other essential services. The more recent IOM reports argue that innovations in the design and implementation of public health policies and programs need to be grounded in an ecological model of population health, based on research on the multifactorial determinants of health, and developed through broader intersectoral collaboration to ultimately improve the health of populations and reduce persistent health disparities.

According to the 2003 IOM report on the future of public health in the twenty-first century, public health advocates need to take action in six areas to move public health to the level at which it should be (IOM 2002a):

1. They need to consider all the factors (physical, environmental, social, and economic) that affect health when implementing population-based programs.
2. They need to lobby for strengthening the governmental public health infrastructure—the backbone of the public health system.
3. They need to build a new generation of integrated, multidisciplinary partnerships that draw on the perspectives and resources of diverse communities and actively engage these partnerships in health action.
4. They must develop systems of accountability to ensure the quality and availability of public health services.
5. Scientific evidence should be the foundation of public health decision making and the measure of success.
6. They must improve communication within the public health system.

The ACA will have substantial effects on public health. While primarily an insurance coverage and healthcare improvement act, it includes many provisions relating to public health prevention and wellness activities. For example, it encourages prevention services by primary care providers by requiring insurance companies to cover the cost of clinical preventive services, provides for the creation of home visitation programs for pregnant teens and new mothers, and proposes student reimbursement for public health programs to shore up the public health workforce. The establishment of the Prevention and Public Health Fund may increase funding for public health system activities and research. The ACA also provides for allocation of funds for expansion (approximate doubling) of funding for federally qualified primary care clinics, which should increase primary care capacity and cover individuals who remain uninsured on a sliding-scale fee basis.

International Perspective on Health Services

Effectiveness, efficiency, and equity concerns with health services and systems are universal, from the wealthiest to the poorest nations. Developed countries are most concerned with macro-level cost control issues, whereas developing nations strive to allocate extremely limited resources to areas that will achieve the greatest health benefit (European Observatory on Health Care Systems 2002). Therefore, while the clinical perspective of effectiveness is more important in developed countries (where the emphasis is on improving the monitoring of process and outcome indicators for measuring clinical effectiveness), the need for a population perspective of effectiveness (which focuses on such issues as health needs assessment and provision of community-based and personal healthcare services) is highlighted in developing countries.

All systems could benefit from more efficient methods of producing, financing, and delivering health services. Highly market-minimized systems in Sweden, the Netherlands, and the United Kingdom have introduced aspects of market competition to improve efficiency and reduce costs. These countries have been relatively successful at controlling health spending as a proportion of GDP. Their focus is making their systems more responsive to consumers, but they are cautious about the threat of market strategies to the equity of their systems. As the most market-maximized country, the United States has been less successful at achieving cost control and equity in health services delivery. The ACA is introducing market-based competitive and government-based regulatory strategies to improve efficiency and control spending while striving to achieve greater equity in health insurance coverage and access to care.

There is concern that too much reliance on market-driven policies has failed to control cost and that equity and efficiency will be enhanced by a more balanced public–private approach (Cutler 2002; Ma, Lu, and Quan 2008; Reinhardt 1998). Limitations on the efficiency and equity achievable in healthcare markets are an opportunity for government entities to improve the allocation of healthcare resources and the provision of health services. Without competitive market price signals, however, alternative methods and information are needed to make efficient resource allocation decisions. An understand-ing of consumer and provider behavior and application of economic evalua-tion methods is needed to guide public and private decision makers. While optimal economic analysis requires extensive information on incentives, costs, health consequences, and people's valuation of resources and health outcomes, evaluation methods can be populated with the best available infor-mation and applied to even the least-developed countries (Marseille, Kahn, and Saba 1998). HSR is needed to examine resource allocation issues and identify strategies that are likely to be more efficient and highlight areas of uncertainty on which more information is needed for a complete assessment.

Though equity in health services delivery and in the distribution of health is a universal goal of health services, systems, and policies, countries differ with regard to the emphasis they place on equity relative to other goals when designing and evaluating systems and policies. In developed countries with large and complex health service systems, the bulk of HSR expenditures for evaluating equity are focused on the operation and performance of the system itself. A particular equity concern, for example, is the universality of insurance coverage. The health reform debates in the United States and other countries typically have centered on methods for ensuring universal insur-ance coverage. Wide variations exist across countries in the availability and means of financing care. The heart of the debate regarding health reform is often related to whether more market-maximized versus market-minimized methods for the financing and delivery of services would be most effective for achieving the equity objective (Blendon et al. 2002; Daniels, Saloner, and Gelpi 2009; Hacker 1996; Skocpol 1996).

In developing countries, equity considerations assume a great impor-tance because of the countries' prevalent health problems, such as environ-mentally related risks, infectious diseases, and maternal and child health needs, and because the countries lack the resources needed to support a complex health services infrastructure. Correspondingly, the focus of equity research and policies concerns fundamental public health and primary care investments. The World Health Organization (WHO) has, through a variety of national and international programs, attempted to better ensure "health for all" and facilitated the development of indicators and data systems for monitoring and evaluating progress toward this goal across countries. WHO has identified five common problems that policymakers in both developed and developing countries face when making choices to improve their health systems: (1) confusion over the goals of health systems, (2) relatively sparse and often conflicting evidence on strategies for improving health system per-formance, (3) a lack of public or private institutions and individuals who are accountable for system outcomes, (4) a societal focus on the development of new technologies and less attention to technology delivery, and (5) the increasingly technical nature of health system debates (Murray and Evans

2003). Since its inception in 1999, WHO's Alliance for Health Policy and Systems Research has aimed to promote the generation and use of health policy and systems research as a means of improving health and health systems in developing countries. The Alliance pursues this goal by developing and harnessing existing methods and approaches to improve the quality of research and its use to address the problems faced by policymakers (Alliance for Health Policy and Systems Research 2011). By fostering a common framework and set of measurement methods for HSR and policy evaluation, the effectiveness, efficiency, and equity perspectives help to remedy many of these difficulties.

Summary and Conclusions

The three HSR perspectives of effectiveness, efficiency, and equity offer a useful framework for distinguishing intermediate structure and process goals from the end goal of improved health and demonstrating how the intermediate goals are the means for achieving the end goal. They are a universal basis of measurement that may be used to develop databases, define problems, and determine best practices for assessing health services and systems performance. The application of the combined HSR perspectives in policy analysis requires policymakers to consider quality, cost, and distributional issues in program planning and to understand the interaction of services with other determinants of health (e.g., intersectoral programs with education and sanitation programs).

The chapters that follow introduce methods of operationalizing and applying the effectiveness, efficiency, and equity perspectives in evaluations of the performance of health services and systems. Chapters 8 and 9 show how the concepts and methods of HSR can be integrated in policy analysis.

EFFECTIVENESS: CONCEPTS AND METHODS

Chapter Highlights

1. This chapter poses two fundamental questions:
    - What is healthcare effectiveness?
    - How should it be assessed?
2. While concepts and methods for determining the efficacy of healthcare are difficult to apply, assessing the effectiveness of healthcare delivery is even more challenging.
3. Effectiveness research is guided by conceptual frameworks, appropriate research design, and good data.

Overview

Several lines of HSR, such as the study of disparities, practice variation, translation research, and medical errors, reveal that healthcare delivery in the United States is far from optimal (Iglehart 2009a; Orszag 2008; Prasad, Cifu, and Ioannidis 2012; Schuster, McGlynn, and Brook 2005). Each new revelation of wasteful use of resources or harm to patients strengthens the case that healthcare delivery and policy should be redirected by evidence of effectiveness and continuous monitoring of performance. The emphasis on evidence draws on the principles and strategies of the scientific method, which relies on testable hypotheses, transparent methods, skepticism/doubt, and measurement.

Sir Bradford Hill (1965), who noted that "all scientific work is incomplete," suggests nine characteristics by which to judge evidence for causal hypotheses:

1. Strength of association
2. Consistency of association
3. Specificity of association
4. Temporality of association
5. Biological gradient (for biological hypotheses)

6. Plausibility of association
7. Coherence of association
8. Experimental manipulation
9. Analogy to related, recognized effects

The arrows flowing from effectiveness to both efficiency and equity in the model of health services research (HSR) and policy illustrated in Chapter 1, Exhibit 1.5 indicate the points where evidence of effectiveness is needed before questions of efficiency or equity can be addressed. The goals of HSR are to generate, evaluate, and promote this evidence.

This chapter describes the conceptual and methodological challenges and standards of healthcare effectiveness research and addresses several considerations relevant to evaluating effectiveness, including

- whether the analysis is at the clinical or population level;
- what theoretical model of healthcare effectiveness is followed;
- whether to include input, process, or outcome measures or a combination of these measures;
- whether a service should be evaluated in terms of prevention, care, or cure;
- the selection of a study design that balances internal validity and generalizability; and
- the selection and use of high-quality data sources.

Several initiatives—including government efforts by the National Institutes of Health (NIH), Agency for Healthcare Research and Quality (AHRQ), and Patient-Centered Outcomes Research Institute and efforts of private organizations, such as the Institute of Medicine (IOM), AcademyHealth, and the Robert Wood Johnson Foundation—are underway in the United States to boost the quality of effectiveness research and increase its impact on healthcare delivery.

Concepts and Definitions

Efficacy Versus Effectiveness

Analysis of effectiveness depends on understanding the difference between efficacy and effectiveness. *Efficacy* measures whether a healthcare intervention works when delivered under ideal circumstances to targeted individuals or populations, while *effectiveness* is the degree to which an efficacious intervention is delivered with fidelity to the intended patient or population at the right time and place. Evidence of effectiveness is concerned with the actual delivery of healthcare (Pronovost and Goeschel 2011). An effectiveness analysis may examine clinical outcomes, but it also must consider those outcomes in context of the extent to which the service was delivered as intended to the targeted population and under the right circumstances (Glasgow, Lichtenstein, and Marcus 2003).

Levels of Analysis

The perspectives of effectiveness analyses differ between the population and clinical levels (see Chapter 1). A framework of effectiveness research, including characteristics at the clinical and population levels, is presented in Exhibit 2.1. Exhibit 2.2 illustrates the determinants of health from the clinical perspective (Donabedian 1966), and Exhibit 2.3 illustrates the determinants of health from the population perspective (Kindig and Stoddart 2003). Accordingly, evaluation of a healthcare system's effectiveness can consider two types of outcomes: clinical outcomes and population outcomes. Effectiveness analyses at the clinical level involve outcomes for the service recipients, while effectiveness analyses at the population level involve outcomes for a recognized community as a whole, regardless of involvement or participation in healthcare interventions (i.e., both service recipients and non-recipients).

Clinical and population outcomes may be generally categorized as three types: mortality outcomes, morbidity outcomes, and health status outcomes. **Mortality outcomes** include such measures as life expectancy for an individual or a population and years of life lost/premature mortality. **Morbidity outcomes** include a wide range of measures, both disease specific and general, that indicate burden or disability from disease or illness in a patient or in some population. They include familiar clinical indicators, such as blood pressure and pain level. **Health status outcomes** include a range of measures that profile health across disease states. Examples include self-rated health, health-related quality of life, and quality-adjusted life years. These measures of comprehensive health status enable comparisons to be made across morbidity states and the relative benefit gained between two interventions to be calculated.

Process measures of health services delivery may be used in place of outcomes in effectiveness analysis. Process measures of health service delivery include the type and quantity of services delivered (e.g., physician appointments, health promotion messages, screenings), satisfaction with services, and assessments of timely and appropriate utilization by patients. The Andersen–Aday model of access to care describes the factors that contribute to whether a person seeks or receives healthcare (see Aday and Andersen 1974; Andersen 1995) and is central to assessing effectiveness (see Chapter 1, Exhibit 1.5). *Potential access* depends on such factors as health insurance coverage and locally available providers. Barriers include low health literacy, time constraints, monetary costs, availability of time off from work, availability of

EXHIBIT 2.1
Framework for Effectiveness Research

	Population Perspective	Clinical Perspective		
		Level of Analysis		
	Community	*System*	*Institution*	*Patient*
Outcomes Measures	• Mortality — Population death rates • Morbidity — Population morbidity rates — Disability rates • Health status — Disease incidence and prevalence rates — Perceived health status	• Mortality — Case fatality rates • Morbidity — Complication rates — Disability rates • Health status — Diagnosis rates — Averaged HRQOL*	• Mortality — Case fatality rates • Morbidity — Complication rates — Disability rates • Health status — Diagnosis rates — Averaged HRQOL	• Mortality — Individual deaths • Morbidity — Adverse events — Disability limitation • Health status — Clinical endpoints — HRQOL
Risk Adjustment	• Demographic characteristics	• Demographic characteristics • Comorbidity rates • Risk adjustment systems	• Demographic characteristics • Comorbidity rates • Risk adjustment systems	• Patient profiles • Comorbidities — Diagnoses

Study Designs	• Observational—epidemiological	• Observational—interorganizational	• Observational—intraorganizational	• Observational—case reports/series • Experimental—RCT** • Synthetic — Meta-analysis — Decision analysis
Data Sources	• Records — Population health information system — Vital statistics — Disease surveillance • Surveys	• Records — Medical records — Discharge data — Claims data • Surveys	• Records — Medical records — Discharge data — Claims data • Surveys	• Records — Medical records — Discharge data — Claims data • Surveys
Example	Chinese-American community screening (Tu et al. 2003)	European national screening program (De Koning 2000)	Public hospital clinic screening program (Thompson et al. 2002)	Patient screening in response to intervention (Eli et al. 2002)

Typical Effectiveness Research Questions by Level of Analysis

Community	What is the contribution of medical care to the health of the population?
System	What is the impact of system-level variables (e.g., provider specialty mix, organizational form, payment mechanism) on the processes and outcomes of medical care?
Institution	What is the impact of the quality of care on the outcomes of medical care?

*Health-related quality of life
**Randomized controlled trial

EXHIBIT 2.2
Conceptual
Model of Health
Determinants
from the Clinical
Perspective

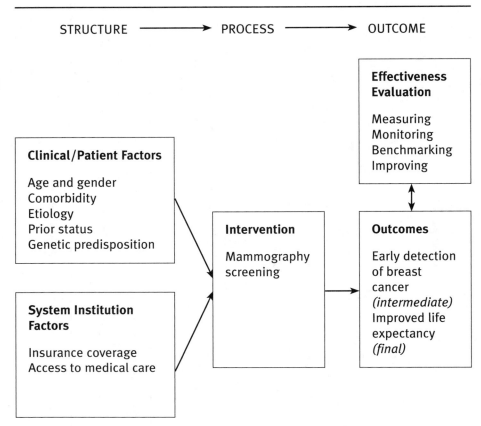

STRUCTURE → PROCESS → OUTCOME

Effectiveness Evaluation

Measuring
Monitoring
Benchmarking
Improving

Clinical/Patient Factors

Age and gender
Comorbidity
Etiology
Prior status
Genetic predisposition

Intervention

Mammography
screening

Outcomes

Early detection
of breast
cancer
(intermediate)
Improved life
expectancy
(final)

System Institution Factors

Insurance coverage
Access to medical care

Source: Adapted from Donabedian (2003, 46–47) and Kane (1997, Figure 1-1, 13).

EXHIBIT 2.3
Conceptual
Model of Health
Determinants
from the
Population
Perspective

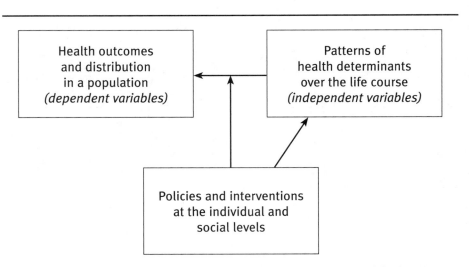

Health outcomes
and distribution
in a population
(dependent variables)

Patterns of
health determinants
over the life course
(independent variables)

Policies and interventions
at the individual and
social levels

Source: Kindig and Stoddart (2003, Figure 1, 382). Used with permission of the American Public Health Association.

day care, and so forth. *Realized access* is participation in the delivery of services, despite any barriers. Exhibit 2.4 presents these dimensions of effectiveness according to the structure/process/outcome model.

If efficacy is established, an effectiveness study may need only to establish that individuals or populations successfully accessed services. For example, an intervention to encourage mammography in a community may evaluate any increase in the proportion of underserved women receiving mammography screenings without evaluating the sensitivity and specificity of those screenings. When evidence of efficacy is less robust, such as when it is sensitive to contextual factors or when the fidelity of an intervention translated from ideal conditions to real-world conditions is uncertain, studies should include both process and outcome measures.

Evidence of Effectiveness

Both efficacy and effectiveness are judgments based on evidence. Evidence is, in its simplest form, observation. The pieces of evidence themselves do not indicate efficacy or effectiveness. Findings from individual studies are typically not sufficient for answering questions regarding the effectiveness of a healthcare service or system. Investigations should be interpreted with respect to noted strengths and limits of the existing body of evidence, and greater weight should be granted to studies that have superior designs and more relevance for the question at hand. All evidence needs to be evaluated in the context of the circumstances under which it was gathered and the situation for which it was sought. Pieces of evidence may contradict each other. Such conflict does not mean that science does not "work" (Lehrer 2010); rather, individual observations should be reviewed to determine whether an evaluative conclusion can be discerned.

Evaluation of evidence involves two key concepts: **bias** (or **confounding**) and **generalizability** (or **ecological validity**). In a study of the effectiveness of an intervention, *bias* concerns the likelihood that other factors account for the observed results. *Generalizability* concerns the degree to which the results can be applied to a target population or circumstance.

Research studies incorporate various designs to address bias and generalizability. Efficacy studies, which primarily address cause-and-effect hypotheses, employ designs that strongly control bias and confounding but often are weak in terms of generalizability. For example, an efficacy study of breast cancer screening may be well designed to address the sensitivity and specificity of mammography in detecting breast cancer in different age groups (Keen and Keen 2008) but would not provide information regarding the likelihood of women in a certain demographic group to adequately follow an indicated repeat mammography screening schedule. An effectiveness study regarding mammography screening might address adherence to repeat

EXHIBIT 2.4
Dimensions of Effectiveness

Structure	Process	Outcome
Effectiveness		
Quantity	Variations in use	Effectiveness
Efficacy	• Quantity	• Mortality
	• Quality	• Morbidity
	• Appropriateness	• Health status
Quantity: the number of physicians, nurses, and other providers as well as the quantity of monetary resources	**Variations in use:** different observed levels of per capita consumption of a service, especially hospital care, office visits, drugs, and specific procedures	**Effectiveness:** actual achieved benefit
Efficacy: maximum achievable benefit	**Quality:** a judgment concerning the process of care, based on the extent to which that care contributes to valued outcomes	**Does it work?*** Does the maneuver, procedure, or service do more good than harm to the people who receive it?
Does it work?* Does the health maneuver, procedure, or service do more good than harm to people who fully comply with the associated recommendations or treatment?	The quality of medical care is the component of the difference between efficacy and effectiveness that can be attributed to care providers, taking into account the environment in which they work.	
	Appropriateness: the extent to which available knowledge and techniques are used or misused in the management of illness and health	

*This question refers to the ability of a particular medical action to alter the natural history of a particular disease for the better, under actual conditions of practice and use.

Sources: Brook and Lohr (1985); Cochrane (1971); Donabedian (2003, 1982, 1980, 1973); IOM (2012); Lohr, Eleazer, and Mauskopf (1998); Sackett (1980); Williamson (1978).

mammography in certain demographic groups (Ryerson et al. 2008) but may or may not assess the clinical outcomes of those mammographies.

A major challenge in effectiveness research design is to limit confounding while not limiting generalizability—for example, deciding whether to recruit a homogeneous participant sample to limit confounders or to recruit a heterogeneous sample to boost generalizability. A study of breast cancer screening that includes a wide age range would be generalizable, but results might be confounded by differences in breast tissue, adherence to repeat mammography, and other age-related factors.

Because healthcare services are delivered in a variety of configurations to the general population, a range of models of effectiveness and study designs are used in HSR.

Conceptual Models of Effectiveness

Structure/Process/Outcome

In biology, analyses differ according to whether they focus on anatomical structure or function. Donabedian (2005, 1966) adapted the structure/function model from anatomy to develop the structure/process/outcome model of health services delivery and effectiveness. This model is reflected in the HSR/policy framework in Chapter 1, Exhibit 1.5. Descriptive studies of effectiveness might illustrate structures, processes, or outcomes associated with health services and systems. Analytic HSR studies may be organized by whether they focus on relating structural aspects of healthcare to outcomes, process aspects to outcomes, or both. The structure/process/outcome model was developed to evaluate effectiveness at the clinical level, such as the effectiveness of quality improvement efforts by a provider of outpatient care, but also can be applied at the population level.

In his model, Donabedian specified seven pillars of quality: efficacy, effectiveness, efficiency, optimality, acceptability, legitimacy, and equity. These aspects of healthcare are incorporated and evaluated in effectiveness research (Donabedian 1990). They also guide planning for the implementation of healthcare services (Schiff and Rucker 2001).

RE-AIM

The RE-AIM framework (Glasgow, Vogt, and Boles 1999) was developed to systematically guide effectiveness analyses based on population outcomes. RE-AIM requires knowledge of the degree of a health or healthcare problem in a given community and involves an assessment of the extent to which an intervention reaches members of that population, is able to promote beneficial outcomes in those reached, and is adopted and sustained. Use of the

RE-AIM framework to evaluate the effectiveness of an intervention involves assessments of

- reach (what portion of the intended population can be reached),
- efficacy (the degree to which the intervention is effective for those who receive it properly),
- adoption (what is required of the providers who deliver the intervention),
- implementation (what is required to deliver the intervention with fidelity and how fidelity is monitored), and
- maintenance (what infrastructure and other resources, such as health insurance reimbursement or professional training, are required for the intervention to be delivered indefinitely).

The RE-AIM framework does not distinguish between structural and process aspects of healthcare, which give the structure/process/outcome model its conceptual strength, but it does overlap Donabedian's seven pillars, particularly acceptability and sustainability of implementation.

Comparative Effectiveness Research

Although not a conceptually distinct model of health services effectiveness, comparative effectiveness research (CER) is a burgeoning perspective focused on reducing variation in healthcare delivery and outcomes across providers, regions, and health systems (Umscheid 2010). As the number of treatment options for different conditions increases, so does the role of advisory guidance, including clinical protocols and disease management programs, in health services practice and policy (Tanenbaum 2009). There is a recognized public and private interest in developing the capacity to manage practice variation without sacrificing individuality and a focus on evaluating the relative benefits of viable therapeutic choices for similar conditions and patients (McClellan et al. 2009). Heterogeneity in clinical care patterns (Wennberg 2004) and increased emphasis on measures of effect size rather than on p values (Cohen 1994) have provided a platform for the trend toward CER. The IOM Committee on Comparative Effectiveness Research Prioritization (2009) has noted that, in addition to measuring efficacy, CER ought to reveal what works best for which patients under what circumstances.

CER requires that the same outcomes be targeted by two (or more) interventions so that relative outcomes can be judged. Further, CER addresses relevant, high-priority issues that have the potential to change practice (IOM Committee on Comparative Effectiveness Research Prioritization 2009). Evidence should be developed and consulted to inform decisions, such as which interventions will be recommended by clinical guidelines, reimbursed by healthcare payers, or encouraged or discouraged by copayment (Teutsch and Fielding 2011).

Other Models

Other effectiveness and service delivery models exist, but they are less recognized or greatly overlap the ones just presented. The Homer/Hirsch/Milstein model (Homer and Hirsch 2006; Milstein 2008) and quantum model (Resnicow and Page 2008) emphasize health and healthcare as dynamic systems and focus on process. The Quality Health Outcomes Model (Mitchell, Ferketich, and Jennings 1998; Sidani, Doran, and Mitchell 2004), similar to the Donabedian model, focuses on the quality of healthcare at the level of the clinical/delivery setting. Some models focus on translation of new knowledge into practice (Estabrooks et al. 2006; Khoury, Gwinn, and Ioannidis 2010). In the RE-AIM model, knowledge translation is part of the adoption assessment; in the structure/process/outcome model, knowledge translation would be a study of process effectiveness.

Some models are suited to analyzing special topics or circumstances. For example, the UCLA model, largely based on the Andersen/Aday model, is used to analyze the effectiveness of community healthcare safety nets on patient access and outcomes (Brown et al. 2004; Davidson et al. 2004).

Study Designs

As noted earlier, a study's design determines the degree to which the results are valid and generalizable. Study design is always a matter of trade-offs, the leading of which is cost, both in dollars and time. Thorough, strong studies are usually more costly than less comprehensive, less rigorous ones. Typically, effectiveness analyses depend on a few optimized studies and draw additional support from a host of less optimal ones.

Available studies may not report all of the information required to judge the validity or generalizability of results. Advocacy and use of reporting standards, such as CONSORT (Consolidated Standards of Reporting Trials, released in 1996) for clinical studies and STROBE (STrengthening the Reporting of OBservational studies in Epidemiology, published in 2007) for observational trials, have increased over recent years (Begg et al. 1996; Fung et al. 2009; Moher, Schulz, and Altman 2001; Simera et al. 2010, 2009; Vandenbroucke et al. 2007; von Elm et al. 2007). This movement has influenced grant proposal review and journal peer review; nevertheless, the burden remains on the consumer of the evidence to be aware of the strengths and weaknesses inherent in a chosen study design.

This review of study design provides a basic overview of the leading parameters by which studies vary. With this information, any two studies can be compared in terms of the degree to which results might be generalizable or biased/confounded by other factors.

HSR studies are categorized as either interventions or observational trials. In intervention studies, the investigator identifies and composes a relevant study sample, introduces ("manipulates") the change of interest, and measures the resulting outcomes with predetermined metrics. In observational studies, no change is introduced; data concerning some aspect(s) of healthcare are gathered from an existing group of individuals or settings and analyzed to evaluate various hypotheses. In an intervention study, measures are selected for their appropriateness and then applied and hypotheses are stated in advance. In an observational study, measures of the relevant concepts are either developed ad hoc from existing data or selected and applied when opportunity permits.

Observational studies typically are more generalizable because they are drawn from actual healthcare populations involved in real-world service delivery rather than from the controlled conditions of an intervention study; however, observational studies do not control factors under analysis and so are more subject to influences beyond the researcher's control. An additional weakness of observational studies is that they often are conducted with compromised measurements. If the observational study is based on administrative data (hospital discharge data or insurance claims data), the measures of utilization and outcome may be proxies that rely on the accuracy of medical recordkeeping and coding. If the observational study is a survey, the measures are a compromise between desired detail and the burden placed on the study participants to provide the detail.

Intervention studies have two leading strengths: the methodological strength of determining appropriate measures in advance (although participant burden is still an issue) and the strength of controlling the interventions introduced to the sample as other factors are held constant or otherwise "controlled" by design aspects, such as randomization. While these design aspects strengthen evaluation of causal hypotheses, efforts to control all potential confounding influences may limit generalizability. For example, studies may need to be limited to one age group to control undesired variance across age groups; the resulting evidence, while valid, might thus be limited to that age group. Recruitment of study samples presents a host of challenges that also may limit generalizability (e.g., biases may influence whether participants are motivated to consent to participation). Clever intervention study design is dedicated to paralleling the "real world" to minimize the inherent artificiality. While they control for confounders, well-designed clinical studies are often too narrowly focused to be predictive of effectiveness in health services delivery. Consequently, they may fail to provide the type of information clinical and policy decision makers need (Glasgow et al. 2005; Khoury, Gwinn, and Ioannidis 2010; Tunis, Stryer, and Clancy 2003).

Good observational studies parallel the design aspects of intervention studies to achieve internal validity, such as by including statistical adjustment for a wide range of confounders. Good intervention studies parallel the desirable aspects of observational studies to achieve generalizability, such as by using a sample that is strongly representative of the general population and including subgroup analyses.

Observational Studies

Descriptive Information

A great deal of HSR related to effectiveness is simply descriptive: What portion of a population with a specific illness is receiving care? How many providers are practicing in a certain geographic area? What is the cost of healthcare for a specific illness? A *needs assessment*, the starting place for designing or improving health services and systems, is primarily a descriptive study of the nature, magnitude, and distribution of health problems that includes some analysis to determine the causes of the problem and the outcomes that should be pursued (Rossi, Lipsey, and Freeman 2003). Data sources include population surveys (for determining incidence or prevalence of a health problem) and reviews of claims data (for describing healthcare utilization or costs). Such data often do not exist, are not complete, or are not sufficiently detailed to adequately diagnose a problem or identify a solution. This situation is changing as the gathering and reporting of descriptive data on basic population health and health services become more common at the national, state, and local levels in the United States. See Chapter 3 for more discussion on the sources of these data.

Case Study

A *case study* could concern a patient who had a novel experience or a health service delivery organization that implemented a change to improve performance. Cases can be individuals, groups of people, organizations, communities, or nations. Observed outcomes and experiences are described, and various factors may be suggested as possible causes. This type of study does not strongly defend apparent connections between predictors and outcomes but proposes they are worthy of additional attention.

Case studies often are guided by one or more theoretical models and serve as educational examples to further illustrate one model or to contrast two models. They also can be used to illustrate phenomena that call for new explanatory models. For example, the field of psychosocial resilience was developed through case studies of individuals who thrived despite their disadvantaged circumstances (Masten 2001), and the field of positive deviance was developed through the study of cases, both individuals and systems, that thrive where others fail to perform well (Marsh et al. 2004). Case studies can serve the "black swan" purpose, noting an occurrence, previously believed to be impossible or exclusionary, that may significantly influence a body of thought (Harris 1987; Taleb 2007).

Case Series

A *case series* is a case study of multiple subjects. The goal is to observe whether some cause–effect relationship is apparent in more than one case or to test a model's suitability for use in multiple circumstances. This type of study could be conducted with a series of patients or a series of healthcare delivery changes, such as those made in response to changing occurrence of a disease in a population, changing demographics, changing federal policy, and so on. Optimally, equivalent data are gathered on each case. This task may be challenging if measures are not set up in advance for collection, as would be the case in an intervention study. In a case series, the greater the consistency of the relationship between predictor and outcome across studies, the more compelling the causal hypothesis will be. A significant limitation of case series is lack of a control group as a reference for other possible influences, such as maturational or secular change. Another limitation is the potential for selective reporting; the researcher may notice or report cases that fit some hypothesis but fail to report other cases that would not support that hypothesis.

Case Comparison

A *case comparison* is a case study that includes a comparison group and some control of coincident influences, such as maturational and secular effects, to evaluate a hypothesis. If outcomes suspected to be attributable to a unique aspect of a case are also detected in the comparator condition, the evidence for the causal hypothesis is weakened. A comparison group can be developed from existing descriptive data for some relevant population. For example, quality-of-life results for some study group can be compared to available norms for demographically similar groups. The manual for the SF-36, a health-related quality-of-life survey (Ware Jr., Kosinski, and Gandek 2002), provides a set of such norms.

Case Control

A *case control* study is similar to a case comparison study but includes a more deliberately formed comparison group. Typically the study group is composed of many cases, and each case is matched, frequently one to one, with a control on the basis of compelling, relevant matching criteria (e.g., sociodemographics, clinical indicators, comorbidities). This observational study design resembles a controlled trial, in which seemingly equivalent groups differ only with regard to exposure to the intervention, but it differs from a controlled trial in that the researcher does not introduce the exposure but rather gleans it from the data. Any candidate factor that statistically differentiates between the cases and controls has elevated suspicion as a causal factor and should elicit further investigation.

A case control study can be conducted prospectively or retrospectively. The prospective strategy typically includes a well-planned set of suspected predictors, while the retrospective strategy is conducted after the fact and so typically has a weaker set of predictors available for analysis. A notable limitation is that, unlike other study designs, each of the two groups (cases and controls) will have its own unique set of selection biases: Cases (whether they be people, clinics, or communities, etc.) are selected for "case-ness," and then controls are somehow selected from the entirety of total possible controls.

Surveys

As noted earlier, use of a survey that includes an intentionally selected set of measures and targets participants of interest is a better means of measuring some aspect of health or healthcare than is use of various existing data. Survey participants can be individuals, institutions, communities, or nations. A large sample can improve researchers' ability to detect true relations and can alleviate the noise of spurious associations. Many hypotheses can be explored, surveys can be repeated over time to analyze trends, and survey results can be linked to other data sources.

Nevertheless, the validity of associations that emerge from survey data may be limited due to lack of control of confounders, unclear temporal sequencing of measures, and inaccuracies in participant self-reports. With regard to self-reports, people tend to report their behavior as better than it really is, which leads to problems such as overreporting of healthful habits and underreporting of unhealthy habits. Furthermore, stigmatized behaviors and conditions are likely to be underreported. Participants also may be weak historians (i.e., have a limited capacity to report past experiences accurately or to report health habits validly because of poor recall or because they had no reason to be aware of certain behaviors or conditions).

A common observational study design in HSR is the cross-sectional survey. In this design, a set of selected measures is obtained from a sample of people, organizations, or other groups and the relationships among these measures are examined. Common patient indicators include vital signs, blood cholesterol levels, demographic characteristics, and self-ratings of health. Organizational indicators commonly include size and for-profit versus non-profit status. Noted relationships between measures indicate possible causal relations; the evidence is only suggestive.

A cross-sectional study may be repeated over time, drawing from a new sample of participants at each iteration. This design may help researchers note trends, but any observed differences could be due to the samples developed rather than to a change in the phenomenon measured. Sampling/

recruitment strategies can improve the similarity between samples drawn at different points in time.

In a longitudinal survey, a study population is established at a baseline point in time and at least one additional measurement is made at a later point in time. Longitudinal survey design makes a stronger case for causality than does a cross-sectional survey because temporal ordering can be established. A great deal of health knowledge has emerged from following cohorts of people, noting incident outcomes such as heart disease, and exploring factors predictive of these outcomes. Longitudinal surveys are particularly valuable for evaluating the influence of various structure and process aspects of health-care coverage on patterns of healthcare utilization. For example, an analysis can be conducted to determine the effect that a change in patient copayment for some service has on the overall pattern of utilization.

A limitation of longitudinal observational studies is that many of the predictors that emerge are correlated with, and logically intermingled with, other factors. For example, education level usually is predictive of health outcomes across time, but a study cannot conclude that some aspect of education leads to better health because education is confounded with income, which might influence health through improved healthcare access. Although which covarying factor is causally linked cannot be established, more elaborate analyses can strengthen the test of such hypotheses. An extensive set of analytic and statistical methods has been developed to address such confounding.

Experimental Studies

The essence of an intervention study (i.e., trial) is the researcher's ability to apply, deliver, or "try" a predictor and then measure whether the outcome of interest changes. The evidentiary power of this type of study is the researcher's opportunity to determine what the predictor is, determine who the recipient is, determine the process and outcome measures to be used, and determine the various ways biases might be controlled or eliminated.

In a simple trial, an intervention is delivered to a patient, a patient population, or some component of the healthcare system (e.g., a hospital, a community, a state) and the outcome is measured. A simple trial's persuasiveness is limited because other factors may account for any change, and a simple trial has no design aspect to control for these confounders. Mere participation in a study may cause a desired outcome when the intervention is actually ineffective. Measurement reactivity, the Hawthorne effect, placebo effects, recruitment biases, selection biases, and expectancy effects are all examples of biases that can cause a desired outcome to occur even when the intervention is ineffective. One advantage of observational studies over trials is that they may not introduce such biases.

An "A/B" trial is an enhanced design that may eliminate some of these biases. The intervention can be delivered to see if it has the desired effect and then be withdrawn to see if the effect goes away, as would be expected in certain circumstances. In an A/B/A trial, the intervention is introduced, withdrawn, and then reintroduced. This design may rule out some biases, especially the effect of coincident factors on the outcome of interest. Quality improvement interventions, such as disease management for some patients or conditions, can readily be tested with an A/B design or an A/B/A design.

A limitation of an A/B/A design is irreversibility: If the intervention is expected to deliver a lasting effect (e.g., the delivery of an immunization, the delivery of some knowledge, a change in practice style), the A/B/A design is not appropriate because the changed outcome cannot be reversed. Some educational interventions use "booster" sessions, in which the teaching or training is reviewed and reinforced at a later date; a trial testing the benefit of a booster session ends up being of the A/B/A design when striving to determine whether that booster session improves long-term outcomes.

In a controlled trial, researchers select a group comparable to the group receiving the manipulation, and both groups' outcomes are assessed. If this type of trial is properly designed, the difference in the outcome between the intervention group and the control group can be attributed to the experimental intervention. Like other study designs, this design has limitations, key among which are those introduced simply by receipt of an intervention; when participants know that they are receiving the intervention, they may experience a placebo effect. More stringent study designs, noted later in this chapter, can reduce these biasing influences. Another problem is possible non-equivalence between the intervention group and the control group (known as *assignment effects*). For example, a researcher may recruit, either consciously or unconsciously, a certain type of patient for the intervention group and then select participants for the control group on the basis of different criteria. An eager researcher might enroll participants who arrive early at the clinic in the intervention group and relegate late arrivers to the control group. An intervention group might be formed first due to pragmatic reasons—for example, a study sample of flu patients would be formed during flu season by certain staff members working at the clinic during that time, and the control group might be formed later, possibly in another season, or by other staff members.

The placebo-controlled study design is the same as the controlled trial, but some comparison intervention is given to the control and intervention groups so that biasing influences (placebo effects, expectancy effects) affect both groups. The control group participants must believe they are being treated as the intervention group or that the comparison intervention they receive has potency. This design strengthens the evidence that observed differences in outcomes between the intervention and control groups can be attributed to the intervention. A placebo- or attention-controlled trial does not control for selection biases, so the sampling/recruitment strategy remains a potential source of bias.

In a randomized controlled trial, the researcher randomly assigns participants (or other units of analysis, whether healthcare settings, communities, classrooms, or school districts) to the intervention and control groups. Randomization limits the impact of selection and assignment effects (mentioned earlier). Again, as in a controlled trial, if a placebo or an attention intervention is not included to provoke placebo or attention effects, whether an observed outcome is due to the intervention or to some other effect will be unclear. In the randomized controlled clinical trial design, after random assignment, the intervention group receives the intervention under investigation and the control group receives some comparison intervention so that biasing influences (placebo effects, expectancy effects) are able to affect both groups.

In any of these trial designs, a range of biases may be introduced simply because the researcher knows who is in the intervention group and who is in the control group. Researchers may favor the intervention they are testing, and participants may want to satisfy the researcher by providing the answers they suppose the researcher wants. These competing explanations of outcomes can be controlled by conducting a *blind trial*, meaning that the researcher, the participants, or both do not know the group to which participants have been assigned. When both the researcher and participants are blinded to treatment or control assignment, the trial is referred to as a *double-blind trial*. When only one of the two is blinded, it is called a *single-blind trial*.

A trial may also involve a third type of blinding. Whoever is conducting the outcomes assessment (i.e., a rater who is not the same person as the researcher) could be blinded to a subject's study group assignment. If the rater is blinded, he will not introduce biases into the outcomes assessment. The rater need not even know what the study hypothesis is.

Unblinding occurs when some aspect of the study, such as a medication side effect or a chance discussion between participants from each group, occurs, thereby revealing study group assignment. A development in drug trials is the use of placebos that provoke side effects in a manner similar to the investigational drug so that the blind is preserved even if side effects are experienced.

Designing a study to maximally limit biases and competing explanations is challenging and requires substantial resources. No study is perfect. Much of the evidence available to support decisions falls well below optimal standards. Many studies do not even report the blinding aspects of their design (Montori et al. 2002). A common conclusion of systematic literature reviews of research on the effectiveness of health services and systems is that well-conducted and well-reported studies are rare.

Optimal trial study design standards are often achieved in prototypical pharmaceutical efficacy trials. In HSR, however, these standards typically are impractical. For example, a test of a physician pay-for-performance experiment cannot be blinded; knowledge of the intervention (i.e., incentives) is the very factor driving outcomes (improved performance). If a policymaker wishes to try a new way of assessing eligibility for public programs, the entire eligibility effort would need to be redesigned and delivered. The staff carrying out the new process likely would be the staff already in place, who are familiar with the status quo. Also, eligibility candidates often have knowledge of the eligibility process, either from past experience or from being informed by others. Such implementation realities make blinding impractical in many HSR circumstances. Instead, the study design would have to be sufficient to evaluate the effectiveness of the novel eligibility process without blinding to control for placebo effects. The majority of health services delivery research is observational, not randomized, and not blinded.

Systematic Reviews and Meta-Analyses

Systematic reviews and meta-analyses may be done of observational studies and of intervention studies. A *meta-analysis*, in its strictest sense, is a technique for mathematically combining the outcomes of similar studies to arrive at an overall representative result. In simple terms, results from contributory individual studies are compiled to determine an average effect. This combined estimate is more confident than that which would be gained if yet another study were conducted.

One challenge with a meta-analysis is deciding on the inclusion/exclusion criteria. Ideally, the criteria for judging study design quality would be determined in advance of the literature search. Otherwise, the process would be subject to various biases, conscious or subconscious. Because the establishment of selection criteria involves discretionary judgment across a range of study characteristics, these decisions affect the eventual sets of studies to be pooled for analysis and so will affect the eventual outcome. Two well-conducted meta-analyses might have differing inclusion criteria and thus arrive at differing results. To some degree, this limitation is addressed by a customary meta-analysis procedure: When essential data for any of the single studies are not included in a study's published results, the authors of that single study may be contacted and asked to provide additional data before the study is permitted to be included in the meta-analysis.

A systematic review is less exacting than a meta-analysis but still provides a nuanced evaluation of a body of evidence. Relevant studies are reviewed with respect to their varying approaches to form an overall conclusion regarding the effectiveness of healthcare (Liberati et al. 2009). Patterns can be sought across studies to account for disparate outcomes. For example, a systematic review of studies involving the same intervention might reveal a strong effect for men or for younger people, a stronger effect when the outcome is measured one way versus another, or a stronger effect when the intervention is delivered by one means versus another. In many cases the result is not one answer but a range of answers. The strength of the evidence also can be rated. Rating helps make a coherent whole of the existing evidence and identifies where future research needs to focus.

Other Study Designs

Several other study designs have been developed that are appropriate for addressing different kinds of effectiveness research questions. Each incorporates elements of the study designs discussed in the previous sections.

Complex Interventions

Real-world healthcare delivery innovations often aim to address healthcare problems with variable, multicomponent interventions implemented in various settings and targeting multiple outcomes. The relevance of these studies depends on clear reporting of these aspects, and the field is increasingly recognizing that such complex interventions require a distinct category of study design (Francis et al. 2011; Lamb et al. 2011).

A recent, well-recognized complex trial has been the STAR*D trial, designed to provide conclusions that have direct implications for real-world practice. Recognizing that different depression interventions work for different patients and that patients prefer a choice of intervention, STAR*D developed a complex treatment protocol including patient choice points and a complex of outcomes, such as depression, treatment side effects, quality of life, and functioning (Sinyor, Schaffer, and Levitt 2010). Design and outcomes were necessarily spread across several publications, and great effort has been devoted to discerning what conclusions have emerged from this study (Nelson and Campfield 2006; Rush 2007). STAR*D was intended to function similarly to a traditional trial. Other complex study designs adhere less to that idea.

Program Evaluation

Program evaluation is a study design for determining whether a unique program, usually a onetime, one-location effort, meets the intended process and outcome goals. The program's uniqueness may stem from a variety of factors; for example, the proposed program might be a pilot, might be a local application of widely recognized interventions, or might have been implemented in response to local circumstances or other circumstances that preclude the use of, or need for, a controlled trial. This design is suited for broad-scope, multimodal interventions, such as those intended to improve some health outcome for a school, community, or healthcare delivery setting. Optimally, the interventions making up the program already have an evidence base as justification for their selection because efficacy testing of component interventions is not a prime intention of program evaluation.

Because the focus of program evaluation is to determine the degree to which a program improved a local situation rather than to test some general healthcare hypothesis, and because stakeholder involvement is usually involved, the intervention should be modified as challenges are encountered and new opportunities emerge.

The design of a program evaluation is based on a "logic model"—an explication of how the program is expected to achieve its results and corresponding process and outcome measures for determining the extent to which the intervention was implemented as planned. Researchers often take a "mixed-methods" approach to evaluation (O'Cathain 2009), using both quantitative and qualitative data to assess adherence to the logic model and whether goals were met and to share lessons learned. Evaluation varies according to the audience for which it is intended and the purposes it is to serve (Rossi, Lipsey, and Freeman 2003).

Practical Clinical Trials

As efforts were under way in the 1990s and 2000s to improve healthcare through commitment to evidence-based practice (Kazdin 2008; Sackett et al. 1996), practitioners were discussing the pragmatic limits of practicing according to the evidence base from controlled trials (Eddy 2005; Timmermans and Mauck 2005). From these discussions, the concept of practice-based evidence emerged. Practical trials (also called *pragmatic trials*) have been advanced as a study design suitable for developing research-based evidence that readily relates to real-world practice contingencies.

The ethos of practical trials is twofold: The sites of delivery are actual clinical settings, and outcomes, including patient preference and quality of life, will have a bearing on subsequent adoption of the intervention if it is proven clinically effective (Tunis, Stryer, and Clancy 2003). Control conditions should be strategically selected to limit confounding factors, and trials should be randomized if possible. The National Institute of Mental Health has supported several major examples of this design, such as STAR*D and CATIE.

Assessments of Collaboratives

A *healthcare collaborative* is a collective effort of local stakeholders in some area of healthcare or community to address challenges so that the sum can function better than the parts could individually (Nowell and Foster-Fishman 2010). In the fragmented healthcare environment, if various actors can work together, healthcare delivery should improve beyond the status quo (Community Care Coordination 2010; Frost and Stone 2009). Thus far, because the nature of collaboratives have been varied and their purposes diverse, the field does not recognize a single model or set of criteria for evaluating the superiority of a collaborative effort over the status quo. However, some characteristics of collaborative evaluation are common: Research designs for evaluating collaboratives are similar or identical to program evaluation design and include strong evaluation of processes, such as communication among partners and shared decision making (Lasker, Weiss, and Miller 2001). Some formal assessment instruments have been developed to evaluate the functioning of the collaborative (Davis 2008; Lasker, Weiss, and Miller 2001).

Because of the uniqueness of a collaborative, and because of the magnitude of healthcare problems that prompts the decision to develop a collaborative, benchmarking performance and determining whether the effort invested is producing a worthwhile outcome are challenging. Processes can be assessed over a time frame similar to that involved in other healthcare research studies, but collaborative efforts may take years to make improvements great enough to be detectable by community indicators. Most outcomes studies report results for less than five years, while outcomes require three to ten years to be detectable (Roussos and Fawcett 2000). As part of its "Quality Information & Improvement" effort, AHRQ has developed tools, guidance, and evaluation resources for local collaborative efforts addressing healthcare issues.

Qualitative Research

Effectiveness studies are usually *quantitative*—that is, they apply numeric measurement of a defined set of factors to determine the mathematically represented relationships between them in terms of amount, degree, or quantity. In healthcare, *qualitative* research has been valuable for revealing social and psychological factors for quantitative study, such as treatment adherence, decision making by provider as well as patient, trust in healthcare, stigma of disease, and conceptualizations of complex disease. Additionally, methods springing from qualitative research are vital to systematic improvement in healthcare because many quality improvement strategies depend on analysis of complex processes and idiosyncratic deviations from normal variation.

Because qualitative research yields evidence that is narrowly focused but rich in depth, results commonly have limited generalizability. The strategy of constant comparison (Glaser 1965) has been developed as a means to increase the generalizability of theories and hypotheses drawn from narrow-scope qualitative findings and has been advanced for this purpose in healthcare (Bradley, Curry, and Devers 2007). Qualitative methods are increasingly being used as adjuncts to the quantitative study designs described earlier in this chapter to assist in the development of interventions, assessment methods, or measures (e.g., designing a survey) or to explore the meaning of findings from empirical analysis (O'Cathain 2009). Through "readers' guides," the *Journal of the American Medical Association* has facilitated the consumption of qualitative research in healthcare (Giacomini and Cook 2000a, 2000b). As noted earlier in this chapter, practical trials, RE-AIM analyses, evaluations of collaboratives, complex interventions, and other study designs require consideration of more than just clinical outcomes; in many cases, these nonclinical outcomes include qualitative and quantitative data.

Other Important Aspects of Effectiveness Research

In addition to identifying the theoretical model and study design of effectiveness research, investigators must consider other significant dimensions on which studies differ.

Prevention Versus Treatment

The study design required to test a prevention hypothesis is different from the study design required to test a treatment hypothesis. A prevention study needs to include a sample of people at risk for some undesired health condition, evaluate the delivery of the protective intervention, and then monitor the study sample over time to detect incidence of the undesired condition. Occurrence of the condition is the outcome. In contrast, a treatment study begins with a sample of people who have experienced the undesired condition, delivers an intervention, and then measures resolution of the condition. Because the incidence of conditions that occur infrequently need to be observed to establish prevention, prevention studies require larger sample sizes. Also, because incidence occurs over time, prevention studies generally require longitudinal time frames.

A challenging aspect of treatment studies is detection of side effects of the intervention in addition to its effects on a medical condition (Chou and Helfand 2005). If side effects occur, only some members of the study group are likely to experience them, so a sufficient research design for detecting side effects includes either a greater sample size or a greater time span for posttreatment monitoring than that required to sufficiently test whether the intervention is effective. Because the incidence of adverse events is not known for a novel intervention, the sample size and surveillance time span required are difficult to determine. For clinical trials, a data safety monitoring board should be in place to evaluate signals of potential harm (FDA 2006).

A Priori Hypotheses or Post-Hoc Hypotheses

A critical aspect of scientific hypothesis testing is specification of the "rules of the game" before the game begins. Changing the rules after starting the game or even after the game is over yields less impressive evidence; biases can be readily introduced, such as by inventing or changing the criteria for membership in a subgroup analysis, changing measures, or changing the statistical analysis applied to the data. Also, a statistically significant result can be found by "fishing"—looking at data in different ways until a statistically significant relationship is detected among many possible relationships. This strategy increases the likelihood of detecting a relationship that occurred by chance (i.e., a type 1 error); such post hoc, exploratory analyses are misleading if not represented as such. A finding from an a priori (planned) analysis should be regarded more seriously than a finding identified after the study was completed.

Type 1 errors are regularly encountered in longitudinal health surveys, in which, as intended, an extensive set of hypotheses may be evaluated after results are gathered. These health surveys purposefully include many potential predictors of outcomes. In this case, findings are considered tentative. Other lines of evidence, such as those noted by Sir Austin Bradford Hill (1965), are necessary to support the validity of such findings. So, when evaluating evidence for any health or healthcare delivery issue, investigators must consider the threat from fishing or multiple testing by assessing whether the hypotheses were stated a priori and how many tests could have been conducted with the given data.

Statistical Control

When striving to identify the degree to which an intervention predicts an outcome, analysts include another possible predictor in the statistical analysis to account for variation in the outcome. For example, if a study is attempting to evaluate the potential for dietary fat to predict the likelihood of developing breast cancer, it is reasonable to suspect that a person's regular level of physical activity might also be a risk factor. Therefore, along with the factor being tested (dietary fat), a measure of physical activity is included in the analysis as a statistical control to account for the variance in the study's observed incidence of breast cancer. If the analysis, controlling for physician activity, reveals a predictive relationship between dietary fat and breast cancer, the inclusion of the control variable eliminates this factor as a confounder, and so the firmness of the conclusion regarding the relationship between dietary fat and breast cancer is not weakened by the observation that dietary fat and physical activity are probably themselves correlated.

Statistical controls strengthen the case for the internal validity of both observational and intervention studies. In the example presented in the previous paragraph, an intervention study could achieve the same control of confounding factors by limiting recruitment to people with the same level of physical activity, but this limitation might interfere with or delay the recruitment of study participants. Intervention studies typically depend on design aspects (e.g., strict exclusionary criteria) to control for confounders, while observational studies, such as longitudinal cohort studies, tend to depend on statistical analyses for this purpose.

The most common factors used for statistical control are those noted for their ubiquitous influence on health habits, health outcomes, and health services utilization. They fall into four general categories:

1. Demographic factors (e.g., employment status, education level)
2. Measures of health status (e.g., body mass index, medical comorbidities, self-perceived health status)
3. Sociocultural factors (e.g., race/ethnicity or religious affiliation, which account for culturally determined dietary customs and other lifestyle choices)
4. Psychosocial factors (e.g., perceived social support, depression, anxiety, health locus of control, motivation to change health behavior)

All of these factors are known to influence health and healthcare and so introduce the potential for bias unless eliminated by study design or statistically controlled. Statistically significant relationships often disappear when one or more of these controls are included. Analyses that include control variables are commonly called *adjusted models*, and comparison with *unadjusted models* (which include no control measures) can demonstrate the degree to which statistical control reduces sources of bias. Knowledge of a specific topic is necessary to be familiar with the control measures that may need to be included in an analysis.

Types of Data

Study results vary according to the source of data. Three major types of data are used in effectiveness research: survey data, administrative data, and medical chart data. As mentioned earlier, survey data are gathered by developing or selecting questionnaires and surveying appropriate subjects. Health surveys are rich sources of representative and comparative data on a wide range of health-related topics. Representative data are used to estimate the prevalence of medical conditions, and comparative data are used to determine the burden of a condition in a population. Furthermore, health surveys provide an evidence base for tracking trends in disease prevalence and treatment practices and for tracking relationships between medical conditions and a broad range of social and health-related outcomes. The sample size of these surveys tends to be large enough to include people with and without common medical conditions for comparison. As samples of the general population, results represent the entire population, including people who may not otherwise interact with the healthcare system, such as those without health insurance coverage. Survey data generally yield the best population-level measurements but are usually more costly and time-consuming to obtain.

An alternative means of exploring hypotheses is the use of administrative and medical chart data. Administrative data are collected from the medical records of healthcare providers and the claims files of insurance companies, generated in the course of managing, paying for, or monitoring the provision of healthcare services. Health encounters create claims for payment, and public and private healthcare providers and insurance plans collect these claims data and include them in administrative databases. Common administrative data sources include national and state hospital discharge databases as well as Medicare, Medicaid, and private insurance claims databases.

Each type of data has its strengths and weaknesses. Survey measures are planned in advance so that data of optimal validity and reliability are collected. However, surveys have several important limitations. First, participation is voluntary, and some populations are not covered. Response rates to general population surveys, particularly those conducted by telephone, have declined significantly over the past several decades—a potential source of nonresponse bias (Galea and Tracy 2007). Adequate coverage of the general population through traditional landline random-digit-dialing sampling methods has become challenging to achieve due to the increased use of cellular telephones. These methods also generally omit other important segments of the population, such as people who are homeless or living in institutions.

Second, population surveys cannot be used to collect data on specific population subgroups. Although population health surveys target large samples, due to the relatively low prevalence of many medical conditions they collect too few data on such cases to identify any rate differences across specific subgroups, such as differences by severity of the condition or by exposure to a given treatment. Finally, surveys rely on self-reported data and are vulnerable to error. For example, these data may overestimate the presence of a medical condition in the population due to reports of symptoms mistakenly associated with the condition. Survey participants' recall of medical care use also may be limited.

A leading strength of administrative data is the speed with which they can be gathered on numerous subjects. Since the 1980s, the federal government has required submission of uniform data on all acute hospital inpatient discharges paid through Medicare and Medicaid (Kanaan 2000). In 2010, a total of 48 states had systems for reporting hospital discharge data, many of which included statewide all-payer, all-patient data on inpatient hospital stays (Love, Custer, and Miller 2010). The trend toward greater use of outpatient care has led 32 states to collect data from ambulatory treatment centers and 30 states to include data from emergency department visits. Hospital discharge data are population based and can be used for analyses that examine patient demographics, the use of codes for diagnosis and treatment, hospital service use, and total costs (Love, Custer, and Miller et al. 2010). The data typically contain diagnosis, treatment, and cause-of-injury codes on each admission or visit; unique personal identifiers can be used to link admissions and visits to individuals for determining admission type, length of stay, acute care charges, primary and secondary procedure codes, sources of payment, and discharge disposition (Iezzoni 2003).

Hospital discharge data have important limitations. They do not include actual payments to the healthcare facility, nor do they collect data on the majority of pharmacy services or ambulatory care services provided outside hospitals (Love, Custer, and Miller 2010). In most cases the data obtained from hospital discharge databases cannot be validated, and coding errors and diagnostic misclassification that result in over- or underdiagnosis are known to occur (Iezzoni 2003). Even when accurately coded, the diagnoses available from such data sets provide limited clinical information and may not be sufficient to determine the subtype of a person's condition or its severity. Finally, hospitalization costs can be only approximated, either by applying hospital cost-to-charge ratios to hospital charges obtained from discharge data or by applying Medicare payment rates to hospital stays (Drummond et al. 2005).

In the process of providing public (e.g., Medicare, Medicaid, Children's Health Insurance Plan) and private (e.g., Blue Cross Blue Shield, UnitedHealth Group, CIGNA) health insurance coverage and paying providers, fiscal intermediaries collect large quantities of claims data. Many of the data elements included in hospital discharge data, such as demographic information, dates of service, service types, diagnosis and treatment codes, charges, and payments, also are included in claims data for every covered visit or service. Claims data are particularly useful because many include information on a comprehensive set of services, including hospital, physician, and medication use, which can be linked to de-identified individuals to track cases, service use patterns, costs, and outcomes over time. Because these data sets often are large and cover many people and services, they can be used for studies of people with major medical conditions and even, in some instances, for studies comparing incident versus prevalent cases or subgroup analyses of different demographic groups or subtypes of a condition (Iezzoni 2003).

As valuable as these data are for research purposes, they have important limitations. Claims data provide no information on populations lacking health insurance coverage or those who avoid seeking care because copayments and deductibles are too expensive, and analyses of where patients receive healthcare if they change their type of insurance coverage are not possible (Love, Custer, and Miller 2010). As with hospital data, accurate case identification from claims data is difficult for several reasons: ICD-9-CM codes are not consistently applied nor sufficiently detailed, and treatment codes are complex. In addition, the methods used to identify cases and services frequently are not validated.

Medical charts are potentially rich in clinical detail, but locating specific data elements in the medical chart and entering those elements into a database (described as *abstracting*) can be difficult and time-consuming and may require specific clinical knowledge. Medical chart data available through electronic medical records are easier to gather. As quality improvement efforts such as pay for performance and the adoption of more clinical care guidelines force clinical care to be documented more extensively, the detailed information in medical chart data will become more readily available to researchers.

Efforts to Improve the Quality and Availability of Data

As noted earlier in the chapter, promotion of study data reporting standards is increasing (Simera et al. 2010), so consumers of research are better able to assess available evidence. Observational studies are encouraged to follow the STROBE standards, and the CONSORT guidelines are recommended for randomized clinical trials. Major efforts by the federal government aim to increase the availability of data for effectiveness research.

Trial Data Registration

Modifications of the Food and Drug Administration (FDA) Act, including those made in 2001, require that investigational drug trials be registered with the FDA (Turner 2004). These records are a source of pharmaceutical trial data, even if the results of the trial are never published. This information was used in a noted meta-analysis (Turner et al. 2008) indicating that the apparent efficacy of antidepressants for depression is smaller when unpublished studies are included. *Publication biases* are those involved in the selection of studies for publication. Research journals may favor "positive" trials (those that support their hypotheses) over "negative" trials, and researchers may be hesitant to publish a study if the results do not match their personal preferences or beliefs.

Data-Sharing Requirements

To foster greater utilization of federally funded healthcare research, in 2003 NIH began requiring recipients of large grants (over $500,000 per year) to develop a plan for sharing resulting data, beyond obvious limits such as those concerning confidentiality or proprietary issues. The National Science Foundation (2011) and the European Science Foundation (2008) have adopted similar policies. Data sharing is motivated by many principles, two of which are prominent. The first is the ethic that data developed with public money should be open to some degree rather than preserved as publicly funded proprietary data. Second, science has an ethos of public scrutiny: Data sources should be elucidated, measurement methods should be shared, and results should be subject to review and replication. This movement has yet to bring about public availability of the majority of healthcare research data (Tenopir et al. 2011), but a trend is developing. Its progression holds great potential for advances in healthcare effectiveness knowledge.

Publicly Available Data

Various efforts, mostly federally funded, have been undertaken to make administrative and survey data regarding aspects of health and healthcare utilization available to the public. Data sets are typically hosted on public websites, accompanied by such supporting resources as data dictionaries and help desks. These data sets serve many functions in healthcare effectiveness research; they are used to benchmark patterns of utilization, summarize community health, and evaluate causal hypotheses.

The Centers for Medicare & Medicaid Services provides access to administrative data of two large healthcare delivery programs. AHRQ's Medical Expenditure Panel Survey, instituted in 1996, is a leading survey of healthcare coverage and utilization by households and by employers who sponsor healthcare coverage. Cohorts participate in interviews over a time span of one year, and new cohorts are initiated regularly, providing an enhanced, short-term longitudinal aspect to an otherwise cross-sectional survey.

The Behavioral Risk Factor Surveillance System, instituted by the Centers for Disease Control and Prevention (CDC) in 1984, is an annual cross-sectional survey of citizens regarding health status and health behaviors, such as exercising and receiving recommended screenings. The CDC's National Center for Health Statistics also provides guidance on numerous other sources of publicly available data sets useful for HSR purposes, including effectiveness purposes.

Summary and Conclusions

The study of effectiveness depends on two factors: the evaluation of efficacy and the evaluation of service delivery. Effectiveness data serve as a foundation for evaluating efficiency and equity of health services, systems, and health policy. Effectiveness can be studied at two levels: the clinical level and the population level. Whether aimed at prevention or at treatment, healthcare studies require an appropriate research design that balances internal validity and generalizability. Models of effectiveness lay the foundation for effectiveness research and are increasingly being incorporated into data-gathering efforts and health services planning and implementation.

Effectiveness data are challenging to digest, especially because results may vary greatly across studies. Understanding of a range of study-related aspects, especially the theoretical framework, study design, and strengths and limitations of the study data, is necessary to provide evidence-based answers to real-world healthcare questions. Meta-analyses and systematic literature reviews are becoming more accepted in the effectiveness research literature. The use of other study designs, such as evaluation of complex interventions and evaluation of collaboratives, is also becoming more common.

Several efforts are working to improve the nature and availability of healthcare effectiveness data. Trends include increased access to trial data, developments in reporting standards, and the growing availability and ease of use of administrative and survey data.

EFFECTIVENESS: POLICY STRATEGIES, EVIDENCE, AND CRITERIA

Chapter Highlights

1. Effectiveness strategies at the clinical level address the structures, processes, and outcomes of personal healthcare services involved in preventing illness and preserving and restoring the health of individuals.
2. Effectiveness strategies at the population level include the personal healthcare and community-based efforts aimed at influencing environmental, social/behavioral, biological, and care-related determinants of health.
3. A blending of clinical- and population-level perspectives and strategies is needed to improve the effectiveness of healthcare services and policies.

Overview

From an effectiveness viewpoint, the basic health policy question is: What policy strategies are most effective for improving and sustaining the health of individuals and the population as a whole? Strategies to improve healthcare effectiveness at the clinical level include

1. enhancing structural factors, such as sources of funding for medical training or hospital construction;
2. implementing process controls, including regulation of professional and institutional performance; and
3. promoting desired outcomes through various methods, including service delivery performance assessment and incentives.

Assessment of these clinical-level strategies' effectiveness involves selecting a theoretical framework by which to define clinical effectiveness in healthcare delivery and setting judgment criteria. Strategies to improve healthcare effectiveness at the population level include

1. ensuring access to healthcare for all segments of the population;
2. improving the quality of the healthcare system overall; and

3. implementing population- and community-based efforts to influence environmental, social/behavioral, biological, and care-related determinants of health.

Assessment of these population-level strategies' effectiveness involves identifying community-wide indicators of the environmental, social, biological, and healthcare status of populations. Strategies for improving health at the clinical and population levels are noted in Exhibit 3.1.

Strategies for Improving Clinical Effectiveness

By following the Donabedian structure/process/outcome model, we assume there are three major categories of efforts to improve effectiveness of healthcare at the clinical level: enhancing structural factors, implementing process-of-care controls, and managing the outcomes of interventions.

Enhancing Structural Factors

Prominent policy-driven efforts have included attempts to expand access via federal health insurance programs. Public insurance programs (Medicare,

EXHIBIT 3.1
Health Policy
Strategies
Related
to Factors
Contributing
to Population
Health

Contributing Factor	Policy Strategy
Population perspective	Population health information systems
Environment	Health protection
Behavior	Health promotion
Human biology	Biomedical research
	Preventive services
Healthcare	
Structure	
Efficacy	Biomedical research
Quantity	Investment in resources
Distribution and	Health planning and regionalization of
organization	services
Process	Organized/integrated delivery systems
Utilization	Enhanced access
Clinical perspective	
Healthcare	
Process	
Quality	Regulation of professional performance
Outcomes	Outcomes assessment and management
	Practice guidelines
	Performance monitoring systems

Medicaid, and Children's Health Insurance Program) were designed to boost effectiveness by increasing access and covered services for otherwise under-served groups.

A major objective of health policy is to improve effectiveness at the clinical level by enhancing the structural aspects of healthcare delivery. The predominant strategy in the early post–World War II era was investment in the structure of healthcare delivery, including the efficacy, quantity, distribu-tion, and organization of medical care resources. This strategy is reflected in the formation of the National Institutes of Health (NIH), the Hill-Burton program, the Health Professionals Educational Assistance Program, public insurance coverage for vulnerable populations, the Comprehensive Health Planning program, and government support for integrated delivery systems.

Arising out of the Marine Hospital Service, NIH was established in 1930 to fund biomedical research as a means of developing a knowledge base of the causes and treatment of diseases. Other agencies merged under the NIH umbrella, including the National Cancer Institute in 1944 and the National Heart Institute in 1948 (Harden 1986), and NIH became the vehicle for establishing new federally supported research initiatives, such as the National Microbiological Institute in 1958.

Further structural policy efforts have included the establishment of the Regional Medical Programs in the 1960s and the Consensus Development Program (CDP) in the 1970s. The Regional Medical Programs, also known as A National Program to Conquer Heart Disease, Cancer, and Stroke, were established to bring, among other benefits, the results of biomedical research to the practice of medicine through such vehicles as continuing medical edu-cation (Komaroff 1971).

Another major policy strategy aimed at structural factors sought to improve the health of the population through increasing the availability of medical care facilities and human resources. Examples include efforts to build community-wide capacity through the Hill-Burton Act of 1946, provision of grants and loans for hospital construction, and efforts to increase the number of healthcare providers through the Health Professions Educational Assistance Act of 1963, which established subsidies for health professional education. Whereas the Hill-Burton legislation was aimed at enhancing the number and the distribution of hospitals, the Health Professions Educational Assistance Act targeted better availability and distribution of doctors, nurses, and other health professionals (Greene 1976). This legislation provided a range of financial incentives, such as funding to medical training sites and loan forgiveness programs for medical graduates, to direct more medical stu-dents toward primary care practice and practice in underserved areas.

A third major structural policy thrust were the Comprehensive Health Planning Act and Regional Medical Programs, which addressed the distribu-tion and organization of medical care through regionalization (Bodenheimer

1969) and formation of integrated healthcare systems (Kissick 1970; Shortell et al. 2001, 2000a, 2000b, 1993). The premise for policy strategies aimed at health planning, regionalization, and integration of medical care is the suggestion that not only the quantity of medical care resources but also their distribution and coordination are important to health. The Comprehensive Health Planning legislation provided grants for both state- and area-wide health planning, and the Regional Medical Programs legislation fostered the development of a technical infrastructure for regional delivery systems (Kissick 1970).

The Health Maintenance Organization Act of 1973 was another attempt to prompt the development of integrated models of healthcare delivery (Wolinsky 1980). This legislation and subsequent private-sector responses attempted to encourage the organization of networks of providers and payers that offer a coordinated continuum of services to a defined population and are willing to be held clinically and fiscally accountable for the outcomes and the health status of the populations they serve (Shortell et al. 2001, 2000a, 2000b, 1993).

A number of efforts to increase the distribution and organization of services also targeted special populations, thereby increasing access to medical care. Examples include the Maternal and Child Health Program, the formation of state and local health departments, the Medicare and Medicaid programs, and the creation of Office of Economic Opportunity neighborhood health centers. Some of these examples are discussed in Chapters 6 and 7 in the context of health equity.

The most recent policy action to enhance regionalization and integration has been the Patient Protection and Affordable Care Act (ACA) of 2010 (Office of the Legislative Counsel 2010). The ACA, to be rolled out over a number of years, is aimed at reforming many different structural and process components of the healthcare system. With respect to the integration of health services, the ACA encourages the formation of *accountable care organizations (ACOs)*. An ACO is a type of payment and delivery reform model that seeks to tie provider reimbursements to quality metrics and reductions in the total cost of care for an assigned population of patients. A group of coordinated healthcare providers form an ACO, which then provides care to a group of patients. The ACA authorized the Centers for Medicare & Medicaid Services (CMS) to create the Medicare Shared Savings Program, which allows ACOs to contract with Medicare (American College of Osteopathic Family Physicians 2010; CMS 2010b; Gold 2011). To motivate providers to form ACOs, the ACA introduced a pay-for-performance reimbursement incentive for ACOs that document achievement of specific process and outcome goals.

Implementing Process-of-Care Controls

Following the establishment of Medicare in 1965, the federal government sought to improve the effectiveness of healthcare by monitoring the decisions of healthcare providers. Factors motivating these efforts included the rising level of Medicare expenditures and pioneering research in practice variation by John Wennberg, who evaluated Medicare delivery to examine the degree to which rural areas might be underserved. While this correlation did not clearly emerge from Wennberg's studies, he did find variation in medical practice across many dimensions. He postulated that this variation is largely driven by physicians' unique backgrounds, preferences, and circumstances rather than by patients' needs. Wennberg and others subsequently promoted changes in the healthcare system to direct care away from idiosyncratic variations in practice style toward recognized, evidence-based patterns. These efforts have been aimed either at individual providers, such as physicians, or at healthcare organizations, such as hospitals or HMOs. Leading strategies have included monitoring rates of service delivery to detect variation and provide feedback to physicians and healthcare systems, boosting the collection of service effectiveness evidence and increasing dissemination of this evidence, and reducing hospitalizations by identifying patients and conditions that can be effectively and safely treated in the ambulatory setting (Wennberg 1984).

One of the first federal efforts to monitor physicians was the formation of the Professional Standards Review Organization (PSRO) in 1972. Partly due to Wennberg's analyses of regional variation in Medicare utilization, overutilization was blamed for escalating Medicare costs, and the PSRO aimed to constrain it through peer review of physician decision making. Physicians strongly opposed this oversight, and the PSRO morphed into state-level professional review organizations, putting more power in the hands of the profession. CMS maintains responsibility for Medicare utilization review strategy.

Managing the Outcomes of Interventions

The third category of strategies aimed at improving the effectiveness of healthcare services at the clinical level—outcomes management—has fostered the development of practice guidelines. Practice guidelines are "systematically developed statements to assist practitioner and patient decisions about appropriate healthcare for specific clinical circumstances" (IOM 1992). The CDP continues to foster regular reviews of the evidence regarding standardized clinical treatment practices across many health topics (Burtram 1994) and disseminates these statements through its website, consensus.nih.gov.

The Agency for Healthcare Research and Quality (AHRQ), along with many health professional associations, has developed and disseminated practice guidelines with the goal of increasing the effectiveness of services for many clinical conditions. Its content and strategy somewhat overlap those of the CDP, but the CDP is more focused on developing clinical efficacy statements on biomedical topics and AHRQ is focused on providing a range of effectiveness resources, including a clearinghouse for clinical practice guidelines developed in-house or by other entities (including NIH) and other sources of evidence concerning health service delivery, such as health information technology.

Another outcomes management strategy that has been sponsored by states, employers, the federal government, professional associations, and provider organizations is the development of performance monitoring systems. One of the most prominent of these systems is the Healthcare Effectiveness Data and Information Set (HEDIS) developed by the National Committee for Quality Assurance (NCQA), a private, nonprofit entity sponsored by the Robert Wood Johnson Foundation. HEDIS, first drafted in 1991, is "a set of standardized performance measures designed to ensure that purchasers and consumers have the information they need to reliably compare the performance of managed health care organizations" (NCQA 2006). HEDIS criteria were reviewed and updated periodically for various reasons, such as to better accommodate Medicare or Medicaid populations. Updates were made in 1993, 1995, 1996, and 1997 (Davis 1997). Since 1995, updates have been less dramatic and have been issued annually (NCQA 2011). Medicare adopted HEDIS standards for its managed care programs. HEDIS also is widely used by state Medicaid managed care programs and many private preferred-provider plans (NCQA 2012).

The eight performance domains of HEDIS include (1) effectiveness of care, (2) accessibility and availability of care, (3) satisfaction with the experience of care, (4) stability of the health plan, (5) use of services, (6) cost of care, (7) health plan descriptive information, and (8) informed healthcare choices.

The ACA will likely bring HEDIS, and possibly other accreditation standards, into effect in healthcare delivery at the institution level because participants in the health insurance exchanges are mandated to adhere to "clinical quality measures such as the Healthcare Effectiveness Data and Information Set" (Office of the Legislative Counsel 2010) (PPACA, Section 1311). Healthcare effectiveness research will focus on demonstrating that desired clinical outcomes result when these standards of care are met.

Yet another example of federal health policy aimed at performance is the development and dissemination of provider report cards. AHRQ published hospital mortality rates for several years, starting in the 1990s. This practice was controversial; hospitals offering the most advanced care were concerned they might be perceived negatively because the cases they treat are more severe than those treated at other hospitals and thus more likely to experience poor outcomes (Fottler, Slovensky, and Rogers 1988; Romano, Rainwater, and Antonius 1999). The practice was discontinued in 2002 partly because quality-based measures did not appear to notably influence the utilization of hospitals (Mennemeyer, Morrisey, and Howard 1997).

As a result of the renewed interest in quality and effectiveness over the past decade, this practice was reinstituted. CMS had been gathering hospital quality indicators since 2004, and in 2008 it launched its Hospital Compare website to share much of this information. The quality improvement trend has also prompted state and private initiatives to benchmark and report quality indicators (Christianson et al. 2010). Whether the availability of these quality data influences the behavior of providers or patients remains to be seen (see the Evidence section that follows this discussion).

To identify evidence-based preventive services, the federal government created the United States Preventive Services Task Force. The first Task Force report, *Guide to Clinical Preventive Services*, was published in 1985; several updates have since been released. Due to the high level of expertise of Task Force members, the transparency of their evidence review process, and their strong methodological approach, the Task Force's recommendations have greatly influenced healthcare practice, training, quality benchmarking, and coverage and payment policies (Garber 2001). A recent illustration of this influence was the controversy around the recommendation made in 2009 that regular mammography-based breast cancer screening for most women (those with no noted risk factor) should begin at age 50 rather than 40 (Squiers et al. 2011).

Comparative effectiveness research (CER), which is discussed in Chapter 2 and promoted in the ACA, is regarded by many as a strategy for promoting more effective care at the clinical level. The 2009 American Recovery and Reinvestment Act (ARRA) provided a onetime funding boost for CER research, predominantly divided between AHRQ, NIH, and the US Department of Health & Human Services (HHS). The ACA promotes CER through the establishment of and permanent funding for the Patient-Centered Outcomes Research Institute (PCORI), a national-level, nonprofit, nongovernmental authority. PCORI leadership includes federal healthcare researchers (AHRQ and NIH), healthcare providers (including manufacturers of drugs and devices), payers, and consumers (Keckley et al. 2011). CER as a policy strategy to improve effectiveness may be limited, however, due to the public concern over the role of government in individual medical decisions (Coleman 2011).

Evidence

Significant policies intending to boost effectiveness at the clinical level have addressed structural aspects of healthcare. Prominent are those aimed at increasing the number and location of hospitals and physicians. The Hill-Burton Act has been credited with financially supporting the establishment of more than 9,000 hospitals (Lipscomb 2002). In addition to increasing the number of public hospitals, Hill-Burton set the stage for racial nondiscrimination in federally funded healthcare. While nondiscrimination was stated as one of the criteria that had to be met to receive federal support under the act, Hill-Burton permitted recipient hospitals to be "separate but equal," meaning hospitals could continue to be segregated but had to provide equal care to all populations. In 1963, the landmark *Simkins v. Moses H. Cone Memorial Hospital* case ruled that federally supported separate-but-equal hospitals were not acceptable (Reynolds 1997). This decision influenced the watershed Civil Rights Act of 1964, in which Title VI discontinued federal support for separate-but-equal hospitals and extended the nondiscrimination requirement to all federally funded healthcare programs. As noted earlier in this chapter, access to healthcare also was improved through the Health Professions Educational Assistance Act of 1963, which helped to almost double the number of annual medical school graduates and boost the ratio of physicians per 100,000 population from approximately 150 in 1970 to approximately 200 in 1980 (Lewin and Derzon 1982).

Policies affecting access to clinical care by promoting access to health insurance coverage have become a significant part of healthcare. It is a challenge to quantify the outcomes attributable to monumental policy innovations aimed at the clinical level, such as the establishment and expansions of the Medicaid and Medicare programs. Legislative intent has been to make coverage more complete and equitable, and enrollment in the millions seemingly is evidence of its effectiveness. Despite this great uptake, overall enrollment in health insurance has not changed much. Data from the National Health Interview Survey note that 78.9 percent of adults under age 65 had private insurance coverage in 1976, and 5.1 percent were covered by Medicare or Medicaid, leaving 14.1 percent uninsured. Across the decades, the portion with private coverage has gradually decreased, while the portion with public coverage has gradually increased. By 2006, 66.3 percent were covered by private insurance and 18.6 were covered by public insurance, leaving 17.0 percent uninsured. Thus, evidence of the effectiveness of these public programs depends on their ability to cover the populace more equitably and improve benefit coverage along the way. Examples of such improvement include the establishment of Medicare hospice coverage in 1982 and prescription drug coverage in 2003.

The evidence regarding policies aimed at improving effectiveness through process controls is mixed. As noted earlier, PSROs were established to encourage optimal outcomes and reduce excessive utilization through a utilization review process. Systematic evaluations of the usefulness of performance reporting systems are lacking. Examinations of selected evaluations of single-focus programs (Blumenthal and Epstein 1996; Epstein 1995) have yielded mixed results. A review of performance reporting systems for hospitals, health professionals, and healthcare organizations by Marshall and colleagues (2000) concluded: "Seven US [performance] reporting systems have been the subject of published empirical evaluations. Descriptive and observational methods predominate. Consumers and purchasers rarely search out the information and do not understand or trust it; it has a small, although increasing, impact on their decision making." Overall, these efforts do not seem to influence patient behavior (Fung et al. 2008), although some analyses (e.g., Mukamel and Mushlin 1998; Romano and Zhou 2004) have found relationships between reported quality and subsequent volume in limited circumstances. Physicians are skeptical about performance data, and only a small proportion uses the information. Hospitals appear to be most responsive to it.

Similarly, reviews of outcome studies (Grimshaw and Russell 1993; Lugtenberg, Burgers, and Westert 2009; Worrall, Chaulk, and Freake 1997) consistently yield mixed evidence regarding the degree to which adoption of clinical care guidelines leads to improvements in effectiveness. In some instances, clinical guidelines, outcomes assessment, and performance monitoring may improve the effectiveness of medical care. In the 1980s, the RAND Corporation was commissioned to evaluate the CDP (discussed earlier in this chapter). This evaluation found that the CDP's statements were widely recognized and disseminated and that they generally influenced physician behavior some, but not all, of the time (Kanouse et al. 1989).

Recommendations from that evaluation led to the 1989–1990 "Improving the Program" effort, directed by the Institute of Medicine (Council on Health Care Technology 1990). A later analysis demonstrated that, for sponsored research between 1998 and 2001, CDP's research agenda–setting function had an influence on NIH research applications and funded projects (Portnoy et al. 2007), illustrating the CDP's power to direct scholarly attention to a specific set of clinical concerns.

Uptake of clinical guidelines may currently be receiving a policy-driven boost from ARRA. The act included financial incentives nearing $50,000 over the four-year span of the program for physicians who transition to an electronic health record between 2011 and 2014, if the purposes for doing so meet "meaningful use" criteria, which include regular reporting of a range of clinical quality and process measures (e.g., tobacco use) that significantly overlap clinical guideline content. ARRA meaningful-use incentives are great—spending for this program is expected to total up to $27 billion over a period of ten years (Office of the Federal Register 2010)—even though there is only modest evidence that policy-based monitoring can lead to improvements in healthcare provider outcomes and healthcare system outcomes.

As managed care rose in the 1990s, HMO enrollees became concerned about the quality of care in managed care plans. In response, many states passed a wave of legislation that mandated more specifically how managed care organizations should practice (e.g., hospitals are not permitted to discharge a woman and her newborn within 24 hours of delivery) (Kuper 1998). Research has not supported enrollees' concerns, however. In his early review of the performance of HMOs, Luft (1978) examined the few outcomes studies available at the time and concluded that HMO outcomes were similar to those of conventional practice. In later updates, when many more studies were available, the conclusion was still equivocal; on average, HMO outcomes were no better or no worse than conventional practice outcomes (Miller and Luft 2002, 1997, 1994). The primary exception noted in several studies was negative outcomes for Medicare enrollees with chronic conditions.

Criteria

The widely recognized structure/process/outcome model developed by Donabedian (1966) offers clinical-level criteria for assessing the effectiveness of healthcare. An overview of the criteria for assessing the effectiveness of health policies is presented in Exhibit 3.2. This model focuses on healthcare delivery processes, such as diagnosis, intervention, communication between providers, and coordination of care, and on healthcare structures, such as facilities, medical staff, and financial arrangements.

The development of effectiveness criteria, such as those promoted by the National Quality Forum (NQF) and AHRQ's Quality Indicators program, has advanced tremendously. These high-profile indicator efforts are widely used in practice, but their adoption generally remains voluntary. NQF, in collaboration with the RAND Foundation, is positioned to be a leading source of outcome criteria for evaluating funding/reimbursement reform under the ACA, including ACO strategies, medical home primary care performance strategies, and global payment strategies (Schneider, Hussey, and Schnyer 2011). Use of these clinical-level effectiveness indicators in private quality assurance efforts is set to shift significantly to use for publicly mandated outcomes reporting.

Population Level

Strategies

Population health strategies are concerned with influencing the nonmedical determinants of population health and improving the accessibility and effectiveness of personal healthcare to ensure effective care is available when needed and the health of the population overall is sustained. These strategies are aimed at healthcare structures, processes, and outcomes. Leading structural efforts have included policies aimed at benchmarking the health of the population and assessing change across time and public policies focused on funding health-promoting activities across the range of social determinants.

Prominent examples of population health strategies come from Canada, where the Lalonde report (1975) set forth an agenda recognizing four categories of influence—environment, lifestyle, human biology, and healthcare service factors—on health. The Canadian population health

Dimensions	Criteria	Indicators	Examples
Population Effectiveness			
Need based	Based on the results of a community health needs assessment	Population health information system	The majority of population databases related to breast cancer in the United States contain data on patients with cancer (e.g., SEER*) and individuals with selected types of coverage (e.g., Medicaid, Medicare).
Comprehensiveness	Reflect an appropriate relationship to the continuum of healthcare services	Full continuum of services	Discontinuities often exist between the systems and services for breast cancer screening and the availability and coverage of breast cancer follow-up and treatment services (e.g., NBCCEDP**).
Clinical Effectiveness			
Precision	Structure/ process criteria specified in advance	Practice guidelines	Practice guidelines for mammography screening vary widely across agencies and organizations (e.g., American Cancer Society, American Geriatrics Society, National Cancer Institute, US Preventive Services Task Force).
Performance	Monitored process and outcome indicators for selected conditions	Performance monitoring system	Performance monitoring systems (e.g., HEDIS***) are often proprietary or used only to track members of health plans.

EXHIBIT 3.2
Criteria for Assessing the Effectiveness of Health Policies

*Surveillance Epidemiology and End Results Program

**National Breast and Cervical Cancer Early Detection Program

***Healthcare Effectiveness Data and Information Set

perspective is reflected by the nation's overall goal of equal access to *health* as opposed to equal access to health*care* (Mhatre and Deber 1992). Following the Lalonde model, Canada addresses the full range of health determinants when formulating health policy (Evans, Barer, and Marmor 1994) and when adopting population health information systems to guide policy development.

While Manitoba and other Canadian provinces were developing the capacity to analyze population health status and health service utilization, population-based surveys were also initiated as a strategy to more fully evaluate the health of the population. Nutrition surveys were carried out between 1970 and 1972, followed by the Canada Health Survey (1978), the Canadian Heart Health Surveys (1988 to 1992), the Canadian Study of Health and Aging (1992), the Canadian Community Health Survey (2004), and the Canadian Health Measures Survey (2007) (Macdonald et al. 1997; Nutrition Committee of the Canadian Paediatric Society 1976; Statistics Canada 2008; Stephens 1986).

Policymakers' request for more analyses of utilization led to the establishment of the Manitoba Centre for Health Policy in 1990 (Marchessault 2010; Roos et al. 1995). Health services researchers at the Centre calculated and published such population health indicators as the percentage of babies born at a low birth weight and the percentage of elderly adults living in nursing homes (Marchessault 2010). Over time, they accumulated data sources, standardized codification methods for patient de-identification, and increased their data storage and data manipulation capacities. As a result, a greater range of analyses became possible, and a greater range of researchers could access the data. This ad hoc assemblage evolved into the Population-Based Health Information System (POPULIS), now called the Population Health Research Data Repository (Roos et al. 1999). Policymakers use this comprehensive database to analyze demographic changes, expenditure patterns, and hospital performance and to compare local and regional information on residents' health status, socioeconomic characteristics, utilization of healthcare services, and other health-related measures.

In the United States, the growing body of knowledge about health determinants was one of the factors that led to the development of an explicit policy strategy of health promotion and disease prevention, beginning with the adoption of the goals set out in the first *Healthy People* report (DHEW 1979). This report, along with the *Promoting Health/Preventing Disease* report published in 1980, firmly established the policy of gathering and benchmarking a health profile of the US population (McLeroy and Crump 1994). The first *Healthy People* effort (HHS 1980) included 15 leading indicators, such as hypertension control, immunization, and control of environmental toxic agents, that had potential for improvement or prevention according to existing knowledge.

Recognizing these influences and the concept of examining health at the population level, various analyses have outlined primary threats to health across the lifespan. A review of current causes of morbidity and mortality by Adler and colleagues (1993) supports the view that the health status of a population is a function of the social determinants of health, including medical and nonmedical influences. In the United States, leading causes of death include tobacco use, poor diet, physical inactivity, and alcohol misuse (Mokdad et al. 2004). These four behavioral factors account in large part for variance in mortality; the burden of all four is equivalent to 14 years of life lost, on average (Khaw et al. 2008).

The United States has reviewed and recommitted to the *Healthy People* concept each decade. In 1990, *Healthy People 2000* was released. This update increased the number of indicator conditions from 15 to 22, included 300 objectives, and added a focused list of leading data needs to prompt population-based data collection efforts (Mason and McGinnis 1990). *Healthy People* 2010, released in 2000, had a somewhat reorganized structure that included ten leading health objectives and an expansion to 28 indicators (HHS 2000).

Following the decadal pattern, HHS convened a panel in 2008 to develop *Healthy People* 2020 (Koh et al. 2011). This release includes a broader framework for affecting health. The social determinants model has been adopted more definitively, and a lifespan development perspective has been incorporated. These foci more strongly emphasize population health and upstream determinants of health along with the organization and delivery of preventive and treatment healthcare services (HHS 2010). The structure was again refined, this time expanded to 26 leading health indicators grouped into 12 topic categories. "Foundation health measures" have been added to four of these categories, including general health status, disparities/inequities, social determinants, and health-related quality of life. Beyond the 12 categories, 42 topic areas were included, each "assigned to one or more lead agencies within the federal government that is responsible for developing, tracking, monitoring, and periodically reporting on objectives" (HHS 2010). These revisions/additions solidify the linkage between desired population-level goals and likely influences on health.

Structural health policy strategies are also directed toward non-healthcare determinants of health, such as the environment. In 1978, the United States initiated policy-based efforts to slow the destruction of stratospheric ozone by reducing the use of chlorofluorocarbons (CFCs), recognizing that a depleting atmospheric ozone layer would contribute to a range of negative health outcomes, including skin cancer and cataracts. The 1990 reauthorization of the Clean Air Act greatly enhanced the effort to control CFC use.

Structural policy has also focused on the health burden of smoking. This burgeoning awareness was a major reason for the creation of the Office of Disease Prevention and Health Promotion in 1976. Other structural health policy strategies directed toward preventive health include promotion of behavioral health programs, such as school-based sex education (Kann, Telljohann, and Wooley 2007) and substance abuse prevention (e.g., Ringwalt et al. 2009).

The Centers for Disease Control and Prevention (CDC) is the primary agency responsible for gathering and managing the data that compose the United States' sources of health indicators. Other federal agencies also track health-related indicators; for example, the Environmental Protection Agency monitors air quality, and the Census Bureau monitors demographics through the decennial US Census and the annual Current Population Survey (Metzler et al. 2008). Private initiatives, such as the Robert Wood Johnson Foundation's County Health Rankings/Mobilizing Action Toward Community Health (MATCH) project and The Brookings Institution's National Infrastructure for Community Statistics, further contribute to the population health indicator data available in the United States (Metzler et al. 2008).

The United States' strategy of coordinated effort toward population health goals has been much less integrated than Canada's, largely because healthcare in the United States is not a matter of governmentally administered universal access. Rather, the public health and monitoring functions in the United States are financed and served by a mix of political jurisdictions, including city, county, region, state, and federal authorities. Many geographic localities' public health functions are divided among more than one local entity, and these entities' tasks may overlap.

One strategy helping to rationalize public health in the United States is the voluntary National Public Health Performance Standards Program (NPHPSP), which was developed in the late 1990s by the CDC in collaboration with seven other organizations, including the Association of State and Territorial Health Officials and the National Association of County and City Health Officials (Corso et al. 2007). Recognizing that the core functions of public health are carried out by three main entities—state-level public health authorities, local governing boards, and local authorities—the CDC developed three evaluation instruments to suit these configurations. After the program was implemented, many of these entities conducted self-evaluations. This activity indicates that the CDC's efforts were having some impact and promoting consistent attention to a recognized core of public health functions across the nation's patchwork of public health jurisdictions and entities.

Following implementation of this federal effort to promote consistent delivery of public health services, the Public Health Accreditation Board (PHAB) instituted accreditation of public health authorities. This private program, largely initiated by the Robert Wood Johnson Foundation, launched in September 2011, and a modest number of public health authorities have already received accreditation. The establishment of PHAB suggests that regulation of public health, initially a federal effort, may remain a largely private matter left to professional organizations, as are many other structural healthcare regulatory initiatives.

At the population level, process-focused policies have mainly been advanced by an emphasis on monitoring the reach of preventive measures and encouraging complete and consistent delivery of these measures. The *Healthy People* efforts have included such process-of-care measures since the first version in 1980. The report was strongly aimed at interventions for people in good health: "[F]ew of the objectives deal with secondary prevention. Objectives relating to the frequency and content of physical examinations and other means of detecting early conditions (such as cervical, breast and colon cancer, diabetes, vision and hearing problems and dental caries) were deliberately excluded from consideration, despite their obvious importance in signaling needs for intervention" (HHS 1980). Examples of processes intended to prevent disease, from the first of the 15 foci—hypertension control—include performance of routine blood pressure checks at healthcare visits and workplace blood pressure screenings. Subsequent versions of *Healthy People* are more inclusive, capturing secondary prevention and other process-of-care priorities.

Outcomes-focused policies have not been exercised at the population level as much as at the clinical level. The *Healthy People* initiatives have intended, as outcomes, to boost state-level attention to the *Healthy People* agenda. McGinnis and Lee (1995), in their midway assessment of *Healthy People* 2000, noted that 41 of 50 states had initiated health promotion plans that were influenced and guided by the initiative.

Noted earlier in the chapter, one example of a population-level outcomes-focused policy has been the federal government's involvement in the initiative to encourage local and state public health authorities to seek certification. The goal of this effort has been to sufficiently address, across all jurisdictions, the ten basic functions of public health (monitor health status, enforce health regulations, educate the public regarding health risks, and so forth). While this effort is a private endeavor, the CDC provided significant guidance at the initiation of the project (Thielen 2004) and through its website offers extensive expertise, guidance, and tools for state and local public health entities striving to achieve and maintain National Public Health Department Accreditation through PHAB. Unlike the common route of many other federal health policies, financial incentives or support have not been part of these outcomes-focused policies (Thielen 2004). A qualitative analysis of many state and local public health entities either involved with this accreditation plan or planning to seek accreditation noted financial support as a desired intervention to promote and accelerate accreditation initiatives (Davis et al. 2009).

Evidence

The population perspective focuses on evidence regarding the health of the population in general; findings on the importance of non-healthcare determinants of health; and the effectiveness of health protection, health promotion, preventive services, and medical treatment. Health policy outcomes at the population level concern the uptake or adoption of promoted or recommended practices by target entities, such as public health authorities.

The indicators of major structure-oriented policies should show evidence of progress across time. The *Healthy People* initiatives have not only described problems but also included and fostered the monitoring of reasonably attainable outcomes indicators. Mason and McGinnis (1990) noted that great progress was made on several of the *Healthy People* 1980 indicators, including lower death rates from heart disease, stroke, and motor vehicle crashes, "three of the leading causes of death among Americans." The portion of these successes directly attributable to the *Healthy People* initiative is unclear, but comprehensive, complex efforts were required to achieve these outcomes, suggesting that a national scope and profile for these problems likely contribute to their amelioration.

An evaluation of progress on the *Healthy People* 2000 goals (McGinnis and Lee 1995) indicated that the data trend for the majority of reviewed objectives was in the desired direction, indicating a likely positive impact of the *Healthy People* initiative overall and fair support for *Healthy People* 2000. While the authors acknowledged that as of the date of publication, sufficient time had not passed for progress to be detected on some measures, they did note improvement in many processes, including immunization coverage and cancer screening. Evaluation of *Healthy People* 2010 likewise showed desirable progress on many key indicators. Klein and colleagues (2006) indicated that of 281 objectives with longitudinal data available for analysis, more than 160 had moved toward the 2010 target or met that target. There is a mixed picture of progress for racial and ethnic population groups; significant health disparities between these groups and the white population continue to exist. Hispanics appear to be faring better than blacks. These developments ought to promote policy efforts to preserve and improve health at a population level, and evidence of success will be in the form of new initiatives and increased efforts for existing health promotion mechanisms that follow the advanced *Healthy People* 2020 perspective.

The *Healthy People* initiative is a leading example of population-based encouragement of quality healthcare processes. As noted earlier, the *Healthy People* indicators have gained the attention of many, if not all, states, and have fostered enhanced monitoring of healthcare processes at the population level. Improvements have included both preventive and secondary prevention measures.

One example of a process-of-care improvement at the population level was documented by Ong and colleagues (2007) using 1999–2004 data regarding hypertension awareness, treatment, and therapeutic control from the National Health and Nutrition Examination Survey. Among adults older than age 60, all three process-of-care indicators notably improved, indicating that, to some measurable degree, providers generally had boosted the process of hypertension management. Such outcomes, however, are not sufficient to declare that these federal-level, population-wide process improvement efforts are due to the federal action. Other lines of evidence can help build the case; for example, surveys of public health authorities indicate they are aware of and influenced by the initiative. A survey of 327 likely users of *Healthy People* 2010, such as local health departments, found that nearly all organizations were aware of the report, and 78 percent reported that they had used the report, mostly for setting priorities and for outreach and collaboration (National Opinion Research Center 2009). The initiative's influence on physicians and healthcare delivery settings has not been assessed.

Population-level outcomes for the national public health accreditation program will be evaluated on the basis of the number and percentage of public health authorities seeking, attaining, and maintaining accreditation. This program was rolled out and piloted in 30 public health authorities in 2009 and 2010 and opened to applicants in 2011. A recent article (Johnson 2011) noted that, following the pilot phase, 17 authorities have signed up for the accreditation process.

The growing body of research on the fundamental determinants of health has resulted in a redefinition of the importance of factors other than medical care as the determinants of health. Over the past two to three decades, a great deal of evidence has accumulated documenting the importance of both the physical and the social environment as determinants of the health of populations. McGinnis and Foege (1993) identified and quantified the major external (nongenetic) factors that contribute to death in the United States using a variety of data sources. The most prominent contributors to mortality in the United States in 1990 were tobacco use, diet and activity patterns, alcohol abuse, microbial agents, toxic agents, firearms, sexual behavior, motor vehicle accidents, and illicit use of drugs, which together accounted for more than half of the deaths. Socioeconomic status and access to medical care were also found to be important contributors. It has been estimated that 60 to 90 percent of cancers are environmentally caused (Blumenthal 1985; Tomatis et al. 1997); as much as one-third of cancer deaths have been attributed to diet (Scheuplein 1992). Specifically, the causes of cancer have been estimated epidemiologically as diet, tobacco use, infection, occupational exposures, and geophysical factors, such as radiation. Environmental risks include food contamination, food additives, water pollution, air pollution, indoor chemicals, occupational exposure, toxic wastes, carcinogens, radiation, and physical agents, such as trauma, accidents, and noise (Tomatis et al. 1997). Besides cancer mortality, environmental factors cause nervous system, endocrine system, and immune system problems; acute poisoning; and birth defects (Misch and Starke 1994).

The social environment, which reflects social class and status hierarchies, income, social ties, and cultural change, has also been demonstrated to powerfully influence the health of population groups (Berkman 2000; Kawachi and Berkman 2001). Position in the occupational status hierarchy has been shown to be a major determinant of the health of individuals in England (Singh-Manoux, Adler, and Marmot 2003). It also has been demonstrated that income, both in the United States and internationally, is a predictor of health status (von dem Knesebeck et al. 2003). In addition, disruptions in social and family ties due to death, divorce, or immigration and major cultural or social changes are clearly related to mortality (Eng et al. 2002).

The extent to which health promotion and preventive services mitigate these risk factors varies. The effectiveness of various prevention strategies (for heart disease, HIV infection, substance abuse, and violence) in US cities over a 15-year period was reviewed by Freudenberg and colleagues (2000), who concluded that most programs reached diverse, low-income residents; employed multiple strategies; and adhered to at least some of the principles of effective health promotion. However, many program interventions were not aimed at changing the underlying social causes of the problems or were not tailored to the subpopulations they targeted, thereby limiting their potential effectiveness. Glanz, Lewis, and Rimer (2002) reviewed cardiovascular disease interventions in communities and found that the interventions only modestly, and in some cases insignificantly, reduced risk factors and mortality. Ford and Capewell (2011) reviewed the contributors to the steady decline in cardiovascular mortality and noted that 44 to 76 percent of the decrease may be attributed to risk factor reduction and 23 to 47 percent may be attributable to medical interventions.

Thacker and colleagues (1994), in a review of methods for assessing the effectiveness of preventive services, presented evidence substantiating the 95 to 98 percent effectiveness of vaccinations on preventing measles, the 20 to 70 percent effectiveness of mammography on preventing breast cancer deaths, and the 50 percent effectiveness of retinal screening and treatment on preventing blindness in patients with diabetes. Bunker, Frazier, and Mosteller (1994), using statistical estimation techniques based on clinical preventive services of demonstrated efficacy, concluded that hypertension and cervical cancer screening as well as childhood immunizations contributed significantly to the increase in life expectancy over the twentieth century in the United States. McKinlay, McKinlay, and Beaglehole (1989) examined the contribution of medical interventions to changes in mortality linked to coronary heart disease, cancer, and stroke, which together account for two-thirds of total US mortality and consume the majority of healthcare resources. Using a combined measure of mortality and morbidity, the authors similarly demonstrated that overall life expectancy has increased over several decades due to medical interventions. Finally, a recent evaluation estimates that the Clean Air Act of 1970, through reduction of auto emissions and other effects, has prevented more than 160,000 deaths (Office of Air and Radiation 2011).

The relationship between the quantity of healthcare resources and outcomes at the population level has been explored in studies with nonexperimental designs using cross-sectional observational data. For example, Berlowitz and colleagues (1998) used this approach to examine outcomes in hypertensive men at five VA sites in New England over a two-year period. The study found that many veterans' blood pressure was poorly controlled. Those who received more intensive medical therapy had better control. Many physicians treating these patients were not aggressive enough in their approach to hypertension.

Criteria

Population-wide health indicators are used to benchmark health status, identify health disparities across sociodemographic groups, and detect changes in health over time (Glouberman and Millar 2003). They describe structural aspects of a population's health.

In 1999, Canada established a framework for monitoring health indicators (Canadian Institute for Health Information 1999) and has since maintained a series of conferences on population health indicators (Canadian Institute for Health Information 2009, 2005). The Canadian indicator model collects data on many of the elements of the population health strategy that has been determined by the most recent conference. Indicators include characteristics of the population; available healthcare services; and environmental determinants of health, such as air quality, water quality, urban location, and exposure to secondhand smoke. The framework has been modified since it first appeared in 1999. The current model is shown in Exhibit 3.3.

In the United States, the *Healthy People* criteria have become the primary indicators of population health. At the time of the first *Healthy People* report, Green, Wilson, and Bauer (1983) noted the underdeveloped state of many indicators and the dearth of information systems for assessing the indicators across time. This rudimentary report was weak as far as monitoring and evaluation was concerned but was nonetheless an original, pioneering effort to develop population-wide evaluation where none had existed before. *Healthy People* 2010 included a set of leading criteria for indicating progress across time: physical activity, overweight and obesity, tobacco use, substance abuse, responsible sexual behavior, mental health, injury and violence, environmental quality, immunization, and access to healthcare. The success of

EXHIBIT 3.3
Health
Indicators
Framework, as
conceptualized
in Canada's
Health
Indicators
Project

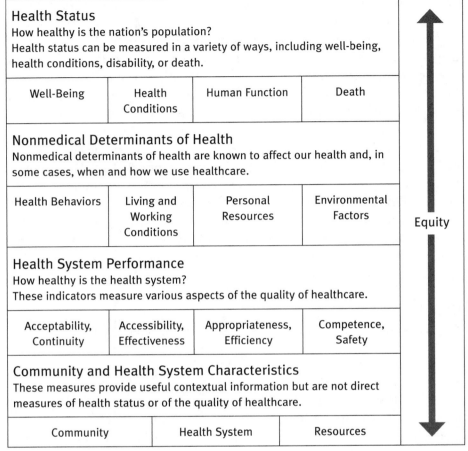

Health Status
How healthy is the nation's population?
Health status can be measured in a variety of ways, including well-being, health conditions, disability, or death.

Well-Being	Health Conditions	Human Function	Death

Nonmedical Determinants of Health
Nonmedical determinants of health are known to affect our health and, in some cases, when and how we use healthcare.

Health Behaviors	Living and Working Conditions	Personal Resources	Environmental Factors

Health System Performance
How healthy is the health system?
These indicators measure various aspects of the quality of healthcare.

Acceptability, Continuity	Accessibility, Effectiveness	Appropriateness, Efficiency	Competence, Safety

Community and Health System Characteristics
These measures provide useful contextual information but are not direct measures of health status or of the quality of healthcare.

Community	Health System	Resources

Equity

Source: Adapted and reprinted, with permission, from a joint publication of the Canadian Institute for Health Information and Statistics Canada titled "Health Indicators 2011."

this population-based effort can be judged by whether it spurred its audiences to adjust priorities and efforts to work toward these goals.

As discussed earlier in this chapter, the CDC developed the NPHPSP to promote uniformity in the organization and activities of public health agencies as they strive to serve the ten core functions of public health. The criterion for success of the effort is whether the standards are influential. The ultimate goal is uniform provision of a core set of public health functions by all public health authorities. The PHAB (2011) criteria are grouped into 12 domains, which include providing education on public health issues, enforcing public health laws, and promoting access to healthcare services.

A conceptualization of a community healthcare management system by Shortell, Gillies, and Devers (1995) offers an integrated set of population-level criteria for judging the effectiveness of specific healthcare and nonmedical, community-based prevention, promotion, and protection interventions and services. They conceptualized a healthcare system that could be delivered by private providers but be based on community health indicators. Healthcare could be delivered in a context of mandates and incentives that would encourage the providers to work toward population health goals as well as clinical service delivery goals. Thus, public policies governing the private delivery of healthcare would be the strategy for achieving population-wide health goals. Their proposed system includes the following stages:

1. Assessment of needs at the community level
2. Development and integration of resources and services across the continuum of care, including health promotion and disease prevention, to meet those needs
3. Development of guidelines and protocols to guide the delivery of care
4. Creation of a monitoring system to ensure the needs are met

The continuum of services displayed in Exhibit 1.1 in Chapter 1 illustrates the range of health services that would need to be considered in this type of system.

Shortell, Gillies, and Devers (1995) anticipated that, to achieve effectiveness at both the population and individual patient levels, healthcare systems' focus would transition from hospital-based care (in which the organization and its income are centered on the delivery of inpatient care) to a predominantly outpatient, community-based system (in which the hospital is relegated to a supportive role). The outcomes criteria they proposed for their community healthcare management system model focuses on seven aspects: (1) management/governance, (2) population-based planning, (3) innovative provider arrangements (to replace the traditional staff and contractor models), (4) clinical reengineering/decision support, (5) commitment to continuous quality improvement, (6) change from a service delivery outcomes model to a population outcomes model, and (7) community health status outcomes measurement. Numerous measures are specified for each of these aspects. The authors emphasized that the general model should be followed but that circumstances may call for flexibility.

Policy-based financial incentives and ongoing outcomes evaluation have emerged as the mechanisms likely to guide healthcare in this population-focused, prevention- and primary care–oriented, continuum-of-care direction (Shortell, Casalino, and Fisher 2010). Population-based outcomes at the community level, leadingly represented by the *Healthy People* series of indicators, have already been developed.

In their quality model of healthcare, Shortell, Gillies, and Devers (1995) did not specify who would sustain a community survey of healthcare processes and outcomes to serve the model's need for ongoing assessment of community health status or how local providers might be incentivized to behave in ways that would lead to detectable progress on community-level indicators. The emerging ACO model instituted by the ACA shares several of the qualities of Shortell's model but thus far does not include this community focus.

Similar structure-, process-, and outcomes-based evaluation criteria have been developed to evaluate the medical home, and a movement to shift primary care to this model is under way. Several medical home certification programs, such as NCQA's, are leading this change. Medical homes are assessed on the basis of numerous criteria. NCQA's standards group them into nine categories: (1) access and communication, (2) patient tracking/registry, (3) care management, (4) support for patient self-management, (5) e-prescribing, (6) medical test tracking, (7) referral tracking, (8) performance reporting and continuous improvement, and (9) advanced e-communications (Carrier, Gourevitch, and Shah 2009).

Policy initiatives aim to connect NCQA certification to reimbursement through federal regulation of health insurance plans. Alongside the burgeoning private certification process, the essential elements of Shortell's model are being implemented, as part of healthcare reform, for Medicare-serving healthcare organizations that want to be designated as ACOs and are willing to vie for payment incentives through the Medicare Shared Savings Program. The proposed rule for this program commented that up to 5 million Medicare enrollees might soon be receiving care from providers participating in ACOs (CMS 2010b), and a press release from HHS (2012) noted that 89 ACOs serving a total of more than one million enrollees had been established as of July 1, 2012.

Healthcare effectiveness may be improved by such policy initiatives that modify providers' funding/reimbursement incentives to favor community health, patient-centered care, efficiency, and long-range quality goals. This mix of population focus and clinical focus could address such problems as the high growth rate of healthcare expenditures, failure to reap the benefits of integrative efficiency, and practice variation. This strategy would favor larger providers that are integrated both vertically and horizontally. However, optimal outcomes would be challenging to identify.

While many quality measures have been developed for integrated care, including for recognized ACOs and for healthcare settings designated as medical homes, Fisher and Shortell (2010) noted that a fair portion of performance measures promote no benefit because they are burdensome to track and are irrelevant to the aim of influencing the value of healthcare delivered. The ACA introduces this new style of healthcare performance assessment in which outcomes are evaluated and incentivized at both clinical and population levels, but the optimal profile of clinical-level and population-level indicators of effectiveness has yet to be determined.

Summary and Conclusions

The development and evaluation of strategies for improving the effectiveness of healthcare services and systems at the clinical level are informed by Donabedian's structure/process/outcome model. With this framework in mind, this chapter has reviewed evidence focused on the question: What policy strategies contribute most to improving the health of the population? Strategies focused on structural and process factors have been evaluated to some extent, and the results are mixed. In general, the evidence reviewed from the clinical perspective suggests that while the point of diminishing returns from further investments in medical care with regard to improving the health of the population may have been reached for some portion of the population, a case should still be made for investments in medical care to improve the health of vulnerable groups, improve the integration of medical services, and reduce variation in medical practice. The health of populations in general, as well as at-risk groups in particular, is most likely to be enhanced, however, by focusing more resources on nonmedical determinants of health, such as the physical, social, and economic environments in which individuals live and work.

The community healthcare management system model proposed by Shortell, Gillies, and Devers (1995) provides a conceptual framework for promoting both clinical-level and population-level outcomes through clinical care settings. Some of these strategies are reflected in the provisions of the ACA, such as incentives to promote the adoption of the ACO model and the medical home model. Methods and measures for evaluating the effectiveness of these models are already established but need to be refined. These methods and measures will help determine whether the healthcare reforms implemented by the ACA achieved intended outcomes.

It is challenging to evaluate evidence of the effectiveness of any health policies aimed at the clinical or population level because controlled designs for testing the purported effects of policy actions, such as publishing clinical guides or population health indicators, are almost impossible to create and because policies of various impact are always being simultaneously introduced or modified. Strong frameworks and strong data analysis are necessary to draw the firmest conclusion that can be supported by available data sources. The development and gathering of indicators at the clinical and population levels have been significant efforts toward achieving empirical evaluation.

EFFICIENCY: CONCEPTS AND METHODS

4

Chapter Highlights

1. *Allocative efficiency* depends on attainment of the "right" (i.e., most valued) mix of outputs. Primary health policy areas that reflect concerns with allocative efficiency include decision making regarding investments in healthcare services versus non-service policy alternatives; coverage of preventive services; and the mix or types of treatment, in relation to health improvements.

2. *Production efficiency* refers to producing a given level of output at minimum cost. For example, inefficiency occurs when physicians provide healthcare services that could be provided just as well by nurses or other less expensive health personnel and when practice does not take advantage of economies of scale, as in the production of laboratory services.

3. Societies have developed need and consumer demand mechanisms for making health resource allocation decisions. *Need* exists when someone is better off with a service than without it; *consumer demand* refers to what consumers are willing and able to buy at alternative prices. Need primarily undergirds regulatory-based approaches to resource allocation, and consumer demand underlies market-based approaches to resource allocation.

4. Analysts use cost-effectiveness analysis, cost-utility analysis, cost-benefit analysis, and comparative systems analysis to examine production and allocative efficiency issues in healthcare.

Overview

The fundamental questions in this chapter are (1) what is efficiency? and (2) how is efficiency measured? Understanding the concepts and methods of efficiency analysis can help policymakers and stakeholders with decisions regarding how to combine limited resources to produce personal and community-based health services of maximum value.

All societies allocate a large portion of their wealth to the provision of health services. The United States leads the world both in level of healthcare spending and in efforts to study the problems of access, quality, and cost of health services delivery. In 1960, 5.2 percent of the US gross domestic product (GDP) was spent on healthcare. By 2009, it had increased to 17.6 percent (Martin et al. 2011). Large variations in medical practice, evidence of the lack of effectiveness of many healthcare services, and renewed interest in disease prevention, health promotion, and non-healthcare determinants of health suggest that the allocation of healthcare resources is not efficient (Deaton 2002; McGlynn et al. 2003; OECD 2009; Thorpe 2005).

In aggregate terms, the efficiency and equity of the US healthcare system compare unfavorably to those of Canada and several Western European countries (Anderson and Squires 2010; Davis, Schoen, and Stremikis 2010). Analysts in the United States have examined those countries to obtain points of reference for US problems and to gain insight into possible solutions. Despite their lower expenditures and broader coverage, other countries face severe problems with their healthcare systems and often look to the United States for innovative healthcare delivery and financing strategies. These countries also look to the United States' extensive HSR base focused on assessing the effectiveness, efficiency, and equity of alternative healthcare services and systems.

Because of the concern about the impact of past and projected healthcare costs on public and private budgets, cost control is a major goal of health policy in countries throughout the world (Zweifel, Breyer, and Kifmann 2009). Although it may not be necessary to restrain the percentage of GDP spent on healthcare (because no one knows what that percentage should be), the high and rapidly growing cost of healthcare raises the question of whether the investment is worth the costs. Ideally, cost containment first would be achieved by eliminating spending on services that were detrimental to or had no effect on patient health. If further reductions were required, services would be ranked and funded according to their yield in terms of health improvement per dollar. Research on the efficiency and effectiveness of health services delivery can help guide these decisions. The State of Oregon, for example, used effectiveness and cost-effectiveness evidence to ground the design of a system for efficiently rationing healthcare (Kitzhaber 2003; Saha, Coffman, and Smits 2010), though the precise mechanisms for making these technically and ethically difficult rationing decisions have inspired substantial policy debate (Eddy 1991; Hadorn 1991; Tengs 1996). Because of the controversy associated with explicit rationing, the 2008 Oregon Health Insurance Experiment tested the use of a lottery system for determining who would and would not have access to Medicaid (see Chapter 3). This experiment found that after one year, relative to the controls, individuals in the treatment group utilized more healthcare services (including preventive care) and had lower out-of-pocket costs, less medical debt, and improved physical and mental health status (Finkelstein et al. 2011).

Researchers have used the Dartmouth Atlas of Health Care to identify low-cost, high-performing health systems at the local and regional levels in the United States (Skinner, Staiger, and Fisher 2006). They have raised provocative questions about whether spending more on healthcare services leads to better health outcomes (Abelson and Harris 2010). Some have suggested that healthcare spending has risen to the point where it may actually cause a decline in health because it diverts resources from other areas, such as education, housing, and environment programs (Evans, Barer, and Marmor 1994; Evans and Stoddart 2003). Others have focused on the low benefit-to-cost ratio of many US healthcare services, the willingness of consumers to pay for those benefits, and the importance of closing distributional gaps in access to care (Chernew, Hirth, and Cutler 2009).

Thus, the questions of how much to spend on healthcare, what mix of healthcare services to provide, and how to provide them are important policy issues. The search for policy solutions that improve efficiency continues because of the nature of health and healthcare, the status of healthcare as a good that many feel should be available regardless of one's ability to pay, the impingement of healthcare costs on public budgets, the lack of consumer information, and other healthcare market imperfections. Efficiency analysis in HSR can help researchers, policymakers, and other stakeholders better understand these problems and the operation of the healthcare system and inform the development of policies that will improve the access, cost, and quality of healthcare.

This chapter introduces the tools and the theoretical underpinnings of efficiency analysis to address the first question posed at the beginning of the chapter: What is efficiency? The concepts of allocative and production efficiency are presented and defined, and the theoretical basis for the need and market demand criteria used in resource allocation and production decisions is discussed. The role of production functions; cost, cost-effectiveness, cost-benefit, and cost-utility analyses; and regional and international comparisons are examined to address the second question: How is efficiency measured?

Conceptual Framework and Definitions

For society as a whole, *efficiency* is defined as a situation in which the welfare of a person cannot be improved without reducing the welfare of another. Efficient service delivery requires that both production efficiency and allocative efficiency be achieved. *Production efficiency* is achieved when a given level of services is produced at the lowest possible per unit cost. *Allocative efficiency* is achieved when "either inputs or outputs are put to their best possible uses in the economy so that no further gains in input or output are possible" (Folland, Goodman, and Stano 2010). As implied in the conceptual framework introduced in Chapter 1 (Exhibit 1.5), improving the health of communities and individuals is the desired and valued end point of societal investments in healthcare services, systems, and policies. These investment decisions also have important implications for the equity of healthcare provision in terms of the fairness of resource allocation (Culyer 1992; Cutler 2002).

Allocative Efficiency

Where healthcare is viewed as an input in the production of health, the focus is on allocative efficiency (i.e., maximizing health given constrained resources). Allocative inefficiency may occur even in a production-efficient health system if the system produces too many or too few services relative to health improvements. Allocative efficiency problems arise in healthcare delivery, for example, when substantial resources are allocated to treatments of minimal effectiveness while more effective services are neglected. Primary health policy areas that reflect concerns about allocative efficiency include decisions regarding (1) investments in healthcare services versus environmental, behavioral, or other community-based, health-related policy alternatives; (2) coverage and payment for preventive versus acute care services; and (3) the "best" mix of services for a given health problem experienced by specific patients.

Healthcare Services Investments

In a broader context of health-oriented social policy, a society may achieve greater health benefits by diverting resources from healthcare services to activities aimed at improving the physical and social environment—for example, air and water quality, education, job training, and community development (Evans et al. 1994). Studies have documented that the marginal product of healthcare service investments in the United States is small for the population as a whole, although it may be higher for population subgroups, such as the elderly and low-income individuals (Finkelstein et al. 2011; Folland, Goodman, and Stano 2010; Manning et al. 1987), and for specific services, such as treatments for cataracts, heart attacks, and depression (Cutler and McClellan 2001b; Skinner, Staiger, and Fisher 2006). Lifestyle factors have been found to be significant predictors of population health, as has education. Grossman (1972) proposed that education improves health. Research documents that better-educated people tend to know what they need to stay healthy and how to use medical and other inputs for better health (Cutler, Lleras-Muney, and Vogl 2008; Cutler and Lleras-Muney 2010; Gerdtham et al. 1999; Lleras-Muney 2002; Oreopoulos 2006; Wolfe and Behrman 1987). These findings present challenges to state policymakers who may be confronted, for example, with deciding the relative value of reallocating state dollars to Medicaid versus public education.

Preventive Services

Another efficiency concern with the US healthcare system is too much spending on treatment of individuals for whom health improvements or survival is remote and too little spending on preventive services, especially population-wide services to reduce air and water pollution (Maciosek et al. 2010; Riley and Lubitz 2010; Shugarman, Decker, and Bercovitz 2009). Typically only a small percentage of national health expenditures are allocated to preventive activities.[1] Thorpe (2005) and Fineberg (2009) have made the case for a more balanced approach to healthcare reform that pays more attention to prevention and control of chronic disease than to extension of insurance coverage.

In the past, studies of effectiveness and cost-effectiveness were used on a case-by-case basis for selecting preventive services to be covered by public and private insurance (Eddy 1980; Gold et al. 1996; Pear 1997; US Preventive Services Task Force 1989). The ACA and associated rules include a systematic approach to investment in prevention and chronic disease management while also broadening insurance coverage in the United States. New health insurance rules prohibit deductibles, coinsurance, and other forms of copayment for preventive services recommended by the US Preventive Services Task Force (Pear 2010a). Services exempted from these charges include immunizations, cancer screening, screening for lipid disorders and type 2 diabetes, and counseling for smoking cessation, among others. Recommendations are based on the quality of the evidence of each service's effectiveness, the net health benefits associated with the service, and the level of uncertainty of outcomes associated with the delivery of the service in primary care settings (AHRQ 2009). This approach is an example of value-based insurance, under which copayments are reduced to encourage use of effective services and are increased for less effective services. The few studies that have been done on this approach to health insurance design show it has limited effects on healthcare-seeking behavior (Chernew et al. 2010). It is being implemented incrementally and will be evaluated as experienced is gained and data are accumulated.

Mix of Healthcare Services

Another area of concern is the misallocation of resources between technical procedures versus services that improve patients' understanding and management of their health problems and of ways they can possibly prevent health problems in the future. Due to the malpractice issue and the prevalence of fee-for-service payment in the US system, physicians have a strong incentive to perform procedures such as surgery and diagnostic tests and a weak incentive to spend time taking patient histories and providing cognitive services (e.g., health education or motivational counseling). Extensive testing produces documentation, which can be used in medical liability lawsuits.

Tests and other procedures also bring in much higher remuneration per unit of time than do cognitive services (Hsiao et al. 1988). Physician ownership of diagnostic equipment, laboratories, and specialty hospitals can exacerbate this problem (Devers, Brewster, and Ginsburg 2003; Hillman et al. 1990; Hollingsworth 2008). This issue was highlighted in a widely circulated article from the *New Yorker*, which compared the cost of care in El Paso, Texas, to that in a similar community in Harlingen, Texas (Gawande 2009). The greater cost of care in Harlingen was attributed to the volume of routine diagnostic and other services associated with Harlingen's entrepreneurial provider culture, where physicians were much more invested in facilities and equipment. Due to this emphasis on procedures, management of patient behavior—a strong component of disease and one of the most important and potentially influential aspects of patient care, education, and counseling—may be neglected.

Production Efficiency

Health is viewed as the final output of the healthcare system, and healthcare services are the intermediate output. Production efficiency (i.e., producing output at the least cost) is of concern for both intermediate and final outputs. Production efficiency is achieved when resources are organized and managed in a manner that minimizes the cost of production and when personnel, supplies, and equipment are paid for at rates that represent their cost in their next best alternative use (i.e., their opportunity cost). Inefficiency occurs when care is not managed in a way that maximizes potential productivity, such as when physicians provide services that could be provided just as well by nurses or other less expensive health personnel and when practice does not take advantage of economies of scale, as in the production of laboratory services. These concepts of efficiency are relevant at the level of the individual patient and practitioner, as well as at the population levels of community and system (see Chapter 1, Exhibit 1.3).

Exhibit 4.1 displays combinations of goods and services that could be produced with society's resources during a given period. The curve AB represents the production possibility frontier. Points on the curve represent the maximum possible outputs of all goods and services, given current technology and the most efficient production methods. If actual production is inside the curve, as at point C, production efficiency is not being achieved. Within the shaded area, improved production efficiency could expand healthcare without reducing the output of other goods and services, and vice versa. However, from any point on the frontier, expansion of one commodity is at the expense of the other. Thus, allocative decisions must be made in terms of the trade-off between healthcare and other goods and services.

The production possibility frontier illustrates only that alternative combinations are possible. It does not identify the efficient combination.

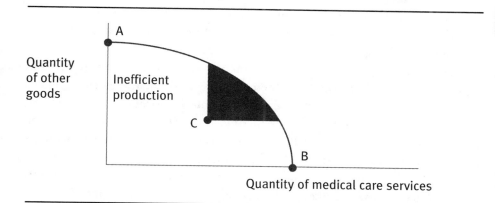

EXHIBIT 4.1
Production
Possibility
Frontier

Quantity of medical care services

Resource allocation is a complex, dynamic process that depends on a mix of private spending decisions and public tax and spending decisions. With a growing economy and technological base, the frontier is continually expanding, and technology itself is the focus of concern. The well-being of society is subject to decisions about the allocation of resources to technology, to healthcare, and to other goods and services.

Both allocative and production efficiency focus on providing guidance for achieving what might be an optimal allocation of resources and associated costs relative to desired outputs (e.g., health and healthcare). The theoretical underpinnings for determining the optimal distribution of resources to produce these desired ends are described in the next section.

Criteria for Optimal Allocation

Examples of resource misallocation and inefficient production of healthcare can be documented (as shown in Chapter 5). Nonetheless, the optimal allocation of resources and production methods is not known. Three major problems confront analysts and policymakers attempting to evaluate healthcare resource allocation issues. The first problem is limited theoretical and empirical information on how to determine the effects of health on *social well-being*, which is defined by Stokey and Zeckhauser (1978) as the sum of individual utilities (benefits) attained by individuals in society. Second is the related problem of limited information on the relationship between healthcare service use and health. The third problem is the uncertainty about market and regulatory systems' capacity to efficiently allocate resources in healthcare delivery (Arrow 1963).

Philosophers have long sought to devise theories and practical guides to define and measure social welfare. Vilfredo Pareto (1848–1923)[2] developed a collection of analytic devices and concepts for evaluating resource allocation decisions, forming much of the theoretical basis of welfare economics. Central to this work is the *Pareto optimum*, which occurs when all mutually beneficial exchanges have been made such that no one person can be made better off without making someone else worse off. With freedom to trade, rational individuals or their proxies make all trades they believe benefit them. However, many Pareto-optimum allocations are possible, depending on the distribution of income. Identifying and achieving the one that maximizes social well-being involves trade-offs between winners and losers and use of a social welfare function. A *social welfare function* describes a decision maker's preferences among alternative combinations of individual utilities (Stokey and Zeckhauser 1978). It describes how the decision maker would trade off gains in utility among some people for losses for others. For example, how is social welfare affected by allocating fewer tax dollars to public education and more to Medicaid for low-income families? To answer this question, the decision maker must aggregate his individual preferences to provide a ranking of welfare, or likely public benefit, for society as a whole.

Arrow (1963) demonstrated that development of such a function at the societal level is not possible. It has been shown in theory, however, that competitive markets can yield Pareto-optimum social welfare (Stokey and Zeckhauser 1978). Informed, rational consumers make mutually beneficial trades, and competitive producers seek efficient methods of production in response to consumer preferences. However, competitive market conditions do not prevail for most types of healthcare services (Rice and Unruh 2009), and societies have developed nonmarket mechanisms (e.g., regulatory approaches) that base resource allocation on the need for services rather than on consumer demand.

Need

Need, as defined by health professionals, is the basis for government-imposed approaches to healthcare resource allocation. Need for medical care exists when someone is better off with a treatment than without it, and the improvement is measured in terms of a person's health (Getzen and Allen 2007; Williams 1974). Unless healthcare professionals deem a treatment to be effective and the patient values its outcome, the treatment is not "needed."

While need is a useful concept for determining the care patients require, the use of need as a basis for resource allocation poses conceptual and practical problems. First, there is no objective basis on which to rank health needs and to compare them with other needs of individuals and populations. Second, even with this restrictive definition, needs appear to be insatiable and thus still must be rationed. New health problems arise (e.g., the obesity epidemic), and the healthcare industry is continually developing new ways to detect and treat diseases and defining new problems not previously addressed by medicine. Third, the relationship between providing healthcare services and reducing health needs is often unclear or even nonexistent (see Chapter 3 for a detailed discussion of this issue). Fourth, health services provided to meet need as defined by health professionals or government agencies may go unutilized because the population does not demand them (e.g., preventive services) (Feldstein 1998).

Consumer Demand

Consumer demand—what consumers are willing and able to buy at alternative prices—is another important criterion for allocating resources. Perceived need may be a major but not sole determinant of demand, depending on the preferences of the individual consumer (convenience may be another consideration, for example). Rational consumers compare the marginal value benefit and marginal cost associated with alternative uses of their limited money and time resources and make allocation decisions in their best interests.[3]

The concept of demand is represented in Exhibit 4.2 as a curve (D). It shows the quantities of a good or service—for example, routine doctor visits (horizontal axis)—that an individual is willing and able to purchase at alternative prices (vertical axis) during a given period. Consumers are assumed to be well informed about prices and services so that they may make choices that maximize their well-being. Numerous factors affect the position and slope of the demand curve, including consumer income, preferences, need, and the prices of other related goods and services. The typical demand curve slopes downward because (1) as price falls, consumers are able to buy more; (2) at lower prices, the service is less costly relative to substitute services (i.e., services that serve the same ends, such as outpatient and inpatient surgery for minor problems); and (3) the marginal value of the service to the consumer falls as more is consumed in a given period. The demand curve represents the marginal value of the service to the consumer at alternative levels of consumption (Q), and the market price (P) represents the marginal cost of the service to the consumer. By consuming at the level (Q') corresponding to the level at which a given price (P') intersects the demand curve (point E'), the consumer maximizes well-being. For quantities of doctor visits that exceed Q', given the price P', marginal cost is greater than marginal benefit (D), making the consumer worse off.

Market demand is merely the aggregation of the individual demands of market participants. While demand is an individual concept and depends on individual behavior, aggregations of individuals form markets. The prices and quantities of goods and services are determined by the operation of supply and demand in markets.

EXHIBIT 4.2
Individual
Demand Curve

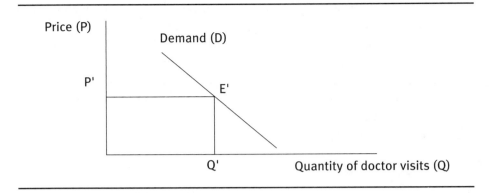

Assumptions of a Competitive Market

In a competitive market, *supply* is the amount of a good or service that suppliers are willing to sell at alternative prices during a given period (see Exhibit 4.3). The curve is positive or upward sloping, meaning that greater quantities are supplied at higher prices. The position of the supply curve depends on technology (i.e., the ability to transform inputs into output), the prices of inputs such as wages and rents, and the objectives of suppliers (i.e., whether they are attempting to maximize profits or services or some combination of the two). For example, technological innovation in electronics has markedly increased productivity and enabled producers to offer the same products at lower prices, shifting the supply curve to the right. Similarly, increases in wages and other input costs require suppliers to charge higher prices for the same number of units, shifting the supply curve to the left. Market supply is the aggregation of the individual supplies of market participants.

Market forces driven by competitive conditions lead to the intersection of market supply and demand—that is, the equilibrium (E') combination of market price (P') and quantity of services (Q') for a given period (see Exhibit 4.4). This model of supply and demand and competitive market forces undergirds the market approach to healthcare policy. By rapidly adjusting to changes in consumer preferences, incomes, resource availability, and technology, competitive markets generally are a flexible mechanism for solving the basic economic problems of what, how, and for whom a good or service is produced. In terms of goods, and possibly routine healthcare, consumers appear to be the best judge of their needs and desires relative to other uses of their resources.[4] Under competitive market conditions, producers who fail to respond to consumer demand, who charge prices greater than the market rate, or who use inefficient production methods are forced out of business, and consumers individually allocate resources to maximize their well-being, shifting the system toward a Pareto-optimum allocation of resources.

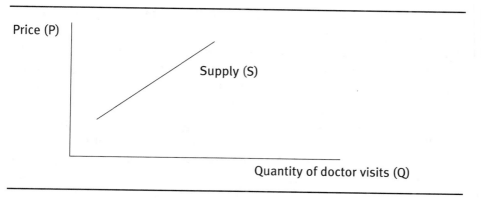

EXHIBIT 4.3
Individual
Supply Curve

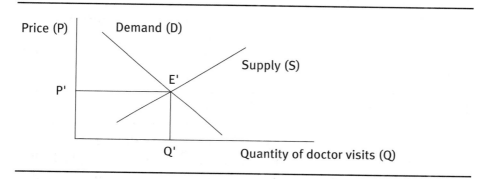

EXHIBIT 4.4
Market Demand
and Supply

Assumptions of Healthcare Markets

Healthcare diverges from some of the fundamental properties of a competitive market. See Rice and Unruh (2009) for a thorough critique of the use of competitive markets to achieve healthcare goals for society. The basic conditions of a competitive market are (1) free entry into and exit from the market by buyers and sellers; (2) many well-informed buyers and sellers, none of whom is large enough to influence market price; and (3) no collusion among buyers and sellers—that is, they act independently. Many healthcare market areas are too small to support competition, especially among specialists and hospitals. Historically, the healthcare market has been characterized by price discrimination and collusion, ostensibly to protect consumers and provide access to those who cannot pay for services. For example, to control medical pricing, the American Medical Association prohibited advertising by its members and physicians developed fee schedules, such as the California Relative Value Scale. Asymmetry of information puts consumers at a disadvantage vis-à-vis providers, and entry by providers is strictly limited by licensing and regulation of the professions and facilities (Fuchs 1972; Kessel 1958; Rice and Unruh 2009).

The competitive model therefore does not fully apply to healthcare because of several inherent market limitations. The market is influenced by significant externalities (i.e., instances in which one person's consumption or production affects another person's well-being). For example, a person who obtains immunizations to prevent infectious diseases benefits others by reducing their risk of contracting those diseases. Private markets tend to underinvest in these types of services because benefits to third parties do not directly influence the demand for them and thus are not considered. Similarly, people seem to care that others have access to basic healthcare and therefore benefit when others gain access to care that otherwise would not be available. Markets have no mechanism for translating this value into the desired result.

Another problem with private healthcare markets is *supplier-induced demand*—that is, the influence that provider interests have on consumer demand. Provider interests may affect consumer demand due to the large disparity of information between provider and consumer and because a third party often pays for a substantial portion of services rendered (Grytten and Sorensen 2001; Reinhardt 1987). Healthcare providers, who generally are not financially disinterested, can have a major influence on consumer demand, greatly diminishing the independent role of consumer choice in the market for healthcare services and insurance (Newhouse 2002). The level of supplier-induced demand may vary among communities, and thus the utilization and cost of healthcare services may differ significantly among otherwise similar populations (Gawande 2009). Due to these problems and monopoly characteristics, such as the lack of free entry and exit to the industry by producers, price collusion among producers, and the potential exclusion of some groups (e.g., low income) from the healthcare market, satisfactory allocation and distribution of healthcare goods and services cannot be assumed.

Despite these issues, efficiency analysis tools grounded in theories of the competitive market provide a conceptual point of reference and a set of criteria and methods for examining the potential for healthcare markets and government regulatory strategies to achieve efficiency—in either the production or allocation of health or healthcare.

Key Methods of Assessing Efficiency

Efficiency analysis typically is divided into micro and macro levels. *Micro-level efficiency analysis* examines the behavior of consumers and firms in markets. It therefore encompasses the clinical perspective of HSR, focusing on patients and providers and how they behave in the local environment (see Chapter 1, Exhibit 1.2). *Macro-level efficiency analysis* examines the economy as a whole and parallels the population perspective of HSR, focusing on aggregate measures of health, social well-being, employment, economic growth, and so forth. Macro-level concerns with healthcare services are measured in terms of the life expectancy of the population, infant mortality rate, disability-adjusted life years, and the growth of healthcare expenditures, particularly in comparison to the growth of other health-producing investments.

Micro Level

The principal methods employed in micro-level efficiency analyses include (1) estimating production functions and costs and (2) performing cost-benefit, cost-effectiveness, and related cost-utility analyses.

Production Functions

Economists have developed a comprehensive model of production efficiency, enabling them to express how the total, average, and marginal costs of a given product or service change under a given set of assumptions about the cost of inputs and technology. For example, inputs for primary healthcare may include nurse and physician time and office facilities and supplies. Inputs are weighted by their market prices and summed to determine the cost of production. Input costs include nurse and physician earnings, rent, and supplies. Outputs may be defined in terms of patient visits and procedures performed and their effect on the health of patients. Production functions describe the relationship between inputs and outputs and depend on the current level of technology. *Technology* is defined broadly as the information and techniques required to transform inputs into outputs. The cost functions are derived from the production function and unit input costs and represent the minimum total and unit costs attainable for alternative combinations of inputs and production unit sizes.

While one theoretically can determine the cost-minimizing mix of inputs for any level of output and the cost-minimizing size of the production unit, the complexity of healthcare services makes this task difficult (Pindyck and Rubinfeld 2008). Even when producers have the "right" combination of inputs and size, they may fail to achieve maximum output because of poor management, low employee motivation, or other unspecified production problems. This situation is referred to as *X-inefficiency* (Leibenstein 1966). X-inefficiency occurs whenever a provider does not produce the maximum possible set of services from given resources. Production and cost functions can be empirically estimated for any production process and level of analysis, although they will be less precise for areas in which output is difficult to define and measure (e.g., healthcare).

Production and cost models have been applied to physician, hospital, and insurance services to determine the extent to which production efficiency has been achieved and how it may be enhanced. Grossman (1972) developed a theory of the demand for health and medical care, applying the production function concept from capital theory to an individual's production of health. Capital theory is concerned with optimal investment in equipment and other fixed assets, given the cost of the initial investment, depreciation, operating cost, interest rates, and the expected value of services provided by the capital over time. Envisioning health as capital stock that yields healthy days over time but also requires investments in medical and other resources due to depreciation, Grossman derived predictions for the role of education, wages, and age in the demand for health and medical care. His model has been successfully applied to numerous important health issues, including child health, obesity, and the role of education and health production (Chou, Grossman, and Saffer 2004; Currie and Moretti 2003; Leibowitz 2004). Similarly, production functions have been applied to the allocative efficiency issue of determining the optimal allocation of resources to improve the health of individuals and communities. Summaries of selected studies are provided in Chapter 5.

Cost-Benefit, Cost-Effectiveness, and Cost-Utility Analysis

Other efficiency analysis methods frequently applied in healthcare are cost-benefit analysis (CBA), cost-effectiveness analysis (CEA), and cost-utility analysis (CUA) (Drummond et al. 2005; Haddix, Teutsch, and Corso 2003; Muennig 2008). (See Exhibit 4.5 for a comparison of these methods.) *CBA* is a systematic analysis of one or more methods or programs for achieving a given objective; it measures both benefits and costs in monetary units. *CEA* is a systematic analysis of the effects and costs of alternative methods or programs for achieving a nonmonetary objective (e.g., saving lives, preventing disease, providing services). CEA is used to determine production efficiency, and effects are measured in nonmonetary units. *CUA* is conducted when effects are weighted by utility measures denoting the preference of a patient or of a member of the general public for, or the overall desirability of, a particular outcome (Drummond et al. 2005; Gold et al. 1996).

CBA determines whether a program is worth establishing, in the sense that its benefits are greater than its costs (i.e., allocative efficiency). For example, do the benefits of breast cancer screening, early diagnosis, and treatment outweigh the costs of providing those services? A broader view might compare the net savings, if any, achieved by providing breast cancer screening services versus other preventive healthcare services (e.g., smoking cessation or obesity reduction programs). Services producing the highest net benefit are most efficient. Societal efficiency decreases when projects' costs outweigh their benefits and increases when projects' benefits outweigh their costs. While ranking all possible competing uses of resources to achieve optimal resource allocation is impractical, services can be compared on an incremental basis.

CEA compares the cost of alternatives for achieving a common objective (i.e., production efficiency) without determining whether the objective itself is worth achieving. For example, what are the costs of mammography

Type of Study	Measurement/ Valuation of Costs in Both Alternatives	Identification of Consequences	Measurement/ Valuation of Consequences
Cost-benefit analysis	Dollars	Single or multiple effects are not necessarily common to both alternatives, and common effects may be achieved to different degrees by the alternatives (e.g., dollars saved as a result of investment in breast cancer screening versus investment in smoking and obesity risk reduction programs).	Dollars
Cost-effectiveness analysis	Dollars	Single effect of interest is common to both alternatives but achieved to different degrees (e.g., different mammography screening reminder systems).	Natural units (e.g., visits, life years gained, disability)
Cost-utility analysis	Dollars	Single or multiple effects are not necessarily common to both alternatives, and common effects may be achieved to different degrees by the alternatives (e.g., quality-adjusted life years added from investment in mammography screening versus investment in smoking and obesity risk reduction programs).	Healthy days or (more commonly) quality-adjusted life years

EXHIBIT 4.5
Comparisons of Cost-Benefit, Cost-Effectiveness, and Cost-Utility Analyses

Source: Adapted from Drummond et al. (2005), Exhibit 1.2, by permission of Oxford University Press.

screening, early diagnosis, and treatment of breast cancer per life year saved? CEA can be used as both a complement to and a substitute for CBA. For example, to evaluate mammography screening, one could use CEA first to determine the most efficient way to encourage women to undergo routine screening, given several available behavioral interventions (e.g., patient reminder systems, provider navigation systems, or a combination of such approaches). These production efficiency results could then be used in CBA to address the allocation question of how much, if at all, society should invest in screening, early diagnosis, and treatment of breast cancer.

Alternatively, one may determine that the program would not have net economic benefits (Cutler and McClellan 2001b) but could yield health benefits and thus should be compared with other programs and societal norms in terms of cost per quality-adjusted life year (QALY) gained. Effectiveness can then be measured in terms of increases in QALYs and compared to other activities on the basis of cost per QALY. Instead of monetary values, life years would be valued, or quality-adjusted, according to utility values—i.e., how people feel about time spent in alternative health states, ranging from states they feel would be worse than death to complete health (Torrance et al. 1996; Torrance and Feeny 1989). For example, complete health could be assigned a utility value of 1, and the condition of late-stage breast cancer could be assigned a value of 0.3 (Kerlikowske et al. 1999). If an otherwise healthy person could avert late-stage breast cancer for one year, the gain would be 0.7 of a QALY. To facilitate this type of analysis, Shaw, Johnson, and Coons (2005) developed cancer-related utility weights for the US population, based on the generic EQ-5D utility instrument.

The application of CBA and CUA in HSR has historically focused on investments in healthcare services as opposed to investments in services aimed at environmental, social, and economic factors that affect health (Blumenschein and Johannesson 1996; Center for the Evaluation of Value and Risk in Health 2011; Cutler and McClellan 2001b; Segal and Richardson 1994). Neither the US Preventive Services Task Force nor the Task Force on Community Preventive Services currently uses cost-effectiveness criteria when recommending clinical and community health services. However, both organizations are collecting information on cost and cost-effectiveness aspects of their deliberations and making the information available to decision makers (Grosse, Teutsch, and Haddix 2007).

In the United States, the economic evaluation of pharmaceuticals and other technologies has become an area of increasing interest due to the growth of managed care and rapidly increasing healthcare expenditures. Out of this focus emerged the field of pharmacoeconomics, in which economic evaluation methods are used to examine alternative drug treatments and to identify the costs and benefits of these treatments (Center for Studying Health System Change 2003; Levy et al. 2010; Sullivan et al. 2009). Australia, Canada, and the United Kingdom have developed guidelines for economic evaluations of pharmaceuticals as a basis for determining which to include in national or provincial drug formularies (Canadian Agency for Drugs and Technologies in Health 2006).

Information from medical effectiveness and outcomes research and clinical guidelines also can be used for economic evaluation of healthcare services. AHRQ established Patient Outcomes Research Teams to carry out broad investigations of alternative services and procedures for managing specific clinical conditions (Deyo 1995). The Obama administration is investing $1.1 billion in comparative effectiveness research (CER) to develop further evidence on the effectiveness of alternative care strategies for specific types of patients (Iglehart 2009b; IOM Committee on Comparative Effectiveness Research Prioritization 2009; Lauer and Collins 2010; Sox 2010). While CEA is not mandated in this legislation, the American College of Physicians (2008) strongly favors including CEA in CER studies, and the need for decision makers at the policy and clinical levels to consider cost relative to effectiveness makes it likely that CEA will become an important component of CER.

In 1990 Oregon policymakers applied a set of community values, including cost-effectiveness, to rank 700 condition-treatment pairs for purposes of determining the level of Medicaid coverage for each. The resulting policy extended basic coverage to more people, but some services judged to be of less value were not covered (Eddy 1991; Hadorn 1991; Kitzhaber 2003). The application of a number of community values in this evaluation (rather than simply efficiency) reflects that the allocation of public resources is ultimately a multi-criterion decision. The rankings recently have been used to develop a proposal for an essential benefits package for a universal coverage plan for Oregonians (Saha, Coffman, and Smits 2010). Low-income residents of the state can now participate in a lottery for a chance to enroll in the Oregon Medicaid program. Research based on the random draw supports the health and economic benefits associated with Oregon Medicaid coverage (Finkelstein et al. 2011).

Macro Level

Principal macro-level efficiency analyses have focused on comparing the performance of healthcare systems in different countries. While comparisons at the system level present significant problems, such as those related to measurement of health outcomes, cultural and demographic differences, and data comparability, they do raise questions about the efficiency and equity of health systems and stimulate inquiry into reasons for major observed differences (Anderson et al. 2003; Davis, Schoen, and Stremikis 2010; Joumard, André, and Nicq 2010; Kanavos and Mossialos 1999; Reinhardt, Hussey, and Anderson 2002).

Researchers at the Organisation for Economic Co-operation and Development (OECD) have collected data and attempted to develop standardized international health accounts for the organization's 30 member countries. Comparisons rely on aggregate measures of life expectancy, infant mortality, and cause-of-death–specific mortality. Simple correlations between healthcare spending per capita and aggregate health measures are examined along with input price differences, the production structure of the health sector (e.g., amount spent on hospitals and doctors), input volumes, administrative costs, and appropriateness of care. Disease-specific comparisons between the United States and Canada have been made for cardiovascular disease, cancer, and psychiatric services (Cutler 2002). Recent OECD research focused on developing a set of indicators for comparing healthcare system performance among OECD member countries (Joumard, André, and Nicq 2010). By grouping countries that have similarly structured healthcare systems and comparing performance data among these groups, researchers can identify the weaknesses and strengths of alternative policies and programs for achieving efficiency.

Many analysts emphasize the need to broaden the policy framework beyond healthcare to include the social and physical environment and to focus more on primary prevention and health promotion services, which are usually underfunded due to the large expenditure on medical care treatment. Healthcare purchasers in some countries (e.g., Canada, United Kingdom, Ireland, Iceland, New Zealand) have established health goals for the population and are searching for alternative ways of achieving those health goals, including preventive healthcare and more effective integration of health and other policy issues, such as education, housing, and social welfare. Methods of allocative efficiency analysis have been applied in decision making regarding these programmatic investments (OECD 2002).

Summary and Conclusions

The principal objectives of this chapter were to (1) define efficiency and (2) describe how efficiency can be assessed. The major types of efficiency analyses—allocative and production efficiency—and the theoretical assumptions underlying them were presented. Allocative efficiency concerns attainment of maximum population health with the limited resources available for that objective during any given period. Policymakers and stakeholders maximize efficiency by choosing the "right" (i.e., most valued) mix of healthcare and non-healthcare investments and production methods that minimize cost.

CBA, CEA, and CUA are used to examine the efficiency of healthcare production and efficiency in the mix of specific healthcare services and programs. Analysts also have developed micro and macro methods of assessing healthcare efficiency. Micro methods include the normative microeconomic theories of markets, including production and cost functions as applied to healthcare, and the concept of the individual- and family-level production of health and investment in health capital. Extensive data on OECD's member countries permit macro-level international comparisons of healthcare spending, healthcare utilization, and population health indicators (OECD 2010b). Chapter 5 provides a selected summary of evidence on the efficiency of the US and other healthcare systems and discusses major policy strategies for improving efficiency.

Notes

1. Spending for environmental activities (e.g., air and water pollution abatement, sanitation and sewage treatment, water supplies) is excluded from the national health accounts (Cowan et al. 2002).

2. For a detailed explanation of Pareto's work, see Kohler (1990), pages 484–519.

3. *Marginal* refers to the next unit of a good or service that the consumer is considering. Marginal value differs from the average total value of all units consumed. A "rational" consumer would not purchase the next unit of a good or service if he perceived the benefit of that next unit to be less than the cost of the unit.

4. Even for sophisticated tertiary care, doctors have long acknowledged, if not always fostered, the patient's right to be part of the decision-making team when contemplating alternative courses of action that include alternative levels of risk, benefit, and cost. Patient values are now being fully integrated with clinical information in patient outcome studies (Epstein et al. 2010; Ware Jr. et al. 1996).

EFFICIENCY: POLICY STRATEGIES, EVIDENCE, AND CRITERIA

5

Chapter Highlights

1. Health systems can be characterized by the degree to which they utilize private markets versus government decision making to allocate resources and determine the production and distribution of health services. *Market-minimized* systems tend to rely on direct government or quasi-government controls to achieve desired results, while *market-maximized* models rely primarily on private markets to allocate resources and use the government to enhance markets and subsidize care for the most vulnerable segments of the population.

2. Efficiency strategies used by market-oriented systems include copayments and other targeted financial incentives, utilization controls, management strategies, managed competition, healthcare reimbursement accounts, and fixed-contribution health plans.

3. To achieve efficiency goals, regulated systems tend to rely on fee controls, supply controls, global budgeting, and other performance-based provider payment strategies; needs-based resource allocation; and limited internal markets.

4. Criteria for evaluating health systems and policies in terms of efficiency focus on successful macro cost control (stabilizing healthcare spending as a percentage of GDP) and dynamic efficiency (finding innovative ways to improve efficiency), as well as allocative and production efficiency.

Overview

Three major questions are addressed in this chapter:

1. What are potential policy strategies for achieving efficiency?
2. What is the evidence regarding the effectiveness of strategies aimed at increasing efficiency?
3. What criteria should be used to judge the success of these strategies?

This chapter describes the theoretical assumptions and specific strategies for achieving efficiency that underlie market-maximized and market-minimized health systems. Evidence is provided regarding the allocative efficiency of the US health system at the population level and its production efficiency (i.e., delivering services at minimal cost) at the clinical level.

Policy Strategies Relating to Efficiency

Anderson (1989) noted that health systems in the developed world vary in terms of their organization and financing along a continuum, from market minimized to market maximized. The *market-maximized side* of the continuum relies on consumer payment for health services. Providers are viewed as essentially autonomous sellers of services who respond to consumer demand and competition. Patients are offered financial incentives to be prudent in their purchases and are assumed to understand their healthcare needs well enough to be able to make such decisions. On the *market-minimized side* of the continuum are (1) highly structured health service and financing systems owned or controlled by government and (2) little or no charge to the patient at the point of service. Charges to the patient at time of use, no matter how small, are regarded as an undesirable barrier that may impede access to needed prevention, early diagnosis, or treatment services.

While most countries seek to achieve equity, efficiency, and overall cost control in their health systems and can be characterized along a market versus nonmarket continuum according to their dominant policy emphasis, each employs a unique combination of strategies to achieve these goals. Market-minimized systems tend to rely on direct government or quasi-government controls and provider incentives to achieve desired results, while market-maximized models allocate resources primarily according to private-market trends and consumer-driven decisions and use the government to subsidize care for the most vulnerable segments of the population. Each country's approach to health policy depends largely on its culture, history, and political situation (Cutler 2002). The theoretical foundations for the market-maximized and market-minimized strategies and implications of each for the formulation of health policy are reviewed in the sections that follow.

With the growth in public payment programs and prospective bundled-payment methods for healthcare services, the United States has taken on more of the characteristics of market-minimized models for paying providers, while countries that have traditionally been more market-minimized have attempted to incorporate some private-market methods to control the rising cost of physician and hospital services and make their systems more responsive to consumers.

Specific Efficiency Strategies

Market-Maximized Models

Paul Feldstein (1998) used a qualitative method to evaluate the allocative efficiency of the healthcare system from a market perspective. The assumption of consumer power in the marketplace and the criterion of maximum consumer satisfaction and well-being formed the basis of his economic evaluation. He examined the sectors of a healthcare system (e.g., insurance, hospital care, and physician care) to assess the consistency of observed behavior with the predictions derived from the economic model of the competitive market. For example, do producers strive to minimize the cost of production, and are the mix and quality of goods and services guided by consumer choices? When he found inconsistencies between the model's predictions and the actual performance of the health system, he examined and altered the basic assumptions of the competitive model to better explain observed behavior. From this study, Feldstein identified structural distortions in the US insurance and healthcare markets that have led to misallocation of resources and inefficient production methods.

Cost-based reimbursement of hospitals prompted non-price competition, excess capacity, and high cost. These problems have been addressed through government control policies as well as market-enhancing reforms. For example, Medicare prospective payment methods were introduced to change the economic incentives for healthcare providers, and managed care health plans were encouraged to compete for health plan enrollees on the basis of value for price. These initiatives have largely failed to improve the efficiency of the healthcare system, and therefore new physician payment, consumer information, and insurance exchange reforms were developed and introduced as part of the 2010 healthcare reform legislation. The political situation in the United States does not permit movement away from a market-oriented healthcare system.

Enthoven (1990) proposed managed competition in the early 1990s as a comprehensive solution to market failure in the US healthcare system. This approach depended on market incentives to motivate health plans and providers to be efficient and responsive to consumer demands and on price incentives for consumers to make prudent choices among health plans. Private sponsors of health benefits (e.g., employers) and public sponsors (e.g., state and federal government agencies) aggressively monitored and managed competition among health plans in the healthcare market. Following the failure of President Clinton's managed competition healthcare reform in 1992, the government and business sectors continued to struggle with healthcare cost, access, and quality concerns.

Aligned with the Committee for Economic Development's Research and Policy Committee (2007), Enthoven (2010) proposed a variation of market-based reform in the debates on healthcare reform preceding the success-ful legislation promoted by President Obama. While the ACA enacted under the Obama administration leaves much of the current fragmented system intact, it does provide for the development of health insurance exchanges to encour-age consumer choice and create price/quality competition among health plans. Exchanges will initially be limited to small employers and consumers who do not have access to employer-based coverage. In the Enthoven model, exchanges would become available to the entire US population over time.

Due to the success of managed care competition in controlling US healthcare costs in the mid-1990s, the private sector and most states expanded enrollment of beneficiaries in managed care and many states estab-lished rules and regulations to protect consumers from some of the negative consequences of market competition (Jensen et al. 1997). States served in the sponsor role for Medicaid managed care patients, and the federal govern-ment established Medicare+Choice to enable Medicare beneficiaries to enroll in competing risk-based health plans. While the Medicare+Choice managed care initiative enrolled up to 12 percent of all Medicare enrollees in 2002, it largely failed to meet its major objectives.

Overall Medicare spending continued to increase. Many health plans withdrew from the Medicare+Choice program, and consumer enrollment declined (Thorpe and Atherly 2002). The program was changed to Medicare Advantage in 2003, and Congress increased payment to Medicare Advantage plans to a level greater than traditional Medicare reimbursement. Enrollment increased from 5.3 million to 11.1 million enrollees in 2010, equal to 24 percent of the Medicare population (Biles, Pozen, and Guterman 2009; Kaiser Family Foundation 2010b; Zarabozo and Harrison 2009). These higher payments for Medicare Advantage enrollees were targeted in the 2009 healthcare reform legislation and 2010 negotiations between the Obama administration and the health insurance industry, and premiums were projected to decrease by 1 per-cent in 2011 (Pear 2010b). While benefits were stable, Medicare Advantage premiums fell 7 percent the first year following the introduction of the ACA and were expected to fall an additional 4 percent in 2012 (Galewitz 2011).

Medicaid managed care fared better, growing from 17.8 million enrollees (56 percent of the Medicaid population) in 1999 to 33.4 million enrollees in 2008 (71 percent of the Medicaid population) as states attempted to improve the quality and efficiency of healthcare delivered to low-income people (Kaiser Commission on Medicaid and the Uninsured 2012). The tight labor market in the late 1990s, reduced capitation payments by govern-ment payers, and the consumer and provider backlash against the constraints imposed by managed care led to less restrictive managed care, reduced govern-ment beneficiary enrollment in managed care plans (Achman and Gold 2002), and renewed double-digit healthcare cost growth (Center for Studying Health System Change 2003; Draper et al. 2002; Lesser, Ginsburg, and Devers 2003).

Private-sector demand for integrated managed care delivery systems declined following this backlash in favor of consumer-driven health plans (Casalino and Robinson 2003; Gabel, Lo Sasso, and Rice 2002). Consumer-driven health plans from Humana and other health insurance firms offered an extensive choice of benefits, premiums, and out-of-pocket payments (Robinson 2002). They featured healthcare reimbursement accounts, in which consumers set aside their own funds for out-of-pocket costs, and extensive information for health plan and healthcare decision making. While these high-deductible health plans put downward pressure on utilization and cost, they may have disproportionately reduced access to care for lower-income individuals (Kullgren et al. 2010). A national employer survey found that consumer-directed health plans dramatically increased their share of employment-based health plan enrollment from 8 percent in 2009 to 13 percent in 2010, likely due to employers' attempts to reduce and shift costs to employees during the economic recession (Claxton et al. 2010).

A dramatic reduction in health spending growth was caused by the economic recession that began in late 2007. The rate declined to 4.4 percent in 2008, the lowest in 48 years (Hartman et al. 2010). Even so, health spending outpaced income growth, increasing the share of GDP spent on healthcare from 15.9 percent to 16.2 percent between 2007 and 2008. This pattern is typical during and after economic recessions due to slower growth in the general economy than in the health sector.

Market-Minimized Models

Williams (1990) contrasted the market-maximized and market-minimized approaches to determining production efficiency. In the latter, government leaders (elected and nonelected) assess allocative efficiency on the basis of such values as the extent to which health systems improve the health status of the population in relation to the resources allocated to the system. Spending priorities are determined by professional judgments of health status and need. European nations with predominantly tax-financed, government-provided health systems have traditionally relied on this top-down approach to resource allocation. Such systems typically promote solidarity and equity over individuals' rights and choice. However, even these systems are increasingly mixing market elements with regulatory controls (Jourmard et al. 2010).

The National Health Service (NHS) in the United Kingdom and the health system in New Zealand largely exemplify the use of needs-based approaches to establishing the allocation of resources to the health sector and the type of services provided. In the 1990s, however, internal markets were developed in the United Kingdom and New Zealand to increase production efficiency (Cooper 1994; Glennerster 1995; Street 1994). The goal was to provide incentives for efficient production and allocation of resources while retaining control of overall spending and tax-based financing of healthcare and maintaining or improving equity in access to care. These markets were designed to separate the responsibility for ensuring that patients receive care from the responsibility for direct provision of care. Under this system, the health authority uses its budget to purchase services from other health authorities, general practitioners, private hospitals, nursing homes, and local government social service departments.

The UK health authorities identify healthcare needs and priorities for their assigned regions and determine the best way to spend funds allocated by the central government to meet them. General practitioner groups, who are also responsible for the healthcare needs of their patients, are incentivized to improve their services and be conscious of the costs of their clinical decisions. Physician groups receive global budgets to provide primary care services and purchase specialty care (e.g., diagnostic services, elective surgical procedures, prescription drugs) for their patients (Audit Commission 2011; Brereton and Vasoodaven 2010; Klein 2006).

The NHS has suffered from underfunding for many years. Hospitals have waiting lists for appointments and low-quality facilities. The UK government attempted to improve the situation by increasing healthcare spending by an inflation-adjusted 6 percent per annum in the late 1990s. Except for some reduction in waiting times for high-profile services (e.g., heart surgery), the market-based reforms discussed earlier and this increased budget allocation did not achieve expected improvements (European Observatory on Health Care Systems 2002; Le Grand 2002). The Labor government in 1996 and the early 2000s instituted further market reforms, and the reforms proposed by the 2010 coalition government promoted decentralization and local accountability, including incentives for improving the quality of primary care (Doran and Roland 2010; Lian 2003; Roland and Rosen 2011). Reduced waiting times, improved health outcomes for major chronic disease, and greater patient satisfaction have been documented, but there is disagreement over the extent to which improvements can be ascribed to market reform versus better reporting and management systems (Thorlby and Maybin 2010).

The United States implemented administered price systems for federal beneficiaries under the Medicare program in the early 1980s. The 1989 resource-based relative value fee scale for physician services was developed to complement the 1983 DRG-based prospective payment system (PPS) for hospitals. The 1997 Balanced Budget Act extended the per case payment system to all types of post–acute care (McCall et al. 2003). Work continues on medical effectiveness studies, guidelines, and incentives for improved quality, and methodological improvements are being made in cost-effectiveness studies so that they yield information that better supports public and private decisions on resource allocation (Bailit Health Purchasing, LLC 2002; Gold et al. 1996; Sox and Greenfield 2009). While these policies improved the status quo, they did not alter the fundamental structural problems with the US healthcare financing and delivery system that led to unsustainable growth in expenditures without commensurate improvements in quality of care.

The strategies employed to ensure efficiency differ across market-minimized policies and systems, but all aim to control the prices and volume of healthcare services through provider payment methods and utilization management.

Payment Methods

Alternative methods of paying physicians and hospitals provide different incentives regarding efficiency (D'Intignano 1990; Newhouse 2002). Market-minimized models tend to enforce global budgets and strict fee controls, while market-maximized models encompass a range of alternatives, including fee-for-service, salary, capitation, prospective payment, and performance-based payment.

Physicians

The United States has many different payment methods and sources operating simultaneously, while other countries have a primary method for hospital and physician reimbursement and funnel payment through relatively few channels. For example, US physicians are paid by local, state, and federal agencies; by more than 1,500 insurers; and by out-of-pocket payments from patients. Methods of payment include fee-for-service, salary, and capitation. Until the 1990s, payment based on usual and customary fees for services was the dominant payment method. Fee-for-service is now based on administered prices for most services covered by private insurance and for government beneficiaries in the Medicare and Medicaid programs. While fee-for-service provides an incentive for high productivity, administered prices tend to be rigid and may be set at levels that exceed the value of the service and thus produce profits beyond the "normal" rate of return on investments (Aaron and Ginsburg 2009; Newhouse 2002). The US government is experimenting with pay-for-performance systems, which are designed to increase the quality and efficiency of care by providing monetary rewards for meeting quality targets for prevention and treatment services. These experiments will be accelerated under the provisions of the ACA in conjunction with the development of accountable care organizations (ACOs), which will earn financial incentives for exceeding expected cost and quality metrics while providing a majority of the care required by Medicare patients. Unlike closed-panel health maintenance organizations (HMOs), patients will not be locked into the ACOs (Rosenthal 2007).

Canada and Germany also pay physicians on a fee-for-service basis, but fees have been strictly controlled. Germany developed negotiated aggregate budgets with a volume control mechanism requiring every office-based physician to invoice her physicians' association quarterly for the total number of relative value service points delivered. The physician's income is calculated by multiplying the service points by the point value. The point value is determined by dividing the regional budget for ambulatory care by the total number of service points submitted (European Observatory on Health Care Systems 2002). An increase in the aggregate number of services causes the per unit payment for services to decline, providing an indirect incentive to control the volume of services. The system has been refined to adjust payments to each physician or group practice according to medical specialty, region, and patient age and sex distribution (Stolpe 2011). German cost control mechanisms have been successful, yielding a 2 percent annual increase in inflation-adjusted health spending per capita, the lowest among all OECD countries between 1995 and 2007 (Joumard, André, and Nicq 2010).

Hospitals

Per diem payment, DRG-based prospective payment, and prepayment are the primary methods of reimbursement for hospital services in the United States. Each method provides different financial incentives and has different implications for efficiency (Dowling 1974; McClellan 1997; Nowicki 2004). Although hospitals traditionally have been paid per diem rates plus fees for individual ancillary services, after the passage of PPS under the Medicare program in 1983 many US payers began to make bundled payments for hospital services. The bundled-payment system was designed to pay a fixed amount per episode of hospital care as defined by diagnostic group. PPS provided an incentive for hospitals to encourage doctors to reduce length of stay and to provide services more efficiently because each hospital could retain any surplus in payments over costs. Peer review organizations monitor the necessity of admissions to offset the incentive to admit more patients, underserve them, and discharge them prematurely.

Canada has global hospital budgets and regional health planning to control the cost of hospital care and the diffusion of medical technology, and many provinces have introduced caps on physician spending. Germany applies target budgeting to hospitals for operating costs. Target budgets are negotiated with sickness funds. Payments are adjusted on the basis of hospitals' progress toward those service targets. Germany's 2000 Statutory Health Insurance Health Reform Act mandated the introduction of a hospital PPS based on DRGs. The reforms were implemented over the period between 2003 and 2009 and now cover all hospital care except psychiatric care (European Observatory on Health Care Systems 2002; Hensen et al. 2008; Stolpe 2011).

Since the 1980s, many countries have focused their efforts to control healthcare expenditures on global budget or sectoral budget caps. The key to cost control in these macromanaged systems is having a dominant source of payment that fixes the budget for a given period. Budget growth is generally limited by economic growth. Thus, the Canadian and German systems rely on macro control of the funds available for physicians and hospitals rather than on a mixture of market incentives and controls similar to that in the United States.

Although regulation and global budgets may control the rate of spending, they do not necessarily ensure improved efficiency. Research has shown that output-based efficiency in a subsector such as hospital care does not correlate well with overall efficiency in improving population health (Joumard, André, and Nicq 2010). In the process of controlling costs, perverse incentives may be created for both allocation and production. More efficient, innovative outpatient delivery may lag because of the lack of incentives to develop new services. Recognition of these issues has contributed to concern about the ability of global budgets and regulation to increase health system efficiency.

Concerns have also been expressed about the ability of these healthcare systems to respond to changing patient needs and demand for healthcare. Spending constraints, for example, have contributed to declining levels of satisfaction with access to care in Canada (Blendon et al. 2002). While Canadians are still more satisfied than the US population with their healthcare (Schoen et al. 2010), these problems have prompted residents to register dissatisfaction with their healthcare system and call for fundamental reforms (Commonwealth Fund 2010). This initiative reflects a much different perspective from that which prevailed in the early 1990s, when Canada was the only developed country in which a majority of the population was satisfied with its healthcare system (Tuohy 2002).

Utilization Management

In contrast to other countries' systems, the US healthcare system has been characterized as micromanaged (Reinhardt 1990). It places emphasis on influencing the behavior of individual providers and patients with a mix of incentives and controls. Managed care plans use elaborate methods for utilization review, selecting contracts, setting capitated payment for providers, and developing practice guidelines. They influence patients' behavior through provider gatekeepers and control of referrals, copayments, coverage limits, restrictions on provider choice, and financial penalties for not complying with plan requirements, as well as provide information services to help consumers choose health plans and healthcare services. Targeted financial incentives for following best practices based on evidence-based guidelines have been used to improve the quality and efficiency of the care process (Bailit Health Purchasing, LLC, and Sixth Man Consulting, Inc. 2011; Strunk and Reschovsky 2002). Competition was introduced through an array of health plan choices for those with public or private insurance (Gabel, Lo Sasso, and Rice 2002).

Recent proposals recommend the development of ACOs to encourage performance measurement and shared-savings payment reform (Fisher et al.

2009). ACOs are provider organizations that are responsible for the total care of patients, including population health outcomes, patient care experiences, and cost per person. ACOs are yet to be fully defined in practice. The concept is similar to integrated managed care, except patients decide whether to use the ACO for their medical care. ACOs must therefore continuously strive to keep patients by providing good care and service. If ACOs keep costs below expected costs, the affiliated physicians and hospitals will share in the financial savings. Since patient choice is a key driver of the system, ACOs represent the use of market forces as opposed to direct regulation of provider behavior.

In macromanaged countries, the key to utilization management is limiting sources of payment and controlling the payment amounts. One example of macro strategy is regional planning to limit the number of healthcare facilities and ensure fair distribution of care, thereby setting constraints on provider practice. In such systems, patients often have to queue for expensive high-technology procedures and equipment, forcing physicians to allocate services according to the urgency of the cases.

Evidence regarding the success of market-maximized and market-minimized models is discussed in the section that follows.

Evidence of Efficiency

Allocative Efficiency

As indicated in Chapter 4, allocative efficiency is essentially concerned with maximizing health, given constrained resources. Three general health policy strategies concerning allocative efficiency were reviewed: investment in (1) healthcare versus non-healthcare services, (2) preventive versus primary versus tertiary services, and (3) alternative types of healthcare services, based on the health improvements they produce. The following sections present clinical-level evidence (derived from health production functions, cost-effectiveness analysis, and other methods) of these alternatives' potential to achieve allocative efficiency. Population-level evidence on the experiences of the United States and other countries is presented and compared to provide a sense of whether market-maximized or market-minimized models of health system design are more successful at achieving allocative efficiency.

Clinical Level
Healthcare Versus Other Investments
A basic conclusion of Chapter 3 was that the contribution personal healthcare makes to population health is modest compared to the influence of human biology, environment, and behavior. Thus, critics have long been concerned that modern, developed countries allocate too many resources to the delivery

of personal health services and too few to broader public health and social interventions at the population level (Fuchs 1974; McKeown 1990; Tarlov and St. Peter 2000).

Folland, Goodman, and Stano (2010) provide an overview of the contributions of healthcare and other health-related interventions to population health, grounded in the concept of a production function for health—that is, the relationship of health inputs to health outputs. They conclude that the production function for health tends to exhibit diminishing marginal returns, particularly in developed countries. For example, while initial investments in primary care may yield large improvements in the health of the population, subsequent investments in tertiary care may yield much smaller improvements, and therefore these resources might yield greater benefits if invested in other sectors, such as primary and secondary education. Historical declines in mortality rates may be most accurately attributed to improved environment and nutrition rather than to healthcare per se. Studies have demonstrated that healthcare's marginal contribution to reducing mortality in the United States does not differ significantly from zero, although it is greater for certain groups, such as the elderly.

Education, as measured by years of schooling, appears to be significantly related to health behaviors and population health (Cutler and Lleras-Muney 2010). This finding argues for a broader focus on other health-related interventions to serve the allocative efficiency, as well as the population effectiveness, objective. Countering this view is research suggesting that innovations in medical treatments for heart attacks, cataracts, depression, and low birth weight have been well worth the investment, as the aggregate dollar value of the benefits has greatly exceeded the aggregate cost (Cutler and McClellan 2001a). The bottom line is that health investment decision makers should allocate resources by considering the marginal expected returns per dollar of investment from healthcare and other areas of population health improvement.

Preventive Services

A Harvard study (Tengs et al. 1995) surveyed the literature on the cost-effectiveness of 587 lifesaving interventions in the United States. *Lifesaving intervention* was defined as any behavioral or technological strategy that reduces the probability of premature death among a specified population. Programs were categorized by sector (healthcare, residential, transportation, occupational, and environmental) and by three levels of prevention (primary, secondary, and tertiary). The 587 interventions ranged from those that save more resources than they consume to interventions that cost more than 10 billion dollars per year of life saved. Cost-effectiveness varied by sector. However, in medicine, primary prevention programs cost only $5,000 per life year saved, compared to about $23,000 for secondary and tertiary programs.

This research was a synthesis of existing studies, so it had significant methodological limitations. The validity of the conclusions was dependent on the accuracy of the data and analyses in the original studies. Due to publication bias, the studies were a nonrandom sample of lifesaving programs, and some benefits and effects were not measured (e.g., efforts to save the lives of some people may have reduced injuries in others, and environmental programs may improve the quality of life as well as save some lives). The study and the accumulating evidence on the cost-effectiveness of healthcare (Center for the Evaluation of Value and Risk in Health 2011) do, however, illustrate the potentially large variation within and between sectors and levels of prevention and, therefore, the potential efficiency gains associated with directing limited resources to programs that achieve the greatest health improvement per dollar of investment.

Economic evaluations of prevention-oriented interventions provide other important evidence to consider in resource allocation decisions. Mammography screening for early detection of breast cancer was underprescribed and underused prior to assessment of its health- and cost-effectiveness. Several studies in Europe and the United States showed that screening and early treatment yielded a cost per life year saved well below the norm of $50,000 per life year saved (De Koning 2000). Due in part to this economic evidence, Medicare began to cover mammography screening for Medicare beneficiaries of all ages. Important current issues are the declining use of mammography screening and underuse of health- and cost-effective colorectal cancer screening in the United States. Research is now focused on the health- and cost-effectiveness of behavioral interventions designed to increase compliance with breast and colorectal cancer screening guidelines (Holden et al. 2010; Lairson et al. 2008; Ramsey et al. 2009). Cost-effectiveness research is expected to grow in importance in response to provisions in the ACA that require insurers to cover and waive copayment for certain preventive services, an intervention deemed cost-effective by the US Preventive Services Task Force.

Mix or Types of Services

The RAND Health Insurance Experiment addressed the allocative efficiency of coinsurance in the context of the US healthcare system. The study examined the effect of copayments on utilization and expenditures for healthcare services and the effect of increases in utilization associated with "free" care on health status. The basic finding was that free care, compared to higher copayment levels, increased expenditures by 50 percent and had no significant effect on the health status of the "typical" person. Similarly, when RAND researchers compared expenditure, utilization, and outcomes among participants randomized into a staff model HMO with those randomized into free fee-for-service care, imputed expenditure was about 30 percent lower for the HMO, without health detriment. The HMO service mix is more conservative and oriented toward primary care, compared to the fee-for-service mix. A caveat to the RAND findings is that enrollees who were sick, poor, or both at the time of enrollment obtained significant health status benefits from increased utilization. Reducing the price of services for the typical consumer to a level lower than the cost of production results in consumption of services for which the marginal value is lower than the marginal cost of production. This scenario is the basic condition of resource misallocation—resources would provide more benefit if allocated elsewhere (Manning et al. 1987).

The RAND experiment established a baseline for the probable magnitude of inefficiencies in the US system and identified some areas for potential savings. For example, Siu and colleagues (1986) found that the introduction of cost sharing had an impact on both appropriate and inappropriate hospital admissions. The percentage of hospital admissions deemed inappropriate (22 percent) was only slightly lower than the proportion of inappropriate hospital admissions for free care (24 percent). This information suggests that significant portions of hospital admissions are inappropriate and potentially avoidable. A follow-up to the RAND studies by McGlynn and colleagues (2003) found that patients receive about half of the recommended care (both treatment and prevention) for their conditions.

These findings are consistent with the landmark research conducted by John Wennberg (2005), who developed the Dartmouth Atlas of Health Care to examine the variation in medical practice in the United States. Using national Medicare data in conjunction with population and healthcare resources information, he showed large variation in medical practice at both local and regional levels that cannot be explained by patient/disease characteristics (Skinner, Staiger, and Fisher 2006). Practitioners in areas that use the most resources may have worse outcomes than do practitioners in regions that practice more conservative and less costly medicine. These findings were instrumental in generating support for comparative effectiveness research and new systems of pay-for-performance provider reimbursement to support the use of evidence-based care (Cromwell et al. 2011).

Other industrialized countries have struggled with efficiency issues, although their solutions have differed from those in the United States. Comparison of US spending, utilization, coverage, and health outcomes with those of other democratic industrialized countries provides an important population-level perspective on the US healthcare system. Although observed differences may be a function of a variety of factors, they nonetheless pose questions, as well as point to answers, regarding ways in which present and future system performance might be improved (Cutler 2002; Rice et al. 2000).

Population Level

The 34 member countries of OECD (2010a) include democratic countries that range from economic powers, such as the United States, Germany, and Japan, to smaller countries with modest economic achievement, such as Greece and Portugal. Exhibit 5.1 provides data on public provision of health insurance coverage and payment for healthcare services in selected OECD countries. Until its market reforms in 1991, the United Kingdom represented the extreme of market minimization with its NHS; government ownership of hospitals; direct employment of hospital physicians, nurses, and allied health workers; and central budgetary control. The United States represents the extreme of market maximization, with mostly private hospitals and physicians and other health workers, numerous private for-profit and nonprofit insurance plans covering a majority of the population, and a plethora of private and public payers with little coordination or regulation of type or amount of payment. Between these two extremes, but leaning toward market minimization, are the Scandinavian countries and France. Countries leaning toward market mechanisms, although far left of the United States on the continuum, are Australia, Canada, Germany, Switzerland, and Japan. Less than one-third of the cost of inpatient and outpatient medical care is covered by public sources in the United States, whereas public coverage is universal or near-universal in the other countries.

Relative to the United States, the Canadian system has greater utilization of inpatient days and doctor consultations (see Exhibit 5.2). Germany has much higher inpatient utilization and doctor consultation rates than do Canada and the United States. Lower rates of utilization in the United States may reflect the out-of-pocket payments often required at the point of service, which traditionally have been the highest among the developed nations. Differences in average length of stay may reflect different policies regarding the use of hospitals for long-term and geriatric care in Germany and Canada (European Observatory on Health Care Systems 2002; Joumard, André, and Nicq 2010).

Compound annual per capita healthcare expenditure in these three countries increased from 7.8 percent to 9.8 percent between 1975 and 1990. The United States experienced the greatest growth, and Germany, the least. Since the early 1990s, growth in spending per capita has slowed from 5.6 percent to 4.3 percent per year. The order of the countries in terms of growth rates (computed from Exhibit 5.3) has remained unchanged. From 1990 to 2008, Canada and Germany more successfully controlled healthcare costs than did the United States in terms of per capita outlays, adjusted for purchasing power parity. Over this same period, the percentage of GDP spent on healthcare also grew much faster in the United States, suggesting the market-maximized US system is less effective at controlling healthcare costs (see Exhibit 5.3).

Country	Inpatient Hospital Care (%)	Outpatient Medical Care (%)
United Kingdom	100[a]	100[a]
Finland	100	100
Norway	100	100
Sweden	100	100
France	99.9	99.9
Australia	100	100
Canada	100	100
Germany	89.2[a]	89.2[a]
Switzerland	100[a]	100[a]
Japan	100[b]	100[b]
United States	26.4[a]	26.4[a]

EXHIBIT 5.1
Public Coverage Against Cost of Medical Care: Selected OECD Countries, 2010

[a]2009

[b]2008

Source: OECD (2012).

Differences in healthcare costs and population health outcomes reflect the differences in organization and utilization of services between the United States and other Western countries. Exhibit 5.4 compares seven of the major industrialized OECD member countries. With 17.4 percent of its GDP directed to health in 2009, the United States spent 5.6 percentage points more than the second-ranked country, France. The US per capita healthcare expenditure was $7,960 in 2009, about two times greater than that in France and Germany, about 1.8 times that in Canada, and 2.3 times more than that in the fifth-ranked country, the United Kingdom. This large expenditure gap apparently was not offset by health outcome advantages in the United States, which had the highest infant mortality and lowest life expectancy among the seven countries. Furthermore, the United States was the only country of the seven in which a significant percentage of the population lacked health insurance. (For a full discussion of the problem of high rates of uninsurance in the United States, see Chapter 7.)

EXHIBIT 5.2
Use of Inpatient Healthcare in Selected Countries, 1991–2009

Year	Bed Days in Inpatient Care (Number per Capita)			Acute Care Occupation Rate (Percentage of Available Beds)			Average Length of Stay in Acute Care (Days)			Doctor Consultations (Number per Capita)*		
	USA	Canada	Germany	USA	Canada	Germany	USA	Canada	Germany	USA	Canada	Germany
1991	0.9	1.4	2.3	66.1	78.6	84.0	7.2	10.0	12.8	—	6.9	5.3
1995	0.8	1.1	2.1	62.8	85.2	81.8	6.5	7.2	10.8	3.3	6.5	6.4
2000	0.7	1.0	1.9	63.9	91.2	81.5	5.8	7.2	9.2	3.7	6.3	7.2
2005	0.7	0.9	1.6	67.4	84.0	74.5	5.6	7.2	8.1	4.0	5.9	7.4
2007	0.6	0.9	1.6	66.6	89.0	76.0	5.5	7.5	7.8	4.0	5.6	7.4
2008	0.6	0.8	1.6	66.4	93.0	76.2	5.5	7.7	7.6	3.9	5.5	7.7
2009	0.6	—	1.6	65.5	—	76.2	5.4	—	7.5	—	—	8.2

*Doctor consultations are defined by the number of contacts with an ambulatory care physician divided by the population. Contacts in out-patient wards are included.

Source: OECD (2012).

	Percentage of GDP			Per Capita Outlays in US Dollars (PPP*)		
Year	USA	Canada	Germany	USA	Canada	Germany
1975	8.0	7.0	8.4	603	479	569
1980	9.0	7.0	8.4	1,101	777	967
1985	10.4	8.1	8.8	1,833	1,259	1,403
1990	12.4	8.9	8.3	2,850	1,735	1,764
1995	13.7	9.0	10.1	3,788	2,056	2,267
2000	13.7	8.8	10.3	4,793	2,519	2,669
2005	15.7	9.8	10.7	6,700	3,442	3,364
2009	17.4	11.4	11.6	7,960	4,363	4,218
2010	—	11.3	—	—	4,478	—

EXHIBIT 5.3
Healthcare Expenditures in the United States, Canada, and Germany, 1975–2010

*Purchasing power parity

Source: OECD (2012).

Allocation Efficiency Summary

Overall, then, the US health system, which represents the market-maximized end of the health policy continuum, appears to be faring poorly in comparison to other countries in terms of allocative efficiency—that is, maximizing health benefits in the aggregate relative to the magnitude of aggregate healthcare expenditures. This finding is reinforced by ongoing international surveys of patients and providers on quality of care, access to care, and efficiency of care. In 2008 the United States ranked seventh out of seven countries in overall performance while spending almost twice as much per person as Canada, the next highest-spending country (Davis, Schoen, and Stremikis 2010). In addition to concern about misallocating resources to services that provide low benefit relative to cost, there is concern in the United States and other countries that healthcare services of a given quality are not being produced at minimum cost; efficiency strategies can also be judged by this criterion. While least-cost production scales and methods are difficult to determine for medical services, several studies have produced evidence of inefficient production. This evidence is reviewed next.

EXHIBIT 5.4
Comparative Expenditures and Health Indicators for Seven Industrialized OECD Countries, 2009

Country	Total Expenditure on Health as Percentage of GDP	Total Expenditure on Health per Capita in US Dollars	Percentage of Population with Public Healthcare Coverage for Inpatient and Acute Care	Infant Mortality per 1,000 Live Births	Life Expectancy at Birth in Years	
					Male	Female
United States	17.4	7,960	26.4	6.5[b]	75.7	80.6
Canada	11.3[a]	4,478[a]	100[a]	5.1[c]	78.3[c]	83.0[c]
France	11.8	3,978	99.9[a]	3.7[a]	78.1[a]	84.8[a]
Germany	11.6	4,218	89.2	3.5	77.8	82.8
Italy	9.6[a]	3,236[a]	100	3.7	79.1[b]	84.5[b]
Japan	8.5[b]	2,878[b]	100[b]	2.4	79.6	86.4
United Kingdom	9.8	3,487	100	4.6	78.3	82.5

[a]2010
[b]2008
[c]2007

Source: OECD (2012).

Production Efficiency

Healthcare services can be provided in many ways by different combinations of personnel, facilities and equipment, production levels, and sites of service delivery. Production efficiency is achieved when production units are of optimal size and the mix of inputs is such that the marginal output per dollar of cost is equal across all inputs. Only then is the cost minimized for a given level of output of health services.

Economists and other health services researchers have conducted numerous studies of production efficiency, concentrating on (1) the administrative costs of health systems; (2) the number and mix of personnel in physician practices and physician payment methods; (3) the optimal number of beds for hospital care, the mix of inpatient and outpatient service delivery, and the effect of payment methods on hospital costs; and (4) the impact of managed care strategies and systems on utilization and cost. Evidence regarding each of these dimensions is reviewed in the discussion that follows.

Administration

It is extremely difficult to measure and compare administrative costs, and critics have argued that US costs are overestimated and comparisons between nations with fundamentally different healthcare systems are not possible (Aaron 2003; Gauthier et al. 1992). Systems that supply and finance care in the public sector, such as those in Canada and the United Kingdom, appear to have lower administrative costs. An estimate based on 1999 data placed such costs at 31.0 percent of healthcare costs in the United States versus 16.7 percent in Canada (Woolhandler, Campbell, and Himmelstein 2004). A 2007 study also showed that the United States and other market-oriented systems, such as those in Switzerland and Germany, have higher administrative costs (Joumard, André, and Nicq 2010). In Canada, administration is simplified by having one or few sources of payment and sets of rules. In market-minimized systems, global hospital budgets and fixed-fee schedules lessen the need to closely monitor provider behavior (Woolhandler, Campbell, and Himmelstein 2003), and costly activities associated with marketing are prohibited or severely restrained. Whether or not a country is able to make fundamental reforms, administrative costs are substantial and may yield ongoing savings if processes can be streamlined and information technologies applied (Bentley et al. 2008; Schoenbaum 2006). In the short term, the ACA is likely to increase administrative costs due to the complexity of the healthcare coverage law, the associated penalties for noncompliance, and the development and regulation of new health insurance exchanges. In the longer term, savings may accrue from electronic medical records and more integrated care generated from payment reform and the development of ACOs. However, whether these gains will be realized is highly uncertain (Eibner, Hussey, and Girosi 2010; Orszag and Emanuel 2010).

Physician Services
Personnel Mix
Studies employing different analytical approaches to achieving optimal use of physician aides have arrived at the same general conclusion: Physicians could raise the productivity of their practices and lower the cost per office visit by employing more aides (Brown 1988; Reinhardt 1975, 1972; Smith, Miller, and Golladay 1972). Adding a nonphysician provider, such as a nurse practitioner, to a managed care practice has been documented to increase a practice's pool of patients by 50 percent (Kindig 1996). Recent studies provide additional evidence on factors affecting physician productivity (Gunning and Sickles 2011; Sunshine et al. 2010). However, physicians practicing alone or in small groups have been reluctant to take on midlevel practitioners despite the potential for improved productivity. As physicians participate in larger groups run by organizations with administrative support and automated records, physicians can profitably hire midlevel practitioners (Kane 2009; Liebhaber and Grossman 2007). Requirements of healthcare reform for improved quality and efficiency coupled with new payment incentives are likely to encourage practices to employ nonphysicians with enhanced skills. For example, the incorporation of electronic medical records into medical practices will require staff or contract workers to have expertise in Internet technologies and the skills necessary to managing quality improvement initiatives.

Economies of Scale
Survivor analysis has also been used to test for economies of scale in physician practice (see Frech and Ginsburg 1974; Marder and Zuckerman 1985). In this type of analysis, the rate of growth in the number of practices of various sizes for a given period is used to judge which practice size is most efficient. The documented growth of large multispecialty group practice arrangements in the United States since the mid-1960s further attests to the production efficiency of this mode of practice (Havlicek 1996; Kane 2009). Medical practice and technology have changed dramatically during the last 30 years, permitting many more surgical and diagnostic services to be provided in the outpatient setting. Capital required to provide more sophisticated outpatient services can be financed and efficiently used in group practice settings. Studies of HMOs have also provided evidence of economies of scale in healthcare (Given 1996; Wholey et al. 1996). In addition to the production efficiencies of group practice, high practice start-up costs, greater competition in a period of growing supply and budget restraints, and national and state health policies that favor ACOs all point to continued growth in the number and size of group medical practices.

ACOs must serve at least 5,000 persons and must integrate care, including complex medical and financial information, across providers. These criteria favor groups that can take advantage of specialization of labor and potential economies of scale.

Physician Payment

The physician payment counterpart to the PPS for hospitals, the resource-based relative value scale, was intended to reduce the rate of increase in physician expenditures in the Medicare program (Sandy et al. 2009). There is some evidence that these policies initially reduced the rate of increase in physician costs and redistributed payments from procedural to primary care services. However, evidence indicates that fee-for-service payment, relative to salaries, increases the number of procedures performed, up to reimbursable levels (Helmchen and Lo Sasso 2010). To address persistent problems of low quality and inefficiency, payers are testing new systems of payment reform, such as pay for performance (P4P) (Cromwell et al. 2011; Fraser, Encinosa, and Baker 2010). These value-based payment systems provide financial incentives for physicians who meet prespecified quality and efficiency targets. Chung and colleagues (2010) assessed the effectiveness of physician-specific P4P among clinics in a multispecialty group practice. While well-established measures of performance improved, little difference was observed between the experimental and control group clinics. Another study found that P4P generated modest improvements in immunization rates for a Medicaid population in New York (Chien, Li, and Rosenthal 2010). With limited evidence of improvements in quality, efficiency, and cost control and skeptical physician groups, P4P in healthcare remains an unproven concept.

Total payments (program expenditure plus beneficiary cost sharing) for Medicare physician services reached $64 billion in 2009 (MedPAC 2010a). From 1997 to 2008, per beneficiary Medicare spending for physician services increased by 90 percent while the physician fee schedule updates totaled 17 percent, indicating that growth in volume of services greatly contributed to spending growth (Hahn 2010; MedPAC 2010a, 2010b). This growth persisted even with negative updates of payment values due to the Balanced Budget Act of 1997, which tied updates to growth in the national economy. The negative updates were not enough to offset the growth in services, so they did not solve the problem of cost growth. The administered price system does not control Medicare physician expenditures, and substantial misallocation of resources may result due to errors of measurement and other problems associated with attempting to set relative prices for more than 10,000 procedures (CMS 2012b; Newhouse 2002). Critics have argued that the price weights are frequently out of date and result in overpayments for procedures that now can be done less expensively. The proposed solution is more frequent reviews, better data on costs, and separation of payment update decisions from the physician specialties affected by the decisions (Reinhardt 2010). Cutler (2006) proposed changing to payment for health improvement rather than for services but acknowledged the difficulty of measuring improvement and the contribution that medical care made to the change in health.

Hospital Services
Economies of Scale

The average number of beds in community hospitals increased over the twentieth century, except for a decline from 172 in 1995 to 166 in 2007 (NCHS 2010). Considerable research has been conducted on the degree to which community hospitals are subject to economies of scale. The methods of hospital cost function analysis have also been somewhat crude because measures of input and output do not account for the complexity of hospital-based care (Berki 1972; Cowing, Holtmann, and Powers 1983). Nevertheless, Feldstein (1998) concluded that slight economies of scale were taking place and determined 200 to 300 beds to be the optimum size of a community hospital. Preyra and Pink (2006) provided evidence that hospitals in Ontario were not large enough to take advantage of economies of scale prior to consolidation in the hospital sector. Rigorous studies controlling for hospital differences and examining long-run cost functions raise questions about the existence of economies of scale and even suggest that large hospitals may be less efficient (Cuellar and Gertler 2005; Fournier and Mitchell 1992; Hansen and Zwanziger 1996; Vita 1990). Valdmanis, Rosko, and Mutter (2008) found that high- and medium-quality hospitals employed too many non-LPN and non-RN personnel and had too many bassinets. High-quality hospitals had too few LPNs, while medium-quality hospitals had too many. These factors had more influence on hospital efficiency than did scale, especially in public hospitals.

A more important issue for hospitals, and one that also raises the quality question, is determining the most efficient size of a given service or department (Getzen 2003; Grannemann, Brown, and Pauly 1986). Luft, Bunker, and Enthoven (1979) and Showstack and colleagues (1987) showed a positive relationship between volume of heart surgeries performed and outcomes. Katz and colleagues (2003, 2002) reported lower mortality and greater patient satisfaction among patients undergoing total hip replacement surgery in high-volume facilities with a large number of surgeons than in lower-volume facilities with fewer surgeons. Jacobs, Rapoport, and Edbrooke (2004) found an inverse association between cost per patient and unit size in intensive care. Several studies have found lower mortality among patients with acute respiratory disease in higher-volume ICUs (Durairaj et al. 2005; Glance et al. 2006; Kahn, Ten Have, and Iwashyna 2009; Kahn et al. 2006; Peelen et al. 2007).

These findings are consistent with a broad literature review of the volume–outcome relationship (IOM 2000). Halm, Lee, and Chassin (2002) found that volume had a positive effect on outcomes across a broad range of care, although results varied greatly and were subject to methodological limitations. The volume–outcome issue is related to the development of "focused factories"—specialty hospitals in the areas of cardiac care and orthopedics (Casalino and Robinson 2003). These hospitals are poised to take advantage of specialization-driven economies of scale and volume-based outcomes improvement. However, when a specialty hospital "creams" highly profitable procedures from community hospitals, the community hospitals may be forced to cut back the public's access to general medical care. Some studies found that specialty hospitals obtained better surgical procedure outcomes than did general hospitals within the same market area (Cram, Rosenthal, and Vaughan-Sarrazin 2005; Cram et al. 2007; Mitchell 2005).

Thus, in cases where higher service volume results in improved outcomes, services can be provided at a lower cost per unit and efficiency improves. Whether by regulation or market competition, such specialized services should be regionalized. Medicare, for example, instituted a program to regionalize heart surgery in "centers of excellence" (later renamed "quality partnerships"), and large, private-sector HMOs, such as Kaiser, traditionally have regionalized delivery of costly, infrequent procedures (Finks, Osborne, and Birkmeyer 2011).

Payment Methods

PPS was initially judged to have successfully contained hospital costs under Medicare without harming patients (Kahn et al. 1990; Russell 1989). However, one result of PPS was rapid expansion of outpatient hospital services, home care, and long-term care. Therefore, hospital cost containment strategies in the 1980s, including PPS, did not affect the underlying increase in healthcare costs in the United States, and reductions in the rate of growth in Medicare expenditures were offset by an increase in non-Medicare spending (Altman and Levitt 2002; Schwartz and Mendelson 1991). Hospital expenditure growth declined to 5.2 percent per annum in 2000 due to the growth of managed care in the 1990s but subsequently increased to 7.8 percent per annum in 2005 as managed care restrictions were relaxed. Following the economic recession, hospital expenditure growth declined to 4.5 percent per annum in 2008, although hospital expenditure growth was already declining in response to the imposition of higher deductibles and the effects of high-deductible health plans (Hartman et al. 2010).

Health Plans

While input mix and economies of scale are important issues, the extent of service use by the US population and the intensity of care provided are more important determinants of healthcare expenditures. These factors have been affected by significant changes in the financial and organizational structure of the healthcare system that have been induced by managed care and related market competition (Glied 2003). Evidence regarding the dynamics and impacts of managed care on state, national, and employer expenditure trends is reviewed in the following sections.

State and National Expenditures

Research suggests that managed care plans reduced the overall rate of growth in healthcare costs in the 1990s by inducing price competition and reducing utilization and costs (Gaskin and Hadley 1997). Other studies suggest that managed care may have lowered cost growth by also reducing the rate of technological diffusion (Baker 2001; Baker and Phibbs 2002) and by increasing production efficiency among tertiary hospitals (Brown III 2003).

Managed care played a leading role in abating cost growth in the heavily market-based US healthcare system (Levit, Lazenby, and Sivarajan 1996). While payers seemed to appreciate the value associated with managed care, consumers and providers did not (Christianson and Trude 2003). Their backlash against these constraints, coupled with a highly competitive labor market in the late 1990s, resulted in relaxation of "tightly" managed care (e.g., patients no longer needed a referral to see a specialist), consolidation of providers, and lower capitation payments for providers (Strunk and Reschovsky 2002). With the relaxation of managed care, the underlying forces of rapid technological development, high consumer expectations, and the aging population unleashed the forces of healthcare cost inflation again, causing national health expenditures to grow at a rate of 7.9 percent per annum in 2005 before declining to 4.4 percent during the recession year of 2008 (Hartman et al. 2010; Truffer et al. 2010). Policy, including provisions in the ACA, has since shifted toward new models, such as ACOs and patient-centered medical homes (PCMHs), that incorporate some aspects of traditional managed care organizations. They focus on primary care, utilize comprehensive electronic medical record information systems, offer indirect provider payment incentives for quality and efficiency, emphasize coordination of care, and take responsibility for the quality and cost of patients' care (Kilo and Wasson 2010; McClellan et al. 2010; Patient-Centered Primary Care Collaborative 2007). One important difference of the ACO/PCMH model is free choice: Patients are not locked into a provider organization, and therefore practices must continually work to keep clients satisfied so they return for needed care in the future. Results from a study of members of the Council of Accountable Physician Practices show these models have positive, if modest, effects on the cost and quality of care for Medicare beneficiaries (Weeks et al. 2010). PCMHs have also been successful in demonstration projects in several places in the United States. By employing dedicated care managers, improving access to care, using data-driven analytic tools, and offering financial incentives, practices have reduced the number of hospitalizations and emergency department visits and the cost of care (Fields, Leshen, and Patel 2010).

Employer Expenditures

Large employers (200 employees or more) slowed the growth of healthcare costs via a managed care and competition strategy during the late 1980s and early 1990s. After the annual percentage growth in employment-based insurance premiums reached nearly 20 percent between 1988 and 1990, the growth rate declined to 0.5 percent in 1996. Following two years of low growth (about 2 to 3 percent), the rate reaccelerated to 13 percent growth in 2002 and 2003 due to the relaxation of managed care. The rate then decelerated again to 3 percent during a period of weak economic growth in 2009. Average annual employment-based insurance premiums reached $13,700 in 2010 (Claxton et al. 2010; Kaiser Family Foundation 2010b; Strunk, Ginsburg, and Gabel 2002).

Production Efficiency Summary

The growth in managed care and competition during the 1990s dramatically altered economic incentives in healthcare. Providers were forced to consider adopting more efficient means of production, reducing prices, and changing their service mix to meet consumer and payer demand. Physician practices modified their personnel mix and scale for greater efficiency; the average size of hospitals increased; and expensive, complex services were regionalized. These changes reduced the rate of cost growth in the mid-1990s. When these trends reversed at the beginning of the new millennium due to the factors discussed in the previous section, the initial reaction was to increase copayments and establish consumer-driven health plans with reimbursement accounts (Gabel, Lo Sasso, and Rice 2002; Robinson 2002). Despite the shift away from tightly managed care, the United States still lags several developed countries with regard to healthcare access, quality, and cost (Davis, Schoen, and Stremikis 2010). These shortcomings motivated the ACA healthcare reform legislation.

Other democratic developed countries appear to be more successful at controlling spending, insuring their populations, and achieving health outcomes. Whether they are truly more efficient is impossible to determine from aggregate data. Even so, attaining cost control and access goals are important social achievements. HSR can play a significant role in US reform by documenting whether the emerging changes in healthcare organization and payment improve the performance of the US healthcare system with regard to these goals.

Criteria for Assessing Policy Alternatives' Ability to Achieve Efficiency Goals

Policymakers strive to design a mix of incentives and controls that will motivate consumers and their physicians to choose efficient amounts and types of health services and encourage providers to adopt efficient practices to deliver those services.

When evaluating policies or programs addressing efficiency concerns, analysts can apply several criteria (see Exhibit 5.5). These criteria are relevant to both population and clinical levels of analysis and concern both allocation and production issues. First, states and nations are concerned about spending an appropriate fraction of gross domestic (or state) product on the healthcare sector. Given the lack of an objective method for determining the allocation of resources that maximizes the well-being of the population, appropriate allocation is a political judgment. For many nations, a guiding principle is that healthcare spending should not increase faster than the rate of growth in national income or wages. This criterion reflects a judgment about the health needs of the population and the effectiveness of additional spending on health services—that is, greater spending on healthcare is not in the best interest of society. Judgment regarding the appropriate share of income to spend on healthcare differs by nation/state and over time, depending on current political and economic circumstances. Spending on any service, such as mammography, depends on health returns per dollar of investment relative to returns from investment in other services.

Second, to achieve allocative efficiency, providers must offer a mix of health services that maximizes positive health outcomes and consumer satisfaction to the greatest degree possible with the share of resources available to be expended on those services. A judgment must be made concerning the existing allocation of resources and whether it should be altered to obtain greater health and well-being for society. The evidence reviewed earlier on the allocative efficiency of the US healthcare system, for example, suggested that it suffers from overinvestment in secondary and tertiary treatment and underinvestment in population health–oriented disease prevention, health promotion, and health protection strategies, relative to the observed, as well as to the likely, health return on these investments. Given that mammography screening is cost-effective and that at least 30 percent of women do not meet recommended guidelines for regular screening (National Cancer Institute 2010), shifting more resources toward screening and away from less cost-effective services may improve allocative efficiency.

Third, production costs for health services should be minimized in the interest of production efficiency. The output of the production process should consider the health of the individuals receiving care, their satisfaction with the method of service delivery, and any health consequences to others who may be indirectly affected by health programs (Joumard, André, and Nicq 2010). Costs should include the direct cost of services plus indirect time costs incurred by participants and other affected parties. Service quality and cost should therefore be compared to those of benchmark organizations deemed to be the most efficient producers of the services in question.

EXHIBIT 5.5
Criteria for Assessing Health Policies' Ability to Achieve Efficiency Goals

Dimensions	Goals	Criteria	Examples
Macro cost control	Spend an appropriate fraction of gross state product on the health sector.	Health spending should not increase faster than the rate of growth in income in the state.	This criterion relates to aggregate spending on healthcare and is therefore not relevant to investments in any particular area of healthcare.
Allocative efficiency	Ensure a mix of health services that maximizes health outcomes and consumer satisfaction to the greatest degree possible with the share of resources available to be spent on health services.	A majority of new health spending should be directed to cost-effective treatments, disease prevention, health promotion, and improvement in the social and physical environments for persons likely to achieve the greatest gains.	The majority of new spending for breast cancer is allocated to basic biomedical research and clinical treatment rather than to breast cancer screening, environmental determinants research, and related interventions.
Production efficiency	Produce health services at a minimum cost.	Produce services at a cost at or below nationally recognized benchmarks of cost per unit of service.	Various types of mammography screening reminder systems (e.g., general patient reminders, tailored patient reminders, provider reminders, joint patient–provider reminders) have yielded different results in terms of increases in the number of screenings relative to costs.
Dynamic efficiency	Search for technological and organizational advances that raise the productivity of given resources.	Encourage research and development of new health services and efficient ways to organize and deliver them.	Significant research is under way to develop and test new technologies for early detection of breast cancer.*

*See, for example, Flobbe et al. (2003) and National Research Council (2001).

There are effectiveness (Vernon et al. 2010) and efficiency studies (Fishman et al. 2000; Saywell Jr. et al. 1999) and related recommendations for the most cost-effective methods of achieving the recommended mammography screening rates among alternative populations of women.

A number of organizations have developed standards of performance, measured performance on the basis of those standards, and provided their results to healthcare providers (Cleverly 1997; Solucient LLC 2004) and health plans (NCQA 2010). For example, the Healthcare Effectiveness Data and Information Set (HEDIS) was developed by the National Committee on Quality Assurance primarily for employers that needed performance information to be able to select health insurance for their employees from among competing managed health plans. The HEDIS instrument was subsequently adapted for use by the Medicaid program. It covers effectiveness of care, availability, satisfaction with care, cost of care, use of services, and plan-descriptive information. HEDIS tracks mammography screening rates for women aged 40 to 69. In 2009, the mean screening rate among women covered by commercial health plans was 71.3 percent, compared to 69.3 percent among Medicare beneficiaries and 52.4 percent among Medicaid beneficiaries (NCQA 2011).

Finally, providers should search for technological and organizational advances that raise the productivity of given resources (i.e., dynamic efficiency). Policies should therefore encourage development of and experimentation with new services and with more efficient ways of organizing and delivering services, such as mammography screening for early detection of breast cancer (IOM 2001; Rijnsburger et al. 2009).

Summary and Conclusions

Three major questions are addressed in this chapter: (1) What are potential policy strategies for achieving efficiency? (2) What is the evidence regarding the effectiveness of strategies aimed at increasing efficiency? and (3) What criteria should be used to judge the success of these strategies?

In response to the first question, national health systems can be positioned on a continuum ranging from market-maximized systems based on consumer demand to market-minimized systems based on government-determined need. The former is characterized by consumer choice of providers and services, voluntary private insurance coverage, numerous private and public payers and types of payment, high out-of-pocket payment, the private practice of medicine, and the private ownership of healthcare facilities, many of which are operated on a for-profit basis. The interaction of supply and demand forces in a market context, however imperfect, guides the allocation of resources for healthcare and non-healthcare services and between health services and other sectors. Market-minimized systems are characterized by services based on public need, universal and public coverage, relatively few sources of payment, low out-of-pocket payments, public practice of medicine or public control of private practice, and public ownership or control of healthcare facilities operated on a not-for-profit basis. Professional and bureaucratic determinations of need and control of supply guide the allocation of resources to and within the healthcare sector. Countries are becoming difficult to categorize because an increasing number are mixing market elements with command-and-control regulations (Joumard, André, and Nicq 2010).

Until recently, the United States eschewed the market-minimizing, macro-control approach (i.e., direct government and community control) that has led to more stable levels of health spending as a percentage of GDP in Canada and Western Europe (European Observatory on Health Care Systems 2002). Considerable evidence exists that the US system fails to achieve maximum value from the resources allocated to healthcare and that it performs less well than many other developed countries' systems. Indicators include evidence on variability in the use of services; a lack of evidence-based best practices (IOM 2001); substantial underinvestment in selected preventive services, including prenatal care; a focus on costly procedure-oriented care that may add little to health at the margin; high rates of spending; and data showing poorer health outcomes among the US population than among other countries (Schoen et al. 2010).

Additionally, numerous studies have documented that hospital, physician, and insurance services are not produced in the most efficient manner in the United States, and comparative data suggest that prices and associated incomes are set higher than necessary to attract resources to healthcare. Evidence includes excess capacity, a lack of attention to personnel mix, limited investment in information technology, and failure to take advantage of potential economies of scale.

The ACA includes both market and regulatory measures for reforming the US health system. Time will tell whether the overall balance will shift toward market-minimizing strategies. The legislation will increase regulation of private insurance, mandate individuals to obtain health insurance coverage, create insurance exchanges to facilitate choice and competition among health plans, and implement new P4P/shared-savings payment methods designed to increase quality and efficiency. The ACA takes a macro approach to increasing access to health insurance via a federal coverage mandate but will continue to test micro market–oriented methods to redesign healthcare delivery systems for increased quality and efficiency. Cost control achieved through the macro approach does not necessarily translate directly into efficiency, but micro incentives have yet to demonstrate long-term cost control, so whether allocative efficiency can be achieved is uncertain.

By examining data comparing the health investment experiences of different countries, US policymakers perhaps can discern new answers to the troubling question of how best to improve the efficiency of the US health system. This effort can begin with a study of alternative models that have been used on a state, regional, or national basis and development of a program to measure their effects on population health costs (Joumard, André, and Nicq 2010; Roos et al. 1999, 1996). Health services researchers and policy analysts can contribute to the fund of knowledge by assessing ways in which other countries have dealt with (1) the role of environmental, social, behavioral, and medical determinants of health in the formulation of health policies; (2) the design of population-oriented data systems directed toward assessing these policies; and (3) the extent to which the effectiveness, efficiency, and equity objectives of health policy have been or are likely to be achieved.

EQUITY: CONCEPTS AND METHODS

6

Chapter Highlights

1. Equity is concerned with maximizing fairness in the distribution of healthcare services (procedural equity) and minimizing disparities in health (substantive equity).
2. Assessments of equity can be based on the distributive, deliberative, or social justice paradigms. The distributive justice paradigm focuses on individuals' rights to healthcare, the social justice paradigm addresses the healthcare and non-healthcare determinants of the health of populations, and the deliberative justice paradigm attempts to balance conflicts between these two perspectives by ensuring full participation of affected parties at all levels of decision making.
3. The principal equity criteria applied from each of these perspectives are distributive justice—freedom of choice and cost-effectiveness of healthcare services; social justice—similar treatment, common good, and need across populations; and deliberative justice—participation of affected parties in decision making.
4. Equity analyses entail gathering data on indicators of each of these criteria and conducting descriptive, analytic, and/or evaluative research to assess the performance or impact of healthcare services, systems, and policies.

Overview

The fundamental questions posed in this chapter are: (1) What is equity in healthcare delivery? and (2) How should equity be assessed? Chapter 7 asks a third question: To what extent has equity been achieved? Provisions in the ACA would substantially reduce the number of uninsured Americans, primarily working-age adults. The ACA also addresses concerns about coverage exclusions and limitations pertaining to particularly high-risk groups. It is hoped that these coverage extensions will help ameliorate disparities in health and in healthcare access and use. However, the extended implementation period for the ACA leaves much uncertainty regarding how, or even whether, provisions will be put into practice. Thus, the health insurance reform debate in the United States continues to accentuate concerns about equity in access to healthcare.

A variety of approaches have been developed and applied in HSR and policy analysis to assess equity. They have focused primarily on potential or realized barriers to accessing healthcare, the extent to which subgroup variations exist in the utilization of healthcare services relative to need, and the conceptual foundations of distributive justice and the associated rights of individuals required to ensure equity (Aday et al. 1993; Aday and Andersen 1981). Many of these conceptualizations, however, have failed to encompass the weight of the empirical evidence regarding the limited role of healthcare relative to other inputs or sectors for improving health and the corollary concerns with the common good and health of populations and communities. They also have failed to acknowledge or accommodate philosophical criticisms of the distributive justice framework and the associated framework of individuals' rights as a basis for judgments of equity, as well as criticisms of the fairness of the deliberative processes and procedures in policy debates on the allocation of public and private resources.

An implicit assumption underlying the perspective on equity presented in this chapter is that the conventional lenses for viewing equity have failed to pinpoint the origins of, or envision other promising remedies for, the persistent health and healthcare inequalities in the United States. An explicit aim is to provide a broader and deeper vision of the foundations of fairness undergirding the formulation and evaluation of health policy. The following discussion presents alternative paradigms, or defining frameworks, of justice and their implications for conceptualizing and measuring equity to address the questions posed at the beginning of this chapter.

Conceptual Framework and Definitions

Contrasting Paradigms of Justice

Three primary philosophical traditions, grounded in different paradigms of justice, can be used to illuminate the correlates and indicators of equity in health and in healthcare: **distributive justice**, **deliberative justice**, and **social justice** (see Exhibit 6.1). These paradigms focus, respectively, on individuals, institutions, and the community (Daly 1994; Habermas 1996; Kolm 1996; Mulhall and Swift 1996). The major theories underlying these different paradigms are summarized in Exhibit 6.3 and discussed later in this chapter.

	Paradigm			EXHIBIT 6.1
	Distributive Justice	Deliberative Justice	Social Justice	
Focus	Individuals	Institutions	Community	
Theory	Liberalism* • Libertarian • Utilitarian • Contractarian	Deliberative Democracy • Discourse	Communitarianism • Community • Egalitarian • Need-based	
Principles	• Personal well-being • Individual freedom	• Public governance • Popular sovereignty	• Common good • Social solidarity	
Issues	What can **I** justly **claim**?	**Who decides,** and **how**?	What is **good** for **us**?	
Policies	Minimalist state: Individuals' rights	Responsive state: Civic participation	Responsible state: Public welfare	
Strengths	• Promotes individual freedom • Protects personal privacy • Applies universal norms	Balances the strengths and weaknesses of distributive and social justice paradigms through rational public discourse (participation and empowerment)	• Promotes social responsibility • Protects public good • Applies community norms	
Weaknesses	• Diminishes the social • Sacrifices public for private • Promotes self-centeredness • Blames the victim	Great variability in the actual implementation of the principles of deliberative democracy at both macro and micro levels	• Diminishes the individual • Sacrifices private for public • Promotes dependency • Encourages paternalism	

EXHIBIT 6.1
Contrasting
Paradigms of
Justice

*Liberalism as the theory base for the distributive justice paradigm is distinct from Liberalism in the modern US political context.

The distinctions between the individual and community perspectives are most deeply lodged in the debate between liberal and communitarian values. The liberal political tradition focuses on the norms of personal well-being and individual freedom. Policies grounded in this tradition have been concerned with protecting or ensuring individuals' rights and its underlying distributive justice paradigm. In this paradigm, rights are benefits to which one has a claim based on what constitutes a fair distribution of benefits and burdens. This perspective considers both negative and positive rights—that is, noninterference and freedom of choice—as well as positive conferment of specific material or nonmaterial benefits. The question of equity posed from this point of view is: What can I justly claim?

This framework argues for minimizing state interference in the organization and delivery of healthcare and maximizing freedom of choice and individuals' rights. This perspective has played a prominent role in policy debates regarding health insurance reform, Medicaid and Medicare reform, and the impact of immigration and welfare reform (Callahan 2001; d'Oronzio 2001; Hanson and Callahan 2001; Office of the Legislative Counsel 2010). The escalating costs of healthcare, the debate over universal healthcare reform at the national level, and the dominance of managed care in both the public and the private sector have raised significant questions regarding to whom and to what extent benefits of coverage might be extended as well as how corresponding costs should be allocated. Increased emphasis is being placed on consumer choice, personal responsibility, experience rating, actuarial fairness, and minimizing the impact of free riders.

Communitarian sentiments are based on norms of common good, social solidarity, and protection of public welfare (Daly 1994; Etzioni 2003a, 2003b, 2000a, 2000b, 1999, 1998). The concept of justice on which this perspective is based is concerned with the underlying social, economic, and environmental underpinnings of inequity. Rather than focusing on conferring or ensuring positive or negative rights or benefits to individuals, this paradigm more broadly considers public health and the social and economic interventions required to enhance the well-being of groups or communities. The question of justice posed from this perspective is: What is good for us?

The social justice paradigm is reflected in traditional public health policy and practice, which emphasizes public welfare and the use of medical police power (e.g., public health regulations, inspections, quarantines) to protect the population's health (Anderson et al. 2009; Beauchamp 1998, 1988, 1985, 1976; Beauchamp and Steinbock 1999; Blacksher and Lovasi 2012; Daniels 2001; Garcia and Fenwick 2009; Perez and Martinez 2008; Powers and Faden 2006). Critics have argued, however, that public health planning and practice have historically focused less on what communities may view as good for them and more on what public health professionals determine communities need on the basis of agency- or administration-driven data-gathering or needs assessment activities (Kretzmann and McKnight 1993; Morgan 2001; Morgan and Ziglio 2007; Robertson and Minkler 1994). In many communities the consequence is that the social, economic, and environmental issues that determine the health of the public are not adequately addressed, and the capacities of affected populations to ameliorate them are untapped or, at worst, undermined.

The distributive and social justice paradigms offer contrasting and complementary strengths as foundations for judging justice. The distributive justice paradigm promotes individual freedom and autonomy, protects personal privacy, and applies nondiscriminatory universal norms to identify basic human rights. On the other hand, the social justice paradigm promotes a balance of social responsibility and protection of the public good and applies community-centered norms and values to formulate program and policy priorities. Both paradigms are central to the healthcare reform debate in the United States, in which considerations of autonomy and individual responsibility often conflict with the goal of achieving the greatest benefit for the broadest spectrum of society at an acceptable cost.

Criticisms of the distributive justice paradigm as applied to healthcare and of the social justice model underlying public health mirror the criticisms that have been raised about liberal and communitarian theories (Daly 1994; Habermas 1996; Mulhall and Swift 1996). It is argued that the dominance of the liberal paradigm in shaping health and social policy in the United States has weakened social and communal sentiments, such as civility and reciprocity; sacrificed considerations of the public good to serve private interests; promoted self-centeredness; and blamed the victim for circumstances that may well have been created by society or others. On the other hand, communitarianism is charged with weakening individual autonomy; sacrificing the ability of the public to make rational, informed choices due to the increasing bureaucratization of what are judged to be paternalistic public institutions; and shifting individuals served by institutions into the role of dependent clients. The tension between these perspectives has helped to shape the healthcare policy debate in the United States for more than 75 years, dating at least to the debate surrounding whether or not to incorporate a national policy for health insurance in the original Social Security legislation (Ball 1995).

Contemporary social theorists, most notably German philosopher Jürgen Habermas, have addressed the weaknesses of the liberal and communitarian traditions by arguing for a new synthesis of the foundations for fairness, based on a theory of deliberative democracy (Habermas 2002, 1996, 1995; Habermas and Fultner 2003). Policies attuned to this perspective address the extent to which norms of civic participation appear to guide decision making. The question of justice posed from this point of view is: Who decides, and how? The foundation for the enlargement of deliberative justice is the growth and promotion of a public sphere of secondary associations, social movements, and civil and political forums for influencing the formal policy-making process. The deliberative justice paradigm recognizes and attempts to resolve conflicts rooted in the other dominant paradigms of fairness through rational discourse on the part of affected groups and individuals. Such discourse is oriented primarily toward mutual understanding. Habermas argues that strategic or technical-rational aims of decision makers at either the macro or the micro level (e.g., implementing a state Medicaid managed care program or achieving patient adherence to therapeutic regimens) are unlikely to be orchestrated and achieved unless affected stakeholders (e.g., providers, patients, taxpayers) have the opportunity to present and have their points of view heard and respected in the process.

A central criticism of the deliberative justice paradigm, however, is that it has been variably implemented in practice. Participation ranges along a continuum from relatively passive, consultative input on the part of patients and affected populations to a dominant, determining role in decision making at either the micro or the macro level. Evidence suggests that fuller participation of patients in decision making about their healthcare has a positive impact (Goss and Renzi 2007; Greenfield, Kaplan, and Ware Jr. 1985; Guadagnoli and Ward 1998; Kaplan et al. 1995; Loh et al. 2007; Marincowitz 2004). However, the impact of public participation in health policy decisions affecting it in terms of health and well-being is not yet confirmed (Boyce 2001; Crawford et al. 2002; Gong et al. 2009; Hubbard et al. 2007; Israel et al. 2010; Minkler 2010; Minkler and Wallerstein 2003; Morgan 2001; Rea 2004; Tomes 2006; Wagner et al. 2000; Zakus and Lysack 1998).

The discussion that follows presents a framework of equity, incorporating elements of the deliberative, distributive, and social justice paradigms and the relationships implied among them as a foundation for guiding HSR on the equity of healthcare provision. The framework attempts to acknowledge and integrate the complementary strengths of each of the paradigms.

A Conceptual Framework of Equity

Exhibit 1.5 in Chapter 1 shows how the conceptual framework for guiding HSR and policy analysis might reflect and integrate the deliberative, distributive, and social justice paradigms. The unshaded boxes represent a conceptual model of equity of access to healthcare developed by Lu Ann Aday, Ronald Andersen, and Gretchen Voorhis Fleming to guide the conduct of national and community surveys of access; this method is rooted in the distributive justice paradigm (Aday, Andersen, and Fleming 1980; Aday and Andersen 1981). The shaded boxes represent components that are reflective of the broader social justice paradigm, grounded in research on the social-structural factors that influence the health and healthcare needs of vulnerable populations (Aday and Andersen 1981; Beauchamp 1998, 1988, 1985, 1976;

Beauchamp and Steinbock 1999; Franzini et al. 2009; Lo and Fulda 2008; Mansyur et al. 2009, 2008; Plowden and Young 2003).

At the topmost level of the original access framework is the influence of health policy on the characteristics of the health delivery system and the population served by it. A dimension in the expanded model (Exhibit 6.2) is the deliberative justice characteristic of health policy that focuses on the institutions and procedures through which policy is formulated and implemented. Placing the governing norm of deliberative justice above health policy in the expanded framework is intended to convey that conflicts between the disparate paradigms of distributive justice and social justice that have tended to guide healthcare and public health policy, respectively, must be effectively addressed if the health and well-being of individuals and communities are to be enhanced. This objective can be achieved by ensuring that those most affected by health policy decisions at both macro and micro levels are involved in shaping them. The deliberative paradigm has not been fully explored as a basis for the equity of health policy. It is, however, implicit in the focus on consumer involvement and community participation in the design and implementation of private and public health programs in the United States and other countries (Minkler 1997; Minkler and Wallerstein 2003).

The unshaded boxes in Exhibit 6.2, which encompasses the delivery system, population at risk, and realized access, define the major distributive justice components of the conceptual framework that has guided much of HSR on access to healthcare (Aday, Andersen, and Fleming 1980; Aday and Andersen 1981). Relevant characteristics of the health system include the availability, organization, and financing of services. *Predisposing characteristics* of the population at risk include those that describe the propensity of individuals to use services, including basic demographic characteristics (e.g., age, gender), social-structural variables (e.g., race and ethnicity, education, employment status, occupation), and beliefs (e.g., general beliefs and attitudes about the value of health services). *Enabling characteristics* include individuals' means of accessing and using services. Individual resources, such as family income or insurance coverage; knowledge of disease or the healthcare system; and organizational resources specific to individuals and their families, such as having a regular source or place to go for care, are examples of such means. *Need* refers to health status or illness as a predictor of health service use. The need for care may be perceived by the individual and reflected in reported disability days or symptoms, for example, or may be evaluated by a provider and reflected in actual diagnoses or complaints.

Realized access refers to the objective and subjective indicators of the actual process of seeking care. The indicators reflect the extent to which the system and population characteristics predict the demand for care (i.e.,

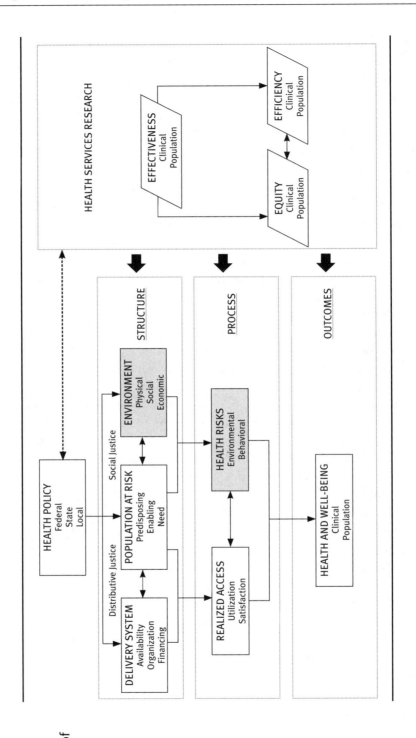

EXHIBIT 6.2
Conceptual
Framework of
Equity

healthcare utilization) and how satisfied potential or actual consumers are with the healthcare system.

As indicated by the shaded boxes in Exhibit 6.2, the social justice component of the model explicitly acknowledges the ultimate outcome of interest that was implicit or assumed in the original model: the health and well-being of individuals and communities. The model acknowledges that the physical, social, and economic environment in which individuals live and work also can influence their access to health and healthcare. The model indicates that the environment directly influences the likelihood of exposure to significant environmental and behavioral health risks (Franzini et al. 2010).

The social justice component of the model may be viewed as focusing on the community level of analysis. It primarily examines the characteristics of the physical, social, and economic environment; the population residing within it; and the health risks the population experiences as a consequence. The distributive justice component of the model relies on individuals as the ultimate unit of analysis. Their attributes and behavior may, however, be aggregated to reflect the characteristics of patients in a given health system or delivery organization or of the population residing in a designated geographic area. The distributive justice paradigm emphasizes the equity of the healthcare delivery system, while the social justice paradigm is reflected in public health and in social and economic policies directly or indirectly related to health.

The goal of health policy, as indicated in the expanded equity framework, is to improve the health of individuals and communities. The ultimate test of the equity of health policy from the social justice perspective is the extent to which disparities or inequalities in health among subgroups of the population are minimized (Lurie 2002). *Substantive equity* is reflected in subgroup disparities in health. *Procedural equity* refers to the extent to which the structure, process, or procedures intended to reduce these disparities are fair according to norms of deliberative, distributive, and social justice. The normative import of these procedural factors for substantive equity can be empirically judged by the extent to which these factors are predictive of inequalities in health across groups and communities. The equity framework (Exhibit 6.2) is intended to provide normative and empirical guidance for assessing both substantive and procedural equity.

Based on the synthesis and integration of the theoretical underpinnings of substantive and procedural equity reviewed here, the answer to the first question posed at the beginning of this chapter—what is equity in healthcare delivery?—may be summarized as follows: Equity is concerned with health disparities and the fairness and effectiveness of the procedures for addressing them. The response to the second question—how should equity in healthcare be assessed?—is: by examining and accounting for health disparities.

The effectiveness of medical and nonmedical investments at producing health is essentially an empirical question. The fairness of the means for doing so is a normative one. The expanded framework, however, implies that health policymaking must take into account norms of distributive and social justice and that conflicts between affected stakeholders grounded in these contrasting norms must be resolved through deliberative discourse if the resultant policies are ultimately to contribute to improving health and minimizing health disparities.

Key Methods of Assessing Equity

Conceptual Frameworks

Conceptual frameworks provide useful analytic guidance for selecting empirical indicators and generating hypotheses about interrelationships between them. The framework Aday and Andersen (1981) developed for the study of access has guided a great deal of research on equity and on HSR in general. Integral to that framework is the value judgment that the system would be deemed fair or equitable if need-based criteria, rather than resources such as insurance coverage or income, were the main determinants of the amount of care utilized. Aday and Andersen, as well as others, have extended this framework to encompass social and environmental aspects and access to healthcare as factors that ultimately influence health and to acknowledge the interdependence of the equity, effectiveness, and efficiency norms in assessing the performance of health policies and programs (Aday 2001; Andersen 1995; Andersen and Davidson 2001; Basu et al. 2010; Bradley et al. 2002; DuPlessis, Inkelas, and Halfon 1998; Gelberg, Andersen, and Leake 2000; Jones, Heflinger, and Saunders 2007; Lurie 2002; Phillips et al. 1998; Guo, Wang, and Yan 2002).

Other useful frameworks have been developed to explore the distributive, social, and deliberative justice paradigms in the context of the growth of managed care, including accountable care organizations (ACOs) (CMS 2010b). In general, frameworks grounded in the distributive justice paradigm may be seen as primarily turning inward, assessing the fairness of the healthcare system for the patients directly served by the system. Social justice–oriented frameworks direct attention outward to assess the equity of health and health risks of the population residing in a community. And as stated earlier, conceptual approaches to equity influenced by the deliberative justice paradigm attempt to develop more effective health policies by enhancing the dialogue between those who design and those who are affected by them. These frameworks, their relationship to the expanded framework of equity (Exhibit 6.2), and the defining focus of each are reviewed in the discussion that follows.

Distributive Justice

Docteur, Colby, and Gold (1996) developed an access framework that identifies a variety of components that are relevant in terms of influencing and assessing managed care enrollees' access to services. The framework includes the structural, financial, and personal determinants of patients' health plan selection; the associated characteristics of the health plan delivery system itself; the influence of these patient and plan characteristics on use of services; the mediators and determinants of the continuity of plan enrollment; and the ultimate clinical and equity outcomes for enrollees and users. Many of the factors that influence plan selection also affect access to care under the selected plan. For example, the factors affecting selection of the Medicare Advantage program (Medicare Part C) or the Medicare Prescription Drug program (Medicare Part D) may also affect access to care under that plan. This framework, then, focuses the lens of distributive justice on the availability, organization, and financing of services under a particular health plan delivery system and the utilization and satisfaction of individuals and families who choose to enroll in it.

Social Justice

A growing body of research documents the influence of fundamental social and economic factors on health and the accompanying need for integrative analytic frameworks to guide more innovative health-centered social and economic policy development (Aday 2005; Albrecht, Freeman, and Higginbotham 1998; Graham 2002; Israel et al. 1998; Link and Phelan 1995; Marmot et al. 2008; Minkler 2010; Spitler 2001; Ward et al. 2011). Aday's (2001) framework for the study of vulnerable populations delineates the social and economic factors that determine health risks and argues for community and individual levels of analyses to explore the correlates of vulnerability to poor health. Her perspective argues for the development of a broader continuum of health services encompassing prevention-oriented services, long-term community-based services, and acute healthcare services (displayed in Chapter 1, Exhibit 1.1) to address the health and healthcare needs of the most vulnerable. The *Healthy People* 2020 objectives, the World Health Organization's "Health for All" database, and accompanying empirical and programmatic emphases also provide guidance for identifying and tracking the indicators and predictors of subgroup disparities in health (NCHS 2010; WHO 2008). Stephen Shortell and colleagues (2000b, 1994) have argued convincingly for the importance of a population health–oriented perspective in designing and assessing organized (i.e., integrated) healthcare delivery systems. However, the de facto implementation of a population health perspective in emerging systems of care varies widely (Kindig and Stoddart 2003). The social justice focus on the health of populations and, by extension, the integrated array of programs and services needed to address the health needs of the most vulnerable provide conceptual and analytic guidance for assessing the extent to which the health of communities as a whole is enhanced in the evolving managed care environment. These issues are discussed in the context of the criteria for assessing the effectiveness of healthcare in Chapter 3.

Deliberative Justice

Community participation and empowerment have ostensibly been central components of the design of social and health programs in the United States as well as in other countries. In many cases, however, the individuals affected by these initiatives have not been fully involved in shaping them. Public health and health promotion professionals are widely criticized for imposing interventions they deem necessary on selected target communities or populations without either soliciting or fully taking into account the wants of the affected groups and individuals (Israel et al. 1998). Program developers may claim that communities have been involved in shaping such interventions when in fact there has been little or only token participation on the part of affected groups.

Habermas's discourse theory provides a template for examining the nature of these exchanges and the aims and actions of the institutional and individual actors involved in them. For Habermas, communication directed toward a mutual understanding between affected parties can best establish the foundations of trust and collaboration needed for solving their common problems, despite their potentially different points of view (Habermas 2002, 1996, 1995; Habermas and Fultner 2003). Opportunities for analyzing the form and quality of participation range from the microcosm of the patient–physician relationship, to the design of consumer-oriented healthcare programs and neighborhood services or community-wide needs assessment and program development efforts, to broader social change–oriented movements that have an important impact on the health of individuals and communities (e.g., environmental justice, AIDS advocacy) (Gellad et al. 2011; Gong et al. 2009; Goss and Renzi 2007; Labonte 1994; Loh et al. 2007; Marincowitz 2004; Stuart, Mudhasakul, and Sriwatanapongse 2009; Thurston et al. 2005; Waitzkin, Britt, and Williams 1994). The fairness of healthcare programs and policies may be judged by whether affected parties have been fully involved in shaping them, which can be assessed through qualitative interviews or more structured quantitative scales of key informants' participation. (Some of these approaches are discussed in the review of selected empirical indicators of equity later in this chapter.)

The discussion that follows reviews how the dimensions of equity reflected in these respective frameworks would be operationalized in HSR to assess the extent to which disparities in health and healthcare have been reduced.

Criteria and Indicators of Equity

Exhibit 6.3 highlights the major theories and related principles of justice underlying the principal justice paradigms from which specific empirical criteria of equity may be derived. Exhibit 6.4 summarizes empirical indicators of equity in relationship to the primary dimensions of the expanded equity framework (Exhibit 6.2) and to the related criteria of justice underlying them. The ultimate test of equity is the extent to which disparities in health are minimized. The challenge to analytic and evaluative public health and HSR is determining how best to design studies to descriptively assess dimensions of procedural and substantive equity and to explore factors that are most likely to influence disparities and the health policy interventions suggested as their consequence. The methods and empirical evidence for assessing how fully the criteria of justice have been realized and their import for reducing health disparities are presented later in this chapter and in Chapter 7.

Participation
Criteria

Habermas's discourse theory is most directly concerned with the extent to which those likely to be affected by decisions participate in shaping them. The defining normative underpinning for Habermas's theory is grounded in his discourse principle: "Only those norms are valid to which all affected persons could agree as participants in rational discourse(s)" (Habermas 1996, xxvi). *Rational discourse* in this case refers to communication directed toward mutual understanding, rather than strictly ends-oriented communication directed toward instrumental (i.e., technical-rational or strategic) or political aims. Habermas's discourse principle is grounded in fundamental democratic ideals, in which the power to govern is ultimately vested in the people and exercised by them directly or indirectly through a system of representation, involvement in a public political sphere, and free elections. The discourse principle characterizes policy or development activities that are oriented toward gaining a reasonable consensus about the definition of the problem and the best possible ways to address it among the stakeholders most likely to be affected by the resulting policy. Communication grounded in mutual respect between stakeholders is essential to ensuring the realization of this principle in the formulation of policy at the micro or macro level. For Habermas, the foundations of trust and collaboration required to successfully address instrumental aims are established through such "communicatively rational" discourse. These norms of deliberative justice would be attended to at the micro level to forge effective patient–physician relationships, shape culturally sensitive service provision at the institutional level, and ensure the full participation of affected populations in the design of health policies and programs at the system and community levels.

EXHIBIT 6.3
Theories
Underlying
Paradigms of
Justice

Theory *(major theorists)*	Justice Principles	Health Policy Focus
Liberalism		
Libertarian *(Robert Nozick)*	**Property:** • *Entitlement:* Individuals are entitled to what they possess, provided they acquire and transfer it through just means. • *Libertarianism:* The state should enforce these property rights and **not** interfere in redistributing assets (i.e., let "the invisible hand" work).	Free market
Utilitarian *(Jeremy Bentham, David Hume, John Stuart Mill)*	**Payoffs:** • *Utility:* Promote the greatest good for the greatest number. • *Consequences:* Gauge the worth of actions by their consequences (i.e., ends justify means).	Cost-benefit/ cost-effectiveness/ cost-utility analyses
Contractarian *(John Rawls)*	**Priorities:** • *Greatest equal liberty:* Every person should have an equal right to the most extensive system of basic liberties available to all. • *Fair equality of opportunity:* Persons with similar skills and abilities should have equal access to offices and positions. • *Difference principle:* Social and economic institutions should be arranged to maximally benefit the **least well-off.**	Social exclusion
Communitarianism		
Community *(Dan Beauchamp, Amitai Etzioni, Alisdair MacIntyre, Michael Sandel, Michael Walzer)*	**Public good:** • *Social solidarity:* The unity produced by or based on community, group, or class interests, objectives, and values is primary. • *Common good:* The well-being of the community as a whole (commonweal) must be protected and ensured.	Public health

Egalitarian (Robert Veatch)	**Personhood:** • *Equal worth:* Principle of equality rests on the assumption of the equal intrinsic worth of **all** human beings. • *Equal opportunity:* Everyone should have an opportunity to access health and healthcare equal, as far as possible, to another person's.	Health and healthcare disparities
Needs-based (Norman Daniels)	**Potential:** • *Normal species functioning:* Meeting health and healthcare needs helps to maintain normal species functioning. • *Fair equality of opportunity:* Society should ensure fair equality of opportunity of access to normal species functioning.	Health and healthcare objectives for the nation
Deliberative Democracy		
Discourse (Paulo Freire, Jürgen Habermas)	**Participation:** • *Discourse principle:* Norms are valid only if all affected persons could agree to them as participants in rational discourse. • *Balance of individual and group interests:* Laws and institutions must balance private and public autonomy (i.e., self- and societal rule).	Participation and empowerment

This philosophical and programmatic thrust and the parallel participatory action research agenda developed by Brazilian social activist Paulo Freire (1995, 1970) are intended to encourage researchers and policymakers to listen to communities more attentively and learn from them. Communication with and the involvement of affected parties in the design and implementation of programs are seen as essential. This emphasis acknowledges that by voicing concerns in their own syntax and semantics, affected parties learn together how best to address their concerns. This perspective is manifest in the formulation and implementation of community-based health education and health promotion initiatives (Aronson et al. 2007; Franzini et al. 2009; Gong et al. 2009; Israel et al. 2010; Minkler 2010, 1997; Minkler and Wallerstein 2003).

EXHIBIT 6.4
Criteria and
Indicators of
Equity

Dimensions	Criteria	Examples of Indicators
Procedural Equity		
Deliberative Justice		
Health policy	Participation	Type and extent of affected groups' participation in formulating and implementing policies and programs
Distributive Justice		
Delivery system • Availability • Organization • Financing	Freedom of choice	• Distribution of providers • Types of facilities and services • Sources of payment
Realized access • Utilization • Satisfaction	Cost-effectiveness	• Type and volume of services used; direct and indirect costs of care • Public, patient, and provider opinions
Distributive and Social Justice		
Population at risk • Predisposing • Enabling • Need	Similar treatment	• Age, gender, race, education • Regular care source, insurance, income • Perceived, evaluated
Social Justice		
Environment • Physical • Social • Economic	Common good	• Toxic, environmental hazards • Social-capital family structure, voluntary organizations, social networks • Human and material capital (schools, jobs, income, housing)
Health risks • Environmental • Behavioral	Need	• Toxic, environmental exposures • Lifestyle, health promotion practices
Substantive Equity		
Health • Individuals • Community	Need	• Clinical indicators • Population rates

Norman Daniels has argued for incorporating the norms of "deliberative democracy" in managed care policies and procedures—that is, participation on the part of affected parties (e.g., patients and providers) must be ensured in decision making regarding the protection of normal functioning of a given population within defined constraints (e.g., limited resources). This perspective would, for example, make explicit the rationale for decisions about covering new technologies, provide an opportunity for public discussion of this rationale, and streamline and make patient grievance and dispute resolution procedures less adversarial (Daniels 2011, 2009, 2008, 2006, 2001, 1998, 1996; Daniels, Kennedy, and Kawachi 2000; Daniels and Sabin 2002; Daniels, Saloner, and Gelpi 2009).

Indicators

Empirical indicators of deliberative justice are developed to express the type and extent of involvement of affected groups' participation in formulating and implementing policies and programs. Arnstein (1969) conceptualized a ladder of citizen participation, each rung representing a gradient ranging from nonparticipation to tokenism to increased levels of citizen power and control. Charles and DeMaio (1993) incorporated this and two other dimensions that reflect (1) the perspective being adopted (i.e., that of a user versus a policymaker) and (2) the decision-making domain (i.e., individual treatment, overall service provision, or macro policy formulation) in constructing a framework for assessing lay participation in healthcare decision making. Promoting lay participation and empowerment has been a particular focus of health education and health promotion activities in the United States, Canada, and other countries. Related indicators with particular relevance in the managed care context focus on the nature and quality of communication between patients and providers, the extent to which norms of "deliberative democracy" guide the development of organizational policies and procedures, and the magnitude of trust healthcare consumers have for providers or organizations (Abelson et al. 2003; Daniels 1996; Davies and Burgess 2004; De Vries et al. 2010; Mechanic 1996).

Critiques of the shift to a population health perspective in Canada and the United States have argued, however, that it has diminished the focus on active engagement of populations and patients in health policy and program development at the macro and micro levels (although see the earlier comments regarding the lack of confirmation that public participation in health policy decisions has a positive impact on health and well-being). Critics argue that the diminished focus on active engagement is due to the fact that, in contrast to the health promotion movement, population health researchers document but do not identify participatory political mechanisms for addressing the fundamental determinants of health and health disparities (Coburn et al. 2003; Hawks 1997; Raphael and Bryant 2002).

Freedom of Choice

Criteria

The freedom-of-choice norm emphasizes the importance of personal autonomy in determining who receives what care. This criterion conforms most closely to Nozick's libertarian theory of justice, which emphasizes that equity is rooted in the freedom to possess and use one's property and resources as one chooses (Nozick 1993, 1990, 1974). From this perspective, people are entitled to what they have as long as they acquire or transfer it through just means—that is, through their own labor or as a result of a gift, an inheritance, or a voluntary exchange with others. Further, the state should not interfere with or attempt to regulate these transactions. Instead, the "invisible hand" governing the free marketplace should be allowed to operate unhindered. The only appropriate intrusions would be to correct situations in which there is clear historical evidence that the property or resources some people possess were not acquired through just means. Such evidence is often difficult to assemble or document, however. This perspective endorses policies that maximize consumer preferences (i.e., choice and satisfaction) in the healthcare marketplace. Proponents of this approach endorse the operation of market-based forces of supply and demand for the allocation of healthcare.

Indicators

Empirical indicators of access based on the freedom-of-choice norm are the distribution and availability of healthcare resources to consumers. For example, personnel-to-population ratios (e.g., number of primary care physicians or specialists per 1,000 population), facility-to-population ratios (e.g., number of hospitals or hospital beds per 1,000 population), and related inventories of healthcare personnel or providers (e.g., HMOs, PPOs) in a given target or market area are indicators of the basic supply of providers and delivery sites available to consumers.

Lists of preferred or participating providers affiliated with health insurance plans (and with developing ACOs) also effectively define the range of enrollees' choices for a regular source of healthcare. Other indicators of the extent to which patients' decisions may be constrained include data on the hours of clinic operation and provider availability at night, on weekends, or in emergencies; the average distance to the nearest medical facility and the available modes of transportation for getting there; and the average time it takes to get an appointment as well as the waiting time to see a physician or other provider once patients are on-site.

For the past half century, the type and scope of benefits provided by major employers and the local public or private arrangements for people who have no third-party coverage have defined the options consumers can realistically afford. Substantial cost-sharing provisions or uncovered healthcare expenses have repeatedly been shown to affect choices about delaying or seeking care (Johnson and Wegner 2007; Rowland and Lyons 1996; Sipkoff 2010; Tu 2004) and decisions about forgoing goals or sacrificing personal resources intended for other uses (e.g., an elderly woman uses her and her husband's life savings ["spends down"] so he can qualify for nursing home coverage under Medicaid) (O'Brien 2005).

These concerns shaped many of the initial design elements in the ACA (Office of the Legislative Counsel 2010), including broad availability of coverage, the individual mandate to purchase insurance, expanded eligibility for Medicaid, and new programs to defray the costs of home health assistance (Kaiser Family Foundation 2012). A number of these elements are controversial, such as the individual mandate to purchase insurance (concern regarding infringement of individual autonomy) and the expanded eligibility for Medicaid (concern regarding drain on societal, i.e., state, resources), reflecting the tension between the distributive and social justice considerations.

Realized Access
Criteria
Utilitarians advocate access to services for which the measured benefits (e.g., health, well-being, productivity) would be maximized relative to the costs necessary to provide them. Utilitarian theory has its origins in the writings of David Hume, Jeremy Bentham, and John Stuart Mill (Culyer 1992; Kolm 1996). It is principally consequentialist or ends-oriented. The value of any decision or action is judged by its consequences; the principal goal is to maximize utility (which incorporates individual preferences). Consideration of the utilitarian theory of judging the rightness or wrongness of actions by the balance of benefits and burdens produced has increased researchers' and policymakers' focus on cost-effectiveness analyses, cost-benefit analyses, and associated cost-utility analyses (discussed in Chapter 4) when they are weighing the types of programs that should be funded and the categories of services to be covered under public or private insurance schemes and when determining whether the services actually being used are appropriate, effective, and satisfactory to consumers.

Indicators
Components of the costs and benefits of care are reflected in the type and comprehensiveness of services received, the direct and indirect costs of those services, and the level of patient satisfaction relative to some standard. The underlying theory and methods for examining cost-effectiveness is examined in more detail in chapters 4 and 5.

More generally, the IOM Committee on Monitoring Access to Personal Health Care Services developed a set of indicators of services likely to have beneficial health consequences if used, including an array of preventive services (e.g., prenatal care, immunizations, breast cancer screening) and timely and appropriate care for acute or chronic illness (IOM 1993). These and other indicators were confirmed in later IOM committee reports documenting the resulting impact of disparities in access to essential preventive and treatment services on disparities in the quality and effectiveness of care by race/ethnicity, socioeconomic status, and urban versus rural place of residence (IOM 2003, 2002b). The *Healthy People* 2010 objectives subsequently encompassed a series of goals regarding the use of preventive services (CDC 2011c), while the 2020 objectives seek better coordination of health promotion and disease prevention guidelines with more effective engagement of individuals in evidence-based prevention strategies (HHS 2010). These objectives provide foundations for systems of monitoring service utilization. For example, the ACA requires coverage of certain preventive services without copayments or deductibles (Office of the Legislative Counsel 2010). Services qualify on the basis of cost-effectiveness as assessed by the US Task Force on Preventive Medicine.

A variety of scales for measuring satisfaction with healthcare, physicians, and hospitals have been employed extensively to develop report cards or other reports on provider performance (Bailey and Gibson 2005; Boudreaux, Cruz, and Baumann 2006; Boudreaux and O'Hea 2004; Robinowitz and Dudley 2006; Schold 2008; Swinehart and Smith 2004). These scales can be used to assess the extent to which effective care has been rendered from the point of view of patients or the general public. Critics of existing measures of patient satisfaction point out the need for the design of instruments that more directly engage those surveyed to better identify the key issues and questions that need to be addressed (Harris et al. 2001).

Similar Treatment
Criteria

From an egalitarian point of view, the perspective that all individuals are of equal worth and should be treated equally is of primary importance. The similar treatment criterion emphasizes that age, sex, race, income, or type or amount of insurance coverage should not dictate that people with similar needs enter different doors (e.g., private physicians' offices versus hospital emergency departments) or be treated differently in terms of the type or intensity of services provided. This criterion is a defining tenet of the egalitarian concept of justice. As Robert Veatch (1989, 1981) pointed out, egalitarianism may focus on either procedural or substantive equality (i.e., similarity in treatment or outcome, respectively). Procedural equality ensures equal opportunity for all individuals to obtain care, regardless of personal characteristics, such as age, gender, race, income, type of coverage, and whether one lives in the city or suburbs. Substantive equality emphasizes minimizing the health status differentials or variations between groups, such as disparities in infant mortality between black and white populations. Considerations of equity from an egalitarian point of view focus on how to narrow or eliminate these disparities in health and healthcare.

Egalitarian norms also have been central to the social justice paradigm in the context of examining varying exposures to health risks as a function of environmental, social, or economic conditions. Research on environmental justice has, for example, documented that toxic and hazardous waste sites are more likely to be located in racially segregated or socioeconomically disadvantaged neighborhoods (Brown 1995; Bullard 2000; Evans and Kantrowitz 2002; Hipp and Lakon 2010; Mohai et al. 2009; Stuart, Mudhasakul, and Sriwatanapongse 2009). "Social exclusion" programs and policies take into account what can happen when people or areas differentially suffer from a combination of linked problems, such as unemployment, poor job skills, low income, poor housing, high crime environments, bad health, and family breakdown. The Social Exclusion Unit in the United Kingdom, for example, was set up by the prime minister to improve government action to ameliorate the impact of these combined and differential risks (Chernew et al. 2010; Goldsmith et al. 2008; McKinney 2010; Office of the Deputy Prime Minister 2004).

Indicators

The norm of similar treatment is used to evaluate intergroup differences that may indicate inequalities in health or access to care. Data on the convenience and characteristics of the places people go for healthcare indicate whether there is differential treatment of individuals in different settings. Nonmedically motivated transfers of patients, or "dumping," principally as a function of fiscal rather than physical diagnostics, are indicative of inequity under the norm of similar treatment. Prior to the passage of the ACA (2010), hospitals that provided a disproportionate share of uncompensated care for the medically indigent population received additional funding from CMS to cover their costs (i.e., Disproportionate Share Hospital funds). The ACA reduces these funds, with the expectation that uncompensated care will be reduced by ACA provisions. How this scenario will play out in practice is uncertain. There are concerns that particular institutions or providers will continue to assume a disproportionate burden of uncompensated care for this population. Health inequalities and the factors that give rise to them also surface as issues under the norm of similar treatment. From this perspective, differential exposure and differential access to resources for services would be judged inequitable to the extent that they produce these inequalities (IOM 2003, 2002b).

Common Good
Criteria
The concept of the common good is grounded in communitarian theory and focuses on the community as the unit of analysis (Daly 1994; Mulhall and Swift 1996). The primary normative referents are the well-being, or welfare,

of communities and the criteria of social solidarity, or unity, and the common good. These norms find expression in more universal modes of financing healthcare; in traditional public health policy and practice, with its emphasis on promoting and protecting the health of the public; and in investments in the institutions and resources, such as families, schools, businesses, and government, that are essential for maintaining the health and vitality of communities. In this context, the focus of interventions is not on altering individual actions and motivations but on the roots of health problems, such as the social-structural correlates of health and healthcare inequalities inherent in the physical, social, and economic environments in which individuals live and work. Health risks in the physical environment include toxic and environmental contaminants transmitted through the air, soil, or water in a given neighborhood or community. The social environment encompasses the social resources/capital available to individuals through family structure, voluntary organizations, and the social networks that bind and support them. The economic environment encompasses both human and material capital resources, which are reflected in the schools, jobs, income, and housing that characterize the community (Aday 2005, 2001; Franzini et al. 2009, 2005; Mansyur et al. 2008; Mooney 1998; Robertson 1998).

Indicators

Empirical indicators related to the common good encompass the array of social status, social capital, and human and material capital resources available to the population at risk in a given area as well as the significant physical environmental exposures that are likely to exist. Health protection was one of the *Healthy People* 2010 objectives, measured by a series of environmentally related health indicators (e.g., unintentional injuries, occupational safety and health, environmental health, food and drug safety) (CDC 2011c), while the year 2020 objectives expand these indicators to include quality of life and well-being and social determinants of health, among others (HHS 2010). The World Health Organization's Health for All effort also set forth indicators for tracking the social, economic, and physical environments and their influence on health (WHO 2008, 2002).

Need

Criteria

Norman Daniels's (1985) needs-based theory of justice identifies factors that are necessary to address minimal human needs for "normal species functioning." In this framework, health policy initiatives are justified in terms of their role in ensuring equality of opportunity for living a normal life. This perspective prompts consideration of what such needs might be and of the minimum set of services that should be provided to meet them. Daniels suggests the following for consideration: adequate nutrition and shelter; sanitary, safe, unpolluted living and working conditions; exercise, rest, and other features of a healthy lifestyle; preventive, curative, and rehabilitative personal medical services; and nonmedical personal and social support services. However, the basis for deciding what goods and services might be included and how they could be fairly distributed remains controversial.

John Rawls's contractarian theory is based on the standard of what reasonable people would decide if they were asked to come together to derive a fair set of criteria for distributing societal goods, operating under the hypothetical assumption that they could by chance be in any position in a society in which such criteria would be applied, including the least socially or economically advantaged (Rawls 2001, 1971; Rawls and Kelly 2001). Rawls reasoned that under these circumstances, the following criteria would be endorsed, in order of importance: (1) maximize everyone's right to equal basic liberties, (2) ensure equality of opportunity for people with similar abilities and skills, and (3) make sure that those who are the worst-off benefit. The first two criteria have a strong egalitarian orientation, and the third emphasizes that those who are worst-off, financially or otherwise, count more than other groups. This perspective focuses on those least able to buy care or be cured.

Daniels's needs-based theory, as well as the difference criterion recognizing the needs of the least well-off, supports a primary focus on meeting basic needs. Assessing who needs care may be both difficult and expensive (Braybrooke 1998, 1987), and economic theory argues that expressed demand is the most rational basis for allocating healthcare resources. Needs may be subjective and ungovernable unless constrained by some sense that people are willing to pay to have their tastes and preferences satisfied. Furthermore, societal or professional consensus may be required to determine which needs to meet when resources are limited. In this context, needs assessments are and have been an important component of public health–oriented planning and program development activities at the community level. Contemporary needs assessments focus on inventorying the assets, as well as the problems, that exist in the target communities of concern (Kretzmann and McKnight 1993; Morgan and Ziglio 2007).

Indicators

Indicators of equity from the perspective of need assess the magnitude of health risks and health disparities in a population. Sometimes survey respondents are asked questions to obtain their subjective perceptions of the extent to which their needs have been met—for example, "During the past year, did you or a family member need to see a doctor but not see one for some reason? If so, why?" Other indicators of need summarize respondents' objective reports of the number of physician visits relative to the number of disability days they experienced in the year (i.e., the use–disability ratio) or compare the number of people who actually contacted a physician for a set of symptoms to the number of people a panel of physicians thought should have seen one (i.e., the symptoms–response ratio) (Aday, Andersen, and Fleming 1980). The quality and outcomes of care are directly linked to the utilization of appropriate services to address identified needs (Chao, Anderson, and Hernandez 2009; Franzini, Mikhail, and Skinner 2010; IOM 2003, 2002b, 1993; Moy, Dayton, and Clancy 2005; van Merode 2010).

The social justice perspective on substantive equity, based in the need criterion, is concerned with subgroup variations in health. The primary goals of the *Healthy People* 2010 and 2020 objectives include increasing the span of healthy life for all Americans, reducing health disparities between and among groups, and creating social and physical environments that promote good health (HHS 2010). Mortality, morbidity, and years of potential life lost or quality years of life gained are illustrative of the types of indicators that can be used to trace trends and subgroup variations reflective of the extent to which needs are actually met. There is an increasing interest in developing summary measures of population health that integrate mortality and morbidity data, such as health-adjusted life expectancy or other quality-adjusted life-year estimates (IOM 1998; Kindig 1998, 1997; Montazeri 2008; Murray et al. 2002; Richardson et al. 2010; Rose et al. 2011).

In summary, an array of empirical indicators might be developed and used to assess the equity of health policy design and implementation. HSR and policy analysis can help to conceptualize and measure these indicators and to determine which factors appear to be most predictive of the ultimate equity outcome of interest—reducing subgroup disparities in health.

Data Sources

As implied in the expanded conceptual framework of equity (Exhibit 6.2), studies of equity could focus on the delivery system as a whole, particular institutions within it, groups of patients, communities that are the target of health policy initiatives, or various combinations of these levels and their interrelationships. Furthermore, studies could be carried out at the national, regional, state, or local level. Such studies may entail collecting primary data, using data collected for other purposes, or using secondary data. Both quantitative and qualitative data may be needed to fully capture the array of factors reflected in the expanded framework of equity. The sources of primary and secondary data that are particularly relevant to examining the various dimensions of equity are reviewed in the discussion that follows.

Community
Environment

At the community level, environmental indicators focus on the community itself or definable geographic areas within it as the unit(s) of analysis. They are explicitly intended to reflect the structural or environmental context that significantly affects the health risks or health of those who live and work in it. The World Health Organization's "Healthy Cities" movement, for example, has identified a range of community-level variables related to air and water quality, housing availability and quality, and economic development that can be used to profile the health and well-being of communities (WHO 2010, 1999). These data are available from planning agencies, business censuses, US censuses on household characteristics, and local public health environmental surveillance systems. Qualitative studies using participant or nonparticipant observation methods may also be useful for profiling the social and environmental context that may affect the health or healthcare of individuals in a designated neighborhood or ethnic group (Devers 2011).

Population

Population-based studies focus on individuals identified by a shared characteristic, such as geographic area (e.g., the US population), life history (e.g., all veterans of the US Armed Forces), or enrollment in a specific system of care (e.g., Medicare). Surveys of these populations are particularly useful for measuring the attitudes or barriers that preclude targeted individuals or subgroups from seeking care. For example, a number of large-scale, national surveys have examined access and trends over time for the US population, including the Robert Wood Johnson Foundation (2010) surveys, the Agency for Healthcare Research and Quality (2013) Medical Expenditure Panel Survey (Cohen 2005; Cohen et al. 1996), the continuing National Center for Health Statistics (NCHS) National Health Interview Survey (Adams, Heyman, and Vickerie 2009), and the Centers for Disease Control and Prevention (CDC 2006) Behavioral Risk Factor Surveillance System. Similarly, the Medicare Current Beneficiary Survey (CMS 2012a), the Consumer Assessment of Health Plans Survey and its Medicare counterpart (AHRQ 2012a), and the National Survey of Veterans (VA 2001) capture representative data on large and important segments of the US population. Such surveys are complex and expensive to conduct, however, and state or local agencies may lack the resources and expertise for conducting them (Aday 1996; Aday and Cornelius 2006). Qualitative or semi-structured interviews and focus groups may also be useful for profiling the health and healthcare experiences of a population at risk as well as inform the design or interpretation of more structured surveys of a representative sample of the target population (Devers 2011).

Public health population surveillance systems, disease registries, national claims or utilization surveys for the population in general (e.g., the National Hospital Discharge Survey) or from publicly financed programs (e.g., Medicare, Medicaid, the Veterans Administration), census or vital statistics data, and synthetic estimates are some of the major sources of secondary data used for profiling the health and healthcare of a population at the state or local level. For example, the Surveillance, Epidemiology and End Results

(SEER) Program of the National Cancer Institute (2011b) compiles cancer registry information on cancer incidence and survival in the United States, and these data have been merged with Medicare data (Medicare-SEER) to provide a comprehensive, utilization-based data set focused on cancer care.

When locality information is available from these national and state data sets, relatively fine-grained analyses of geographic-specific access and utilization can be constructed. In other instances, data gathered at the national level on utilization rates for certain age, gender, or racial groups can be used to compute estimates at the state or local level given the age, gender, and racial composition of the state or community. Researchers also are increasingly using geographic methods to identify and analyze the impact of environmental and contextual factors on health and healthcare disparities and access (CDC 2011a; Cinnamon, Schuurman, and Crooks 2008; Comber, Brunsdon, and Radburn 2011; Graves 2008; Ricketts III et al. 1994). Managed care plan enrollment files are a source of data on the denominator of individuals residing in a given geographic area who are eligible to use plan services, and combined with healthcare use data, this information can highlight plan characteristics that affect access to care (Morgan et al. 2009).

Healthcare System

Descriptors at the system level focus on the availability, organization, and financing of services as aggregate, structural properties. Secondary data sources most often are used for this type of analysis. The National Center for Health Workforce Analysis, for example, has compiled a database called the Area Resource File, which contains an array of health and healthcare data by county or metropolitan statistical area (Health Resources and Services Administration 2011). The American Medical Association, the American Hospital Association, and other groups routinely publish directories and, in some instances, offer computerized data on the characteristics and distribution of medical personnel. NCHS collects data on the characteristics and utilization of hospitals, nursing homes, and outpatient healthcare practices. CMS and the Health Insurance Association of America also periodically publish information on the amount and distribution of expenditures by major public (i.e., Medicare and Medicaid) and private third-party payers. Organizations such as the Agency for Healthcare Quality and Research (AHRQ), CDC, and CMS make nonsensitive public-use files available for download at no cost (or at a relatively small cost), enabling researchers to characterize use of the healthcare system in the ways best suited for their needs (AHRQ 2012b; CDC 2011b; CMS 2013d), while the Dartmouth Atlas of Health Care provides summaries of healthcare resource use. These data sources are particularly useful for describing the delivery system at the national, state, and local levels (CMS 2013a; Dartmouth Atlas of Health Care 2013; HHS 2010; NCHS 2010).

The Community Tracking Study, conducted by the Center for Studying Health System Change (ICPSR and Robert Wood Johnson Foundation 2011; Williams et al. 2006) with support from the Robert Wood Johnson Foundation, was a major data collection and analysis effort that drew on site visits, consumer surveys, and secondary data sources to monitor and understand the dimensions and impact of healthcare system change in more than 60 randomly selected communities and a random subset of 12 intensive study sites throughout the United States.

Public health departments, researchers, and private providers (e.g., national managed care organizations) considering entering a market may want either more current or more detailed information on the types of services being provided or the profile of clients seen by facilities in a given area. The National Center for Quality Assurance (2011) HEDIS data system provides a profile of the organizational and financing features of participating plans, while CMS maintains the Medicare and Nursing Home Compare databases listing characteristics of plans and nursing homes participating in Medicare and Medicaid (CMS 2013b, 2013c). If data are not available through these sources, the interested party could collect primary data based on interviews with key community informants, telephone requests to providers for brochures describing their services, or full-fledged surveys of providers. See Chapters 4 and 5 to review indicators from the OECD and other sources for describing and comparing the healthcare systems in different countries.

Institutions

Secondary data used most often by institutions and organizations to assess access to a particular facility include enrollment data, encounter data, claims data, and data from medical records. Medical records, increasingly in the form of electronic medical records, can be used to examine the scope of care provided to patients and answer questions regarding the equity of healthcare quality that cannot be easily addressed using claims data, such as Medicare and Medicaid claims files (Kahn and Ranade 2010; Smith 2008; Tang et al. 2007). Financial records indicate the level of uncompensated or undercompensated care a facility provides and for what types of patients and services. Other institutional sources, such as clinic logbooks or emergency department referral records, are used in studies of the magnitude and profile of unscheduled walk-in visits and of nonmedically motivated transfers within an institution. Finally, administrators, providers, or patients could be surveyed to gather institutional operations data relevant to access or availability issues.

Patients

Patient surveys are major sources of primary data for evaluating access and outcomes at the institutional level (Morgan and Sail 2012). They tap individuals' subjective perceptions of their experiences at a given facility (e.g., how long they had to wait to be seen), which may or may not agree with more objective institutional records or data sources (e.g., average clinic waiting time estimates). These subjective perceptions are more reflective of people's satisfaction with and loyalty to a facility than are objective, records-based indicators. A variety of standardized instruments have been developed and utilized for this purpose, such as the Community Assessment of Health Plans Survey, HEDIS, and Press Ganey satisfaction questionnaires (AHRQ 2012a; Bindman and Gold 1998; NCQA 2011; Press Ganey 2013). Focus groups and ethnographic interviews of patients also may help to explain problems providers have encountered in dealing with certain types of patients or in designing culturally sensitive or consumer-oriented services.

Patient origin studies use patient address and zip code information to determine the areas from which most patients are drawn. Patient record data also could serve as a basis for generating profiles of the demographic composition (i.e., age, sex, and race) or the major presenting complaints of patients seen at the facility. When population-based enrollment and utilization files can be linked with institutional information, the resulting combined data can be a powerful tool for assessing access at the community level (CMS 2013d; Dartmouth Atlas of Health Care 2013; Morgan et al. 2009). A variety of research designs that focus on different components of the conceptual framework of equity and their interrelationships (Exhibit 6.2) also may be employed to assess equity at the community, institution, and system levels.

Study Designs

Three major types of HSR designs may be drawn on to define and clarify the objective of equity and programs' and policies' success at achieving it: descriptive, analytic, and evaluative (Aday and Cornelius 2006).

Descriptive Research

Descriptive research focuses primarily on profiling the discrete indicators of equity. In effect, these indicators reflect data that are collected to operationalize the dimensions represented in Exhibit 6.2. (Also see Appendix 7.1 on page 185.) They also can be used to make normative assessments of procedural or substantive equity, based on the criteria of equity they are deemed to most directly express (Exhibit 6.4). Descriptive analyses may, however, be viewed as essentially identifying the symptoms of a problem. More probing analytic research is required to diagnose the underlying etiology and likely health and healthcare consequences of a problem.

Analytic Research

Analytic research is directed toward understanding hypothesized cause-and-effect relationships among the structure, process, and intermediate outcome components of the model (Exhibit 6.2) and ultimately toward achieving the primary outcome of interest—improving the health of individuals and communities. The hypotheses to be explored in such studies are implicit in the arrows between components of the expanded equity framework (Exhibit 6.2). These studies are useful, for example, for illuminating the impact of policy-relevant variables, such as the type and extent of insurance coverage, on the use of services and associated clinical outcomes. Nonrandomized data, such as the population-based data sets typically used to study access to care within health systems, have recognized limitations when it comes to inferring causality (Shadish, Cook, and Campbell 2002). Over the past few years, a variety of statistical techniques have emerged to reduce potential bias and strengthen causal inference from these data, including propensity score methods, marginal structural models, and instrumental variable analyses (Johnson et al. 2009).

A particular challenge for public health and health services researchers with respect to future analytic research on the equity objective as defined in this chapter is identifying the mutable factors that are most predictive of improved health. Evaluating access to healthcare for problems that healthcare cannot address does little to prevent or remedy them. Analytic research on the correlates and consequences of health and human functioning can help to address questions regarding whether investments in healthcare or in other systems or services are the most relevant bases for allocating societal resources.

Evaluative Research

Evaluative research assesses how well programs and services developed and implemented on the basis of descriptive and analytic research have achieved their desired equity objective. Evaluative studies rely primarily on experimental or quasi-experimental designs to determine program or policy outcomes. Evaluations of Medicaid and Medicare managed care demonstrations, for example, have provided useful information for assessing the access, quality, and cost impacts of these models for low-income enrollees as well as informed the design of state and federal Medicaid managed care policies and the Medicare Advantage program (Hurley and McCue 2000; Jones III, Jones, and Miller 2004; Keenan et al. 2009; Shimada et al. 2009).

Summary and Conclusions

The answer to the first question posed at the beginning of this chapter—what is equity?—may be summarized as follows: Equity is concerned with health disparities and the fairness and effectiveness of the procedures for addressing them. The response to the second question—how should equity in healthcare be assessed?—is: by examining and accounting for health disparities.

This chapter has reviewed major paradigms of justice and their implications for an operational framework for the conduct of HSR on equity. The health of individuals and populations is the ultimate dependent variable in the framework and the corollary bottom line for assessing the impact of health policy. The distributive justice paradigm evaluates the characteristics of the system and population that contribute to differentials in the distribution of healthcare. The social justice paradigm examines the factors in the social, economic, and physical environment that contribute to disparities in the prevalence of poor health. The deliberative justice paradigm provides the blueprint for the design of more effective health policies at the macro and micro levels by ensuring that parties affected by such policies participate in shaping them.

The conceptual framework of equity presented in this chapter points to more focused, expanded, and explanatory HSR to assess equity. The framework fully addresses the linkage and integration of concepts and methods from research on effectiveness, efficiency, and equity to assess system performance. HSR, based on this framework, would be more focused on improving the health of patients and communities as the ultimate goal of health policy. The resulting research agenda related to this substantive objective must, by necessity, be grounded in the concepts and methods that underlie the population perspective on enhancing the health of populations and the clinical perspective on improving the outcomes of patients. HSR would be expanded to encompass broader epidemiological, ecological, and related public health theories, methods, and research questions to identify the medical and nonmedical factors that contribute to health. It would draw on studies of allocative efficiency that determine the types and mix of inputs most likely to be productive of health and address the corollary concerns of production efficiency regarding the most efficient means for producing these inputs. And finally, HSR would be more explanatory, in that greater emphasis would be placed on analytic and evaluative research to generate and explore relevant hypotheses regarding the array of factors, and the relationships between them, that are most likely to contribute to the health of individuals and populations. The conceptual framework of equity presented in this chapter (Exhibit 6.2) is intended to guide the development of this more explanatory and health-centered HSR agenda.

Chapter 7 reviews the available evidence to address a third question: To what extent has procedural and substantive equity in health and healthcare actually been achieved in the United States? The distributive justice paradigm has primarily served to guide HSR on equity; the arguments and evidence presented in Chapter 7 are intended to document that norms of deliberative and social justice also must be taken into account if the ultimate health policy goals of improving health and narrowing health disparities are to be achieved.

EQUITY: POLICY STRATEGIES, EVIDENCE, AND CRITERIA

Chapter Highlights

1. The principal policy strategies, grounded in the distributive, social, and deliberative justice paradigms, respectively, are to (1) enhance access to medical care, (2) reduce health disparities, and (3) ensure affected parties' participation in policy and program design.
2. The evidence is mixed regarding the extent to which health disparities have been reduced. Wide variations in healthcare coverage and access exist, health disparities persist, and the norm of participation is neither routinely nor fully considered in the health policy formulation and implementation process.
3. The application of the equity criteria (introduced in Chapter 6) in assessing the incidence, screening, and treatment for breast cancer demonstrates that major procedural and substantive equity issues exist.

Overview

This chapter highlights alternative policy strategies for enhancing the equity of healthcare that are grounded in the conceptual framework introduced in the previous chapter (Exhibit 6.2) and assembles empirical evidence to determine the extent to which health disparities have been reduced in the United States. Findings from HSR and public health research are presented regarding the correlates and indicators of equity derived from the distributive, deliberative, and social justice paradigms. The criteria for assessing health policy in terms of the equity objective are defined and illustrated in the context of breast cancer prevention and treatment.

Policy Strategies Relating to Equity

Three primary policy goals are the focus of strategies for enhancing the equity of healthcare provision: (1) enhancing access to medical care, (2) reducing health disparities, and (3) ensuring affected parties' participation in policy and program design. The distributive justice paradigm and its attendant concern with ensuring equity of access to medical care have tended to dominate equity assessments of health policy in the United States since the mid-1960s. This perspective has focused most notably on the availability, organization, and financing of medical care services by providing support for major federal investments in the training of medical care providers, the construction of healthcare facilities, and the coverage of the poor and elderly through Medicaid and Medicare, respectively, culminating in 2010 in major national health insurance reform in the form of the Patient Protection and Affordable Care Act (ACA) (Office of the Legislative Counsel 2010).

The population perspective on the health of communities as a whole, and on the medical and nonmedical factors that give rise to health disparities, challenges health services researchers and policy analysts to consider broader conceptions of equity rooted in the social justice paradigm. Population health concerns have traditionally been the domain of public health policy and service provision. The US and international public health communities have undertaken a number of major programmatic initiatives, such as the *Healthy People* 2020 objectives (NCHS 2011) and the CDC's Healthy Communities Program, to attempt to ameliorate health disparities, yet disparities persist in the United States and other countries. Population effectiveness research supports public health, social policy, and economic policy investments as necessary for enhancing the health of communities and of the individuals residing within them. Research has identified indicators of quality medical care that can be monitored at a population level—for example, indicators of primary and secondary preventions as well as treatment of acute conditions as described by Jencks and colleagues (2000).

The discussion that follows presents evidence regarding the equity of healthcare provision, based on the respective paradigms of justice and accompanying policy strategies.

Evidence Relating to Equity

Review of the evidence begins with the end point for assessing the equity of the healthcare system on the basis of the expanded equity framework (Chapter 6, Exhibit 6.2): the extent to which subgroup health disparities persist. This focus is defined most directly by the social justice paradigm. In the following discussion, evidence regarding the magnitude and correlates of substantive equity reflected in these disparities is presented first to set the stage for assessing the extent to which this ultimate and defining equity objective has been achieved. A review of the evidence regarding the distributive equity of health services provision follows, focusing particularly on whether the evidence indicates amelioration or exacerbation of health disparities. Finally, evidence related to the deliberative justice paradigm is inventoried and broader HSR and policy agendas are delineated. The distributive and deliberative justice dimensions point primarily to evidence regarding procedural equity. The import of these factors for substantive equity is reflected in their likely contribution to minimizing health disparities.

The bulk of the HSR evidence regarding the equity of healthcare provision is rooted in the distributive justice paradigm. In contrast, evidence regarding the social justice dimensions of equity is drawn primarily from public health and related social science research documenting the predictors and indicators of population health and health disparities. Although the deliberative justice paradigm has not been as explicitly employed in the evaluation of healthcare services or public health policy as have the distributive and social justice paradigms, it finds expression in assessments of the role of healthcare consumers in clinical decision making, the cultural sensitivity of care, and community participation in the design of healthcare programs and services.

Social Justice

The social justice dimension of equity looks at the physical, social, and economic environment; health risks; and associated health disparities between groups. The US Public Health Service and the *Healthy People* 2010 and 2020 objectives provide a framework and a set of indicators for monitoring progress toward the goal of health equity. The findings with respect to selected indicators and environmental and behavioral predictors of health disparities in the United States are reviewed in Chapter 1.

Many disparities between groups persist (Aday 2001; Moy, Dayton, and Clancy 2005; NCHS 2011, 2010). For example, the rates of teenage pregnancy, preterm and low-birthweight babies, inadequate prenatal care, and infant and maternal mortality are twice as high among African-American women as among white women. Life expectancy from birth is almost five years longer for non-Hispanic whites compared to that for African Americans, although life expectancy from age 65 is only 1.5 years longer. The prevalence of chronic disease increases steadily with age, as do the incidence of death and the magnitude of limitation in daily activity due to chronic disease. At any age, men are more likely to die from major chronic illnesses such as heart disease, stroke, and cancer than are women, although elderly women living with chronic illness have more problems carrying out their normal daily routines. African Americans—particularly African-American men—are more likely to experience serious disabilities and to die from chronic illness than are whites. Early in the course of the AIDS epidemic, homosexual and bisexual males were most likely to be affected. In recent years, more and more mothers and children are at risk because of intravenous drug use among women and their sex partners. Higher proportions of African Americans and Hispanics than of whites are likely to be HIV positive, to develop and die of AIDS, and to have contracted the disease through drug use or sexual contact with drug users. Young adults in their late teens and early 20s—particularly men—are more likely to smoke, drink, and use illicit drugs than are their younger or older counterparts. Native American youth are much more apt to drink, use drugs, and smoke than are white and other minority youth, and death rates attributed to cirrhosis and other alcohol-related conditions are higher among Native Americans than among whites and other minorities. Minority substance users are also more likely to develop life-threatening patterns of substance abuse, as evidenced by the higher rates of addiction-related deaths among minority groups. A disproportionate number of medical emergencies and deaths due to cocaine abuse occur among minorities, particularly African Americans.

The physical, social, and economic environments to which individuals are exposed can have a profound effect on their health and healthcare. The movement of businesses and industries out of central cities has contributed to high unemployment rates, particularly among young, inner-city minority males. The percentage of families headed by only the mother has increased among all racial and ethnic groups. Men's wages are higher than women's wages on average, and the average salaries of working African-American women are lower than those of white women and African-American men. The national minimum wage has not kept pace with inflation, and the real purchasing power of the average welfare benefit has continued to decline, further exacerbating the economic burden on female heads of households with dependents. In addition, men are generally made better off financially by divorce or separation, whereas women's economic situations usually worsen (Bryan and Martinez 2008; DeNavas-Walt, Proctor, and Smith 2010; US Census Bureau 2001).

Although more African-American men have entered the workforce in recent years, the rates of unemployment among young African-American men remain high. Lack of employment opportunities; poverty; and the associated problems of crime, substance abuse, and violence plague many inner-city neighborhoods. The socioeconomic status of Hispanic and Native American families resembles that of African Americans more than that of whites. Nonetheless, the reduced number of jobs in the manufacturing and industrial sectors, the growth in the number of minimum-wage and part-time jobs in the service sectors, and the increased tax burden on low-income and middle-class taxpayers have also caused many working poor families—including white families and those with two breadwinners—to experience increased economic difficulties. These aspects of the social and economic environment can have profound consequences for the health and health risks of the most vulnerable (Aday 2001; Bernstein 2009; Martin-Moreno et al. 2010; US Census Bureau 2011, 2001).

Amid these indicators, it remains a challenge to determine the essential meaning of factors such as race and poverty and the dynamics through which these factors operate to influence health. A particular criticism of the application of these variables is that they are typically used as attitudinal, biological, or behavioral descriptors of individuals—especially in studies based on large-scale surveys or databases—while insufficient attention is paid to the social-structural, cultural, and environmental contexts that fundamentally shape these individuals' behavior, especially including health behaviors and access to healthcare. As a consequence, the focus of health policy informed by such research is aimed at intervention at the individual level, not at the broader social and economic conditions or at the systems of opportunity that influence the health risks of socially and economically disadvantaged populations (Franzini 2008; Franzini et al. 2005; Franzini and Fernandez-Esquer 2004; Krieger 2002; LaVeist 1994; Lillie-Blanton and LaVeist 1996; Link and Phelan 1995; Mansyur et al. 2009; Williams 1994).

Evidence from the United States and other countries documents that health disparities based on social and economic disparities among groups persist and have, in fact, widened in some cases. Aday (2001) pointed out the importance of public health, social, and economic policy considerations in addressing the fundamental origins of poor physical, psychological, and social health among vulnerable populations (e.g., persons with HIV/AIDS, the mentally ill, alcohol and substance abusers, families living with physical or emotional abuse, the homeless, immigrant and refugee populations). The challenge to both the medical care and the public health communities is to create and extend the partnerships between them and with other sectors to more effectively address persistent or widening subgroup disparities in health.

Distributive Justice

The distributive justice paradigm has dominated the conceptualization and measurement of the equity of the US healthcare system. Illustrative examples and estimates of indicators of equity based on the distributive justice framework are highlighted in Appendix 7.1. The presentation and discussion of findings in the context of this paradigm focus principally on trends in potential access indicators, their relationship to predicting people's actual utilization, and their levels of satisfaction with care, as well as likely health consequences.

Delivery System

Availability

Potential Access

The number and distribution of providers and, more important, the effect of service availability on the decision to seek care have been and continue to be a focus of health policy efforts. Post–World War II policies supporting medical personnel training and new hospital construction led to overall increases in the number of providers and facilities. These increases were mirrored in steady rises in the traditional provider-to-population and facility-to-population ratios. While many of these policies continue in modified forms to the present day, wide variability nonetheless persists in the geographic distribution of providers. Many areas are facing critical shortages of nurses. Ongoing changes in the financing and management of healthcare, most recently the advent of accountable care organizations (ACOs), have also affected the overall availability of and need for different types of physicians by increasing the demand for primary care physicians and diminishing the use of specialists in many areas (CMS 2010b).

An issue related to availability is the increasing unwillingness of providers to see patients who are publicly insured or uninsured. Physicians' refusal to see Medicaid clients creates significant barriers to care for low-income, pregnant women, particularly those residing in rural and inner-city areas with large minority populations (Grayson 2004; Greene, Blustein, and Remler 2005; Kemper and Clark 2005; Mullan 2002; NCHS 2011; Perloff et al. 1997; Quast, Sappington, and Shenkman 2008; Salsberg and Forte 2002; Silverstein and Kirkman-Liff 1995; Simon, Dranove, and White 1998; Sochalski 2002).

Realized Access

Provider-to-population ratios alone do not determine actual rates of use. Insurance coverage and the availability of a racially and ethnically diverse provider workforce may be equally important as (or even more important than) overall physician supply in influencing access to care, especially in high-risk, underserved communities. There is heightened concern over the effect of a number of national and local trends on the availability of providers and the resultant utilization patterns of residents in rural and inner-city communities. These trends include the buyout and conversion of not-for-profit community hospitals by for-profit healthcare corporations; closures of rural hospitals and of financially stressed safety-net providers serving poor, inner-city populations; and reluctance on the part of primary care providers to relocate to or remain in these same areas (Ballance, Kornegay, and Evans 2009; Claxton et al. 1997; Cunningham 2002; Grumbach, Vranizan, and Bindman 1997; Hixon and Buenconsejo-Lum 2010; MacDowell et al. 2010; Rabinowitz et al. 2010; Ricketts III 2002; Robert Graham Center 2005; Sequist 2011; Stenger, Cashman, and Savageau 2008).

Health Impacts

The effect that the trends discussed in the previous paragraphs will have on actual patterns of service use and health depends to a large extent on whether alternative and appropriate service delivery arrangements subsequently become available to the populations previously served by the displaced providers (e.g., through reconfiguring a formerly inpatient-oriented, rural hospital to a primary care or emergency care service provider). The shortage of nurses in many communities has raised concerns about the quality of hospital nursing care. The lack of an adequate system of primary care in general, and maternity and prenatal care services in particular, for low-income, inner-city women and for poor minorities living in isolated rural counties or communities has been found to contribute to their lower rates of use of effective preventive and illness-related care. HSR has documented higher rates of avoidable hospitalizations and ambulatory care–sensitive conditions (i.e., disease occurrence that could have been prevented with adequate primary care) among racial/ethnic minorities and in medically underserved areas with lower socioeconomic status (Agabiti et al. 2009; Biello et al. 2010; Billings, Anderson, and Newman 1996; Bindman et al. 1995; Davis, Liu, and Gibbons 2003; Epstein 2001; Gaskin and Hoffman 2000; IOM 1993; Jiang et al. 2005; Moy, Barrett, and Ho 2011; NCHS 2011).

Organization

Potential Access

The organization and financing of healthcare in the United States increasingly reflect a tiered system of benefits. In descending order of coverage depth, beneficiaries include the privately insured middle and upper classes, including the elderly who have Medicare combined with supplemental insurance; the elderly who have Medicare only; the poor, Medicaid-eligible indigent and working-class population; and individuals and families with neither public nor private coverage. Such disparities have always been a fact of life in the US healthcare system. They emerge as a particular paradox today, however, because as the overall public and private commitment of expenditures for medical care has continued to rise, so has the number of Americans who have no or inadequate protection against these burgeoning increases. The US healthcare system has been characterized as a "medical-industrial complex" in reference to the large network of private corporations engaged in the business of supplying medical care to patients for a profit, such as chain hospitals, walk-in clinics, dialysis centers, and home health care companies. The diverse and evolving forms of medical practice are linked to methods of paying for care. Organizational models include group practice–based health maintenance organizations (HMOs); individual practice associations, which usually contract with multiple payers; individual and group practice physicians; preferred provider organizations (PPOs); point-of-service plans; and the emerging ACOs. It is important to realize that most medical care financed through the public sector (i.e., through Medicare and Medicaid) is, by design, delivered by private-sector providers.

As of 2010, HMOs and PPOs accounted for the largest portions of the population enrolled in managed care (MCOL Research 2013). However, the organizational distinctions between managed care arrangements are becoming increasingly obscure. All have attempted to develop systems of cost-conscious medical practice and methods of reimbursement. Managed care organizations (MCOs) have historically limited consumer choice of providers to participating physicians and emphasized primary care and less use of specialists, although it is now common for plans to enable enrollees to self-refer to specialists (Anthony 2003; Forrest et al. 2001). Competition among MCOs has also reduced cross-subsidies ("cost shifting") to safety-net providers that serve large numbers of uninsured or medically indigent and either threatened or led to the closure of many safety-net institutions, such as community health centers and Medicaid-dependent hospitals. To address these trends, the ACA increases emphasis on community health centers, increases payments for primary care, expands eligibility for Medicaid, and mandates that, with a few exceptions, everyone has to buy health insurance that meets certain minimum standards (Office of the Legislative Counsel 2010). While these changes are expected to reduce the burden of uncompensated care on safety-net hospitals, policy changes also include reductions in federal payments to disproportionate-share hospitals, which are used to offset the costs of those hospitals' care for the uninsured. Consequently, the net effect of these changes on safety-net hospitals has been subject to debate (Felland, Grossman, and Tu 2011; Katz 2010; Katz and Brigham 2011; Wang, Conroy, and Zuckerman 2009).

The growing number of elderly—particularly the oldest old—and the impetus for shortened lengths of hospital stay resulting from implementation of prospective payment (e.g., payment based on DRGs) are placing increased financial pressures on families and other home- and community-based long-term care (LTC) arrangements (Boucher et al. 2006; Mayes 2007; Mayes and Berenson 2006; Rayburn 1992). The deinstitutionalization movement in mental health care leading to the discharge of large numbers of mentally ill patients also has greatly increased the burden of care on community-based mental health services provision (Aday 2001; Bazzoli et al. 1999; Burns et al. 2000; Deb and Holmes 1998; Dranove and White 1998; Felt-Lisk, McHugh, and Howell 2002; Gaskin, Hadley, and Freeman 2001; Lamb and Weinberger 2005; McAlearney 2002; Penrod et al. 1998; Relman 1980; Talbott 2004).

It is important to note that the US healthcare financing system historically has prioritized coverage of care for acute medical conditions. Preventive care, mental health care, and LTC have, until recently, been treated differently. Coverage for mental health care is changing due to the passage of legislation, such as the Medicare Improvements for Patients and Providers Act of 2008, which mandated equal copayments for mental health and medical care under Medicare, and provisions in the ACA and earlier acts, which mandated coverage for increasing numbers of preventive services (110th Congress 2008; Smaldone and Cullen-Drill 2010). LTC remains problematic. LTC is explicitly not covered by Medicare (although short-term skilled nursing care is) and is rarely covered by private medical insurance, leaving LTC costs to be covered by Medicaid, private LTC insurance, and individuals out of pocket. The rapidly growing demand for LTC services has led to stark, income-based disparities in access and increasing reliance on the Medicaid program, which already finances more than 40 percent of all LTC in the United States (Catlin et al. 2008). In 2006, LTC costs accounted for 36 percent of all Medicaid spending, a sobering statistic for state legislatures struggling to balance state budgets amid revenue shortfalls and rising Medicaid expenditures. This percentage is expected to grow as the demand for LTC increases (Kaiser Commission on Medicaid and the Uninsured 2008).

Realized Access

The major concerns underlying the realized-access impact of the corporatization of medical practice relate to the fact that private and for-profit institutions are less likely to serve the poor and medically indigent and that large-scale, bureaucratic, publicly supported providers are less flexible in their financing of new service arrangements. Public hospitals have been more subject to closure or purchase by for-profit entities in an increasingly competitive healthcare environment. MCOs primarily have enrolled employed individuals, especially employees of large firms. Employers and insurers typically have restricted enrollment and coverage for employees' dependents and for particularly vulnerable or high-risk populations (e.g., persons with AIDS), and coverage, copayments, and enrollment restrictions have increased along with the steady increase in premiums for employer-based insurance. Both not-for-profit and for-profit private institutions are less likely to serve patients without insurance and have much lower rates of uncompensated and undercompensated care than publicly supported institutions have—teaching hospitals in particular. States have responded by enacting laws to ensure access and to improve the accountability of MCOs for the quality and appropriateness of care for managed care enrollees in general and for the most vulnerable enrollees in particular (Gosfield 1997; Marsteller, Bovbjerg, and Nichols 1998; Proenca, Rosko, and Zinn 2000).

Health Impacts

Users of publicly supported facilities, such as public health clinics, hospital outpatient departments, and emergency departments, often may have to wait hours to be seen when they are ill or injured or may be told that it will be weeks or even months before they can get an appointment for a routine or prevention-related visit (e.g., for prenatal care). Both situations place these individuals at risk of serious health consequences. Even among an insured population, such as Medicare beneficiaries, individuals may not have the same access to health services due to differences between MCO and FFS care policies. Data from the Consumer Assessment of Health Providers and Systems surveys indicate that MCO-enrolled beneficiaries are healthier than their FFS counterparts, and MCOs are better at delivering preventive care. In contrast, FFS-enrolled beneficiaries have better access to other types of services and reported slightly greater satisfaction with care overall. While physical and mental health outcomes did not differ for the average MCO and FFS patient, elderly, poor, and chronically ill MCO patients experienced poorer physical health outcomes (Berk, Schur, and Cantor 1995; IOM 1993; Keenan et al. 2009; Landon et al. 2004; Pourat, Kagawa-Singer, and Wallace 2006; Shimada et al. 2009).

Financing

Potential Access

Since the 1940s, private health insurance has assumed a larger role in financing healthcare through employer-based coverage. The advent of Medicaid and Medicare in the mid-1960s led to a significant increase in the proportion of personal healthcare expenditures paid for by the federal government, while the proportion of out-of-pocket expenditures borne by households and individuals has declined dramatically (see Appendix 7.1). As the costs of care continued to rise, public and private third-party payers became increasingly interested in reducing the amounts they had to pay for medical care. The primary cost control shift came in the form of fixed, predetermined (i.e., prospective) rates of reimbursement by service or diagnosis, such as DRGs, and greater consumer cost sharing.

Medicaid expansions and the Children's Health Insurance Program have attempted to expand public coverage to a large number of uninsured families and children in many states. Nonetheless, as discussed later in this chapter, the number of uninsured Americans has remained large, adding impetus to the push for healthcare reform in 2010. A number of key provisions in the ACA, such as the expansion of Medicaid eligibility and the individual mandate for insurance coverage, were specifically targeted at reducing the number of uninsured (Blackwell and Tonthat 2003; Choi, Sommers, and McWilliams 2011; Hofer, Abraham, and Moscovice 2011; Levit et al. 2003; Office of the Legislative Counsel 2010; Pande et al. 2011; Racine et al. 2001; Rosenbaum et al. 1998; Shields, McGinn-Shapiro, and Fronstin 2008; Yu and Dick 2009).

Realized Access

The presence and extent of insurance coverage have been demonstrated to be important predictors of the utilization of medical care services in numerous national and local studies of access. Lack of insurance and related barriers have historically diminished minorities' use of preventive services and medical treatments that could improve health and reduce the associated burden of illness (Kaiser Commission on Medicaid and the Uninsured 2010, 2002; Patel, Bae, and Singh 2010; Weissman et al. 2008).

Insurance coverage and regular sources of care have increasingly been combined in various types of managed care arrangements. Managed care enrollees have lower hospital admission rates and shorter lengths of stay than do those covered under FFS arrangements. Research suggests that they have comparable or somewhat higher physician office visit rates, lower use of expensive tests and procedures, and greater use of preventive services. With regard to access to services, however, racial/ethnic disparities persist among managed care enrollees. Expanded coverage is important to addressing disparities overall, but barriers to equity may still exist (Cook 2007; Haas et al. 2002; Hargraves, Cunningham, and Hughes 2001; Keenan et al. 2009; Lin et al. 2005; Miller and Luft 2002; Phillips, Mayer, and Aday 2000; Shimada et al. 2009; Trivedi et al. 2005).

At a systemic level, hospital utilization and expenditures show that admission rates, total days of care, and average length of stay have declined since the introduction of prospective payment (e.g., DRG-based reimbursement for hospital services), although these trends are confounded with trends that were already underway in the organization and delivery of medical care prior to the introduction of DRGs, such as increasing emphasis on ambulatory care. (See Chapters 1 and 5 for discussion of these trends.) The tendency to discharge Medicare patients when they reach the limit of reimbursable days under DRGs exposed deficiencies in the system of post-hospitalization care for the chronically ill and elderly in many communities, such as inadequate discharge planning, an insufficient number of nursing home beds, lack of community support services, and corollary stresses on patients' families.

Health Impacts

The RAND Health Insurance Experiment documented an inverse relationship between the amount of physician and hospital services consumed and the amount of consumer copayment: The more consumers had to pay, the less medical care they consumed. The office-based medical use rates for children in particular were likely to be lower for those in cost-sharing plans than for those in free-care plans. Although the RAND Experiment documented minimal overall negative health consequences resulting from plan cost-sharing provisions, the negative effects it did find were primarily among low-income, chronically ill individuals. Medical care expenses tend to absorb a much higher proportion of the total income of low-income families than that of families with higher incomes. Policies that encourage greater cost sharing by consumers will undoubtedly reduce the overall use of services, although research suggests that consumers do not discriminate among the services they forego. The resultant economic and health effects are most likely to fall on the poorest and sickest (Anderson, Brook, and Williams 1991; Angelelli et al. 2002; Chandra, Gruber, and McKnight 2010; Chernew and Newhouse 2008; Gross et al. 1999; Newhouse 2004).

Population at Risk

At the population level, equity is grounded in the similar-treatment norm: Variations in medical care utilization should be primarily a function of need rather than of demographic or organization-related healthcare factors. It is particularly important to probe differences in healthcare use and satisfaction with care that are related to an array of predisposing, enabling, and need factors to gain a better understanding of the origins and consequences of health and healthcare disparities.

Predisposing Factors

Age is significantly associated with medical care service use, primarily because it is an important indicator of acquired morbidity. With respect to **gender**, women generally use more health services than do men; to some extent, this difference is a function of their obstetrics-related care needs, their greater longevity, and the perception that it is more socially acceptable for women to engage in help-seeking behaviors. As noted earlier, however, substantial availability, organizational, and financial barriers exist for certain categories of women—especially low-income, uninsured, or Medicaid-eligible women—seeking prenatal and maternity care services. Many women have lost Medicaid benefits as a result of changes in the welfare system, a trend that is exacerbated by states' reliance on service cuts (e.g., in Medicaid) as the preferred mechanism for addressing state budget shortfalls (Hanson 2003; Ross and Marks 2009; Salganicoff et al. 2002; Short and Freedman 1998; Zerzan et al. 2007). **Education** is an important predictor of the use of preventive services. Better-educated people are, for example, more likely to have had a general physical, immunizations, tests, and procedures for preventive purposes, and better-educated women are more likely to have sought care early in their pregnancy. Although racial and ethnic disparities in health and healthcare persist, studies indicate that disparities apparently attributable to race/ethnicity may be partially attributable to geographic disparities instead, emphasizing our need to better understand the influence of regional and community characteristics on access and use of healthcare (Escarce and Goodell 2007; Fiscella et al. 2002; Gilbert et al. 2002; Gresenz, Rogowski, and Escarce 2009; Lambrew 2001; Mayberry, Mili, and Ofili 2000; Mead et al. 2008; Mueller et al. 1999; NCHS 2011; Williams and Mohammed 2009). The influence of predisposing factors such as age, gender, education, and race/ethnicity on utilization has remained relatively stable over time (see Appendix 7.1).

Enabling Factors

Having a regular source of medical care is a strong and consistent predictor of service utilization, particularly the initial decision to seek care. Having an identifiable provider may be particularly important to motivating the use of routine preventive care. According to the 2009 National Health Interview Survey (NHIS), 5.6 percent of children (i.e., aged 0 to 17) and 19.5 percent of adults did not have a usual source of care. Among those who did, private doctors' offices were visited most frequently, followed by health centers and similar sites, such as company or school clinics, and hospital outpatient and emergency departments. Blacks, Hispanics, the poor, males, and residents of large metropolitan areas were least likely to have a regular source of care. If they did have a regular source of care, they were more likely to use clinics or hospital outpatient and emergency departments (NCHS 2011).

In 2009, the percentage of people who saw a doctor during the year was lower among people from families with incomes below the poverty level (80.6 percent) than among those with incomes above the poverty level (86.4 percent). On the basis of subjective perceptions of health, reported days of limited activity due to illness, and limitations in major activity due to the presence of a chronic condition, NHIS survey data indicated that people with lower incomes were in much poorer health than were people with higher incomes. Since the introduction of Medicaid and Medicare, the rates of hospital discharges, days of care, lengths of stay, and the mean number of follow-up visits to physicians have tended to be greater for those with lower rather than higher incomes, reflecting perhaps their greater need and their greater tendency to delay seeking care until the health problem has worsened (NCHS 2011). Along these lines, evidence that healthcare use by previously uninsured adults increases dramatically on enrollment in Medicare was cited in support of the ACA's mandate that all individuals purchase insurance (Hofer, Abraham, and Moscovice 2011; McWilliams et al. 2009, 2007).

Once entry to the system is gained, having an established provider is a less significant predictor of the subsequent number of visits to a physician or length of hospital stay. With the advent of managed care, the identification of a regular provider is increasingly linked to enrolling in a particular health plan. Uninsured individuals are more likely to lack a usual source of care and confront more barriers to access and have lower rates of preventive services use (Cunningham et al. 2007; DeVoe et al. 2011, 2003; Ettner 1996; Hoilette et al. 2009; Kuder and Levitz 1985; Lambrew et al. 1996; Merzel and Moon-Howard 2002; Xu 2002). Almost 17 percent of the US population (an estimated 50.7 million) lacked public or private insurance in 2009. The number of people who were uninsured over a two-year period is even greater. Young adults, children under age 18, Hispanics, blacks, and the poor are more likely to be uninsured at some point in a given year. The percentage of uninsured is higher among blacks and Hispanics than among other racial groups (DeNavas-Walt, Proctor, and Smith 2010). The rate of uninsurance or underinsurance in the United States was a central theme leading to the passage of the ACA.

Most of the uninsured historically have been workers or the dependents of workers who do not receive health insurance through their jobs—for example, workers in small firms or in industries, such as service and agriculture, that do not provide coverage. Even when coverage is offered by employers, the high costs of the plans have inhibited low-wage workers from purchasing coverage. Among those who are insured at a given point in time, some may be inadequately protected (or not protected at all) against the possibility of large medical bills. Those who are uninsured for some period are at higher risk of going without needed medical care than are those who are continuously insured (Andrulis et al. 2003; Collins et al. 2004; Gabel et al. 2002; Gould 2009; Holahan, Hoffman, and Wang 2003; Marquis and Long 2001; Rowland, Hoffman, and McGinn-Shapiro 2009; Schoen and DesRoches 2000; Shen and Long 2006; Vistnes and Selden 2011). As mentioned earlier, the ACA contained several provisions aimed specifically at reducing the rate of uninsurance, balancing the responsibility between individuals (i.e., the mandate that individuals have insurance), employers (i.e., the requirement that firms greater than a specified size provide insurance), and public systems (i.e., expansion of Medicaid and premium assistance for low-income individuals) (Hofer, Abraham, and Moscovice 2011; Office of the Legislative Counsel 2010).

Need

Assessments of need may be based on patients' self-perceptions of their health as well as on medical professionals' clinical diagnoses and evaluations. Providers' and patients' evaluations of needs may not always agree. Nonetheless, need—however measured—is an important predictor of the use of services and, in particular, of the volume of services consumed. Need is generally the most important predictor of the number of physician visits a person makes after an initial visit and of the number of days of care once a patient is admitted to a hospital. The utilization of services may be deemed equitable to the extent that services are distributed on the basis of need. However, for prevention-oriented or discretionary services, such as dental care, need continues to be a less important predictor of utilization than are other factors, particularly enabling factors such as income and insurance coverage (Aday, Andersen, and Fleming 1980; Al Snih et al. 2006; Andersen 1995; Andersen and Davidson 2001; Andersen et al. 1987; Blackwell et al. 2009; Brown et al. 2009).

There is evidence that enabling factors potentially responsive to policy intervention and predisposing and need factors explain many of the differences in realized access between racial/ethnic groups (Al Snih et al. 2006; Blackwell et al. 2009; Brown et al. 2009; Iversen, Chhabriya, and Shadick 2011; Morgan et al. 2009). Surveys of public and patient opinion regarding the performance of the medical care system in different countries confirm that US residents are more critical of the system as a whole and much less satisfied with their own particular care experiences than are people in other countries, including, for example, Australia, Canada, New Zealand, and the United Kingdom (see Appendix 7.1). In 2010, 27 percent of US residents thought the system had so much wrong with it that it should be completely rebuilt, whereas around 3 to 20 percent of people in the other countries had the same sentiment about their nation's system. US residents also tended to report more problems with paying medical bills and negotiating insurance coverage and payment. However, US residents were more satisfied with their access to specialty care. Minorities indicate they confront more barriers and rate the healthcare system less highly than do white Americans (Blendon et al. 2002; Schoen et al. 2010). Satisfaction with healthcare also varies by age, gender, and race/ethnicity. However, as with realized access, potentially policy-sensitive predisposing, enabling, and need factors (e.g., insurance, education, knowledge, health status) may explain a substantial portion of the racial/ethnic differences regarding satisfaction (Cook 2007; Katz and Brigham 2011; Keenan et al. 2009; Morgan et al. 2009; Riley et al. 2008; Shimada et al. 2009; Taira et al. 2001; Trivedi et al. 2005; Weech-Maldonado et al. 2001).

Deliberative Justice

As indicated in the previous chapter, individual and community empowerment and participation have been important components of many international and national health initiatives. However, there are no standardized or widely applied indicators and scales for measuring this key dimension of deliberative justice. Voter turnout rates and public opinion polls regarding levels of perceived confidence in the US population's ability to influence public officials provide macro-level evidence of the presence and magnitude of civic participation. The failure of the Clinton administration's healthcare reform initiatives in the early 1990s was attributed to the dominance of technical-rational experts in the policy formulation process and the lack of a clear public consensus in support of comprehensive reform (Hacker 1996; Skocpol 1996). In contrast, or perhaps in reaction, the discussion leading to the passage of the ACA was explicitly more open, although much of the public discussion was inconclusive, and much of the public's influence on the development of policy was exerted through advocacy groups (Staff of the Washington Post 2010).

Effective implementation of models of deliberative democracy, in which vulnerable populations such as African Americans have full and fair representation in the committees addressing racial/ethnic disparities, has been suggested as an innovative means to productively address persistent disparities. A number of different methods have been utilized to measure participation at the micro and macro levels. Attitudinal scales can be used to assess organization and community members' sense of control or influence over the decisions that most directly affect their health and well-being. Surveys are useful tools for assessing the capacity of health departments to engage in community-based, participatory public health and the magnitude of de facto community mobilization around a public health intervention. Key informant interviews and social network analysis also yield useful data for mapping the extent of community involvement in health program design (Aronson et al. 2007; Bartholomew et al. 2011; Cheadle et al. 2001; Dunet et al. 2008; Gong et al. 2009; Hendryx et al. 2002; Israel et al. 2010, 1994; Parker et al. 2003; Stone 2002; Wagemakers et al. 2010; Wickizer et al. 1993).

A number of practices have been used by MCOs to limit the involvement of both patients and providers in decision making, including "gag rules" that inhibit providers from discussing selected treatment options with patients, "cram-down rules" that compel providers to participate in a state-mandated managed care program to receive benefits through other payer arrangements, selective or misleading plan marketing to potential enrollees, time constraints on patient–provider visits and failure to provide cultural-competency training that could affect patient–provider communication, and adversarial or obstructionist consumer grievance and dispute resolution procedures. While there has been pushback from patients and physicians against many of these practices (e.g., gag rules, misleading plan marketing), they are sentinel indicators of likely deliberative justice concerns. Some of these practices or failures also may have been present in FFS Medicaid provider arrangements; however, Medicaid eligibles' options are likely to be constrained as a function of mandated enrollment in what might be a limited number of competing managed care plans in a given area (Daniels 2001; Holahan and Yemane 2009; Lin et al. 2005; Martin 2011; Quast, Sappington, and Shenkman 2008; Shimada et al. 2009).

Possible future directions for research in the area of community or consumer participation in health policy design would be to extend the conceptual and methodological development of indicators of deliberative justice; to use them in evaluating the performance of policies and programs at the national, community, system, institutional, and patient levels; and to examine their importance in influencing access to health and healthcare on the part of the individuals and of the communities they were intended to serve.

The weight of the evidence indicates that disparities have not been substantially reduced. The evidence of the successes of the broad policy strategies for enhancing equity outlined earlier may be viewed at best as mixed and at worst as falling far short of desired equity objectives. The bulk of the evidence regarding the goal of enhancing access to medical care is rooted in the distributive justice paradigm of individuals' rights to medical care. Although substantial investments in the organization and financing of medical care services have been made at federal, state, and local levels, wide variations in access to care and coverage persist across regions and subgroups of the US population, and the costs and effectiveness of the care provided continue to present challenges to policymakers who must decide what rights should be ensured and at what cost to whom.

The *Healthy People* 2010 and 2020 objectives provide a template for examining the extent to which the social justice goals of minimizing health risks and health disparities have been achieved. Evidence of subgroup variation (or lack thereof) indicates whether the desired health promotion, health protection, and preventive services goals have been achieved. The data routinely gathered to monitor progress toward these objectives show that progress has been made toward some of the goals but that disparities persist—or have widened—in the areas addressed by the rest.

Although evidence is emerging regarding the importance of participation by affected parties in health policy and program design, the deliberative justice paradigm has been largely unexamined as a component of the fairness of the policy formulation and implementation process. The challenge to the public health and HSR community is to determine how best to conceptualize and measure norms of deliberative justice so that the presence and impact of this innovative benchmark of fairness can be more explicitly assessed.

The available evidence suggests that the major health policy strategies directed at achieving both procedural and substantive equity have, as a whole, fallen short. The ACA was a major initiative directed at ameliorating some of the principal contributors to inequities (e.g., lack of health insurance, scope of benefits). However, the ACA provisions have a long implementation period and are still evolving (Kaiser Family Foundation 2010a).

The next section reviews the specific criteria for evaluating equity in the context of breast cancer prevention and treatment to set the stage for the policy example in Chapter 9, which focuses on evaluation of a specific policy alternative—increasing mammography screening rates among low-income, uninsured women.

Criteria for Assessing Health Policies in Terms of Equity Promotion

Exhibit 7.1 summarizes the criteria for assessing health policies in terms of whether they promote equity and provides illustrative examples of the application of these criteria to breast cancer screening and treatment.

EXHIBIT 7.1
Criteria for
Assessing
Health Policies
in Terms
of Equity
Promotion

Dimensions	Criteria	Indicators	Examples
Procedural Equity			
Deliberative Justice			
Health policy	Participation	Ensure that affected groups participate in formulating and implementing policies and programs.	*Population:* Medicaid screening policies have been influenced but not driven by women's health advocacy interests. *Clinical:* Clinical guidelines do not provide explicit guidance for interactive patient–provider consideration of the role of risk factors and age in deciding on whether or how often to screen.
Distributive Justice			
Delivery system • Availability • Organization • Financing	Freedom of choice	Maximize the availability and minimize the constraints on patients' choice of providers and services.	*Availability:* Fewer mammography screening facilities are available in rural and inner-city areas, which have a disproportionate representation of older and minority women. *Organization:* Certain types of providers may be more likely to recommend screening, but substantial variability exists across provider settings. *Financing:* Out-of-pocket costs for treatment and lack of insurance are burdensome to many (especially low-income) women.

Realized access • Utilization • Satisfaction	Cost-effectiveness	Enhance access to prevention and treatment benefits and services that are most likely to be cost-effective.	*Utilization:* The use and adherence rates for mammography, one of the most effective breast cancer screening procedures, still fall far short of the *Healthy People* 2010 objectives. *Satisfaction:* The quality of the doctor–patient relationship, including patient-centeredness and empathy, as well as cultural barriers to care affect satisfaction with medical care in general and particularly women's satisfaction with well-woman and related healthcare services.
Distributive and Social Justice			
Population at risk • Predisposing • Enabling • Need	Similar treatment	Minimize disparities in access to benefits and services across subgroups, particularly among those most at risk.	*Predisposing:* Mammography utilization and adherence rates decline with age and are lower for minority women and women in rural areas. *Enabling:* Having a regular source of care enhances mammography screening rates, though other barriers (e.g., lack of insurance, limited access to screening services) may influence screening rates. *Need:* Death rates and rates of late-stage diagnosis are higher among elderly and black women.

(continued)

EXHIBIT 7.1
(continued)

Social Justice			
Environment • Physical • Social • Economic	Common good	Emphasize primary prevention (disease prevention and health promotion).	*Environment:* Social determinants research documents the influence of social and economic context and related exposures to environmental risks on risk of breast cancer. Specific environmental risk factors have not yet been fully documented, though genetic risk factors influence recommendations regarding mammography screening intervals.
Health risks • Environmental • Behavioral	Need	Emphasize environmental and behavioral risk reduction.	*Health risks:* Smoking and obesity have been found to be associated with higher risk of breast cancer, though mammography screening guidelines do not explicitly take these factors into account.
Substantive Equity			
Health • Patients • Community	Need	Reduce morbidity and mortality overall as well as disparities between subgroups.	*Health:* The percentage of breast cancers diagnosed at a late stage is much higher among black and Hispanic women than among white women. Rate of death due to breast cancer is much higher among blacks than among other races.

The deliberative justice norm of participation focuses on affected groups' involvement in formulating and implementing policies and programs. Participation may be viewed at the macro level as affected populations' role in shaping national or state policy and at the micro or clinical level as patients' engagement in clinical decision making related to their care. For example, Medicare and Medicaid breast and cervical cancer screening policies have been influenced but not driven by women's health advocacy interests. Clinical guidelines do not provide explicit guidance for interactive and effective patient–provider decision making on whether and how often to screen, given the patient's risk factors and age. Research has, however, suggested that women's participation in the decision to be screened leads to higher mammography adherence rates (Abbaszadeh et al. 2007; Phillips et al. 2010, 1998; Platner et al. 2002). The norm of freedom of choice, grounded in the distributive justice paradigm, argues for maximizing—and minimizing the constraints on—patients' choice of providers and services. This criterion is documented most directly through evidence on the availability of providers and services, the accessibility of services within specific organizational and service delivery contexts, and the affordability of services as a function of the cost and extent of third-party financing.

Substantial barriers impede the availability of breast cancer screening and related treatment services. Mammography screening facilities are less available in rural and inner-city areas, which have a disproportionate representation of older (over age 50) and minority women. Select types of MCOs may be more likely than FFS providers to recommend screening, but substantial variability exists across provider settings. Although private and public insurers may cover mammography screening, other factors—disruptions in eligibility, out-of-pocket costs related to deductibles, copayments, or resulting treatment costs—are burdensome to many (especially low-income) women (Feresu et al. 2008; Lee-Feldstein et al. 2000; Lin et al. 2005; McAlearney et al. 2007; O'Malley, Forrest, and Mandelblatt 2002; Perkins et al. 2001; Trivedi, Rakowski, and Ayanian 2008). However, the expansion of Medicaid eligibility under the provisions of the ACA may alleviate the financial burden of treatment, especially when combined with programs such as the Texas Breast and Cervical Cancer Services (TBCCS), which are explicitly directed at getting eligible women diagnosed with breast and cervical cancer enrolled in Medicaid (Texas Department of State Health Services 2013).

The cost-effectiveness norm focuses on enhancing access to prevention and treatment benefits and services that are most likely to be cost-effective. The cost-effectiveness criterion is discussed more fully in Chapter 5. Rates of utilization of services that have been documented to effectively prevent or remedy health problems, as well as patients' preferences and levels of satisfaction with care, provide useful input for judgments of the extent to which cost-effective services are being provided. *Effective access* exists when the use of select services improves health status. The definition of *efficient access* is linked to the improvement in health status relative to healthcare costs (Andersen 1995; Andersen and Davidson 2001; IOM 1993).

Mammography screening has been documented to be the most effective technology to date for detecting early-stage breast cancer (Feig 2002; Humphrey et al. 2002; National Cancer Institute 2011a; Smith et al. 2010). Although the rates of mammography use and adherence have increased over the past decade, they remain short of the *Healthy People* 2010 objectives, especially among Hispanic, multiracial, and low-income women (see Appendix 7.1). The quality of the doctor–patient relationship, including patient-centeredness and empathy, and cultural barriers to care affect satisfaction with medical care in general and particularly women's satisfaction with well-woman and related women's healthcare services (Bibb 2001; Copeland, Scholle, and Binko 2003; Donelan et al. 2011; Foxall, Barron, and Houfek 2001; Parchman and Burge 2004; Ramirez et al. 2000; Robertson, Dixon, and Le Grand 2008; Sheppard et al. 2008; Valdez et al. 2001).

The similar-treatment norm argues for minimizing disparities in access to benefits and services across subgroups, particularly among those most at risk. Variations in rates of service utilization and health outcomes are sentinel indicators of likely problems with the equity of healthcare services delivery. The predisposing, enabling, and need dimensions of the equity framework (Exhibit 7.1) provide guidance for identifying potential equity issues related to the similar-treatment norm. *Equitable access* exists when predisposing factors (e.g., age, gender, need) account for most of the variation in use. *Inequitable access* exists when system factors and predisposing social characteristics (e.g., race/ethnicity) determine who receives care (Andersen 1995; Andersen and Davidson 2001). The roles of enabling factors, such as income and insurance coverage, are at the heart of the philosophical debate about healthcare reform. More precisely, the debate is not about the relationships between insurance, income, and access but rather about individual versus collective responsibility for ensuring equitable financial access to healthcare services (see Chapter 6 for a discussion of theoretical paradigms underlying perceptions of fairness). The similar-treatment norm and related evidence regarding subgroup variations in breast cancer prevalence and screening rates will be central to evaluating mammography screening policy for women aged 40 to 64 (see Chapter 9).

Death rates and rates of late stage of diagnosis are higher among elderly and black women. Nonetheless, mammography utilization and adherence rates decline with age and are lower among minority women and among women in rural areas. Having a regular source of care enhances mammography screening rates, although other barriers, such as lack of transportation and limited access to screening services, may influence screening rates, especially among women most at risk (Amey, Miller, and Albrecht 1997; Bloom et al. 2001; Coughlin et al. 2002; Harper et al. 2009; Hirschman, Whitman, and Ansell 2007; Khan et al. 2010; Kim and Jang 2008; Legler et al. 2002; Lorant et al. 2002; Miller and Champion 1997; Qureshi et al. 2000; Selvin and Brett 2003).

The norms of common good and need, grounded in the social justice paradigm, emphasize primary prevention (disease prevention and health promotion) and related environmental- and behavioral-risk reduction. Public health and clinical research on the risk factors for the development of breast cancer has not yet identified clear primary breast cancer prevention strategies. Social-determinants research documents the influence of social and economic context, and related exposures to environmental factors, on risk of breast cancer. Specific environmental risk factors have not yet been fully documented, although genetic risk factors influence recommendations regarding mammography screening intervals. Smoking and obesity have been found to be associated with higher risk of breast cancer, although breast cancer clinical risk assessment protocols and related mammography screening guidelines do not explicitly take these factors into account (Anglin 1998; Caplan et al. 2000; Chlebowski 2000; Dal Maso et al. 2008; Ferrante et al. 2010; Gonzalez and Riboli 2010; Johnson-Thompson and Guthrie 2000; Kono 2010; Sprecher Institute for Comparative Cancer Research 2013; Steiner, Klubert, and Knutson 2008).

The bottom line to achieving substantive equity is reduction of morbidity and mortality overall as well as reduction of disparities between subgroups. The *Healthy People* 2010 objectives provided explicit benchmarks for judging whether substantive equity has been achieved. As documented in Chapter 1, the rates and distribution of breast cancer in the United States continue to fall short of these objectives. The percentage of breast cancers diagnosed at a late stage is much higher among black and Hispanic women than among white women. Rates of death due to breast cancer are much higher among blacks than among other racial groups.

In summary, major procedural and substantive equity issues exist with respect to incidence, screening, and treatment for breast cancer. In Chapter 9, effectiveness, efficiency, and equity criteria are integrated and applied to evaluate the breast cancer screening component of the Texas BCCS Program, which provides screening and diagnostic services for the low-income uninsured population in Texas under the auspices of the National Breast and Cervical Cancer Early Detection Program.

Summary and Conclusions

The health policy goal of equity has not yet been achieved in the United States. Significant health disparities persist between racial, ethnic, and socioeconomic groups. Vulnerable populations remain at risk of receiving less, or less than adequate, healthcare. Both public and private policymaking appears to eschew rather than elicit the views of affected stakeholders. A core argument of this book is that the ultimate measure of success of US health policy is the level of improvement in the health of the population. This and the previous chapter provide a conceptual blueprint and methodological tools for designing health policy directed toward achieving this objective more effectively.

APPENDIX 7.1
Highlights
of Selected
Indicators of
Equity of Access
to Healthcare

Potential Access
Delivery System

Availability: Distribution of Providers (Boukus, Cassil, and O'Malley 2009; Kaiser Family Foundation 2011b; NCHS 2012)

Active physicians per 10,000 civilian population (2009)

USA = 27.4	Washington, DC = 73.8	Texas = 21.6	Alaska = 24.2

Employed nurses per 100,000 resident population (2011)

USA = 874	Washington, DC = 1,728	Texas = 720	Alaska = 755

Percentage of nonfederal patient care physicians providing charity care

1997	2001	2005	2008
76.3	71.5	68.2	59.1

Percentage of nonfederal patient care physicians receiving revenue from Medicaid

1997	2001	2005	2008
87.1	85.4	85.4	—

Percentage of nonfederal patient care physicians not accepting new patients, by patient insurance status

	1997	2001	2005	2008
Medicaid	19.4	20.9	27.1	28.2
Uninsured	—	16.2	—	—
Medicare	3.1	3.8	3.4	13.7
Private	3.6	4.9	4.3	4.4

Organization: Types of Facilities (NCHS 2012, 2005; Kaiser Family Foundation 2011a)

Community hospital beds per 1,000 civilian population (USA)[1]

1960 = 3.6	1970 = 4.3	1980 = 4.5	1990 = 3.7	2000 = 2.9	2008 = 2.7	2009 = 2.6

Health maintenance organizations (all plans, USA)

1976 = 174	1980 = 235	1990 = 572	1998 = 651	2000 = 568	2004 = 412	2011 = 564

Inpatient and residential treatment beds in mental health organizations per 100,000 civilian population (USA)[1]

1970 = 263.6	1980 = 124.3	1990 = 128.5	1995 = 110.9	2000 = 74.8	2004 = 71.2	2008 = 78.6

Financing: Sources of Payment (NCHS 2012)

Percentage distribution of selected expenditures for health services and supplies (USA)

	1987	1990	1995	2000	2005	2009
Public						
Federal government	16.6	17.3	21.1	18.9	22.4	27.3
State and local government	15.2	15.3	16.3	16.5	17.3	16.3
Private						
Employer contributions to private health insurance premiums	16.2	17.9	17.2	18.4	18.2	16.0
Other employer contributions	7.3	6.8	6.6	6.6	5.5	4.8
Employee contributions to private health insurance premiums and individual policy premiums	8.5	9.4	9.8	9.7	10.2	10.0
Other employee contributions	6.9	6.3	7.0	7.2	6.2	6.5
Out-of-pocket payments	21.3	19.2	14.3	14.7	13.1	12.0
Other private funds	8.1	7.9	7.7	8.0	7.2	7.1

Population at Risk

Enabling: Regular Source of Care (Bloom, Cohen, and Freeman 2011; Schiller et al. 2012)

Percentage distribution of regular care by race, income (2010)

	Race					Poverty Status[2]		
	White	Black	Hispanic	Asian	Two or More Races	Poor	Near Poor	Not Poor
Children 0–17 years								
No regular source of care	4.7	5.0	8.9	6.7	4.7	6.8	7.0	3.0
Location of care for those with regular source								
Doctor's office	75.4	69.2	58.0	76.2	77.1	58.2	67.5	83.4
Clinic	22.8	27.3	39.1	21.1	20.6	38.7	29.6	15.4
Emergency department	0.6	0.8	1.0	N/A[3]	N/A[3]	0.8	1.2	0.2
Hospital outpatient	0.7	2.1	1.0	1.4	N/A[3]	1.6	0.9	0.5

Adults 18+ years								
No regular source of care	15.8	17.6	29.7	18.4	24.3	27.8	24.1	12.1
Location of care for those with regular source								
Doctor's office or HMO	77.1	67.9	59.4	79.4	65.4	56.1	65.6	81.0
Clinic or health center	18.9	22.8	33.3	16.7	27.9	33.4	27.0	15.9
Hospital emergency or outpatient department	1.9	7.0	4.2	N/A[3]	4.1	6.6	4.1	1.5

Enabling: Insurance Coverage (NCHS 2012, 2011)

Percentage of US population under age 65 without insurance[1]

	1984	**1990**	**1995**	**2000**	**2004**	**2007**	**2010**
	14.5	15.6	16.1	17.0	16.4	16.6	18.2

Percentage of uninsured by race/ethnicity, income (2010)

	Race				Poverty Status[2]		
	White	**Black**	**Hispanic**	**Asian**	**Poor**	**Near Poor**	**Not Poor**
	17.6	20.6	32.0	17.1	30.3	32.4	11.5

Percentage of individuals who in the past year (2010):

	White	**Black**	**Hispanic**	**Asian**	**Poor**	**Near Poor**	**Not Poor**
Did not get or delayed medical care due to cost	14.5	17.4	15.4	8.0	23.4	24.0	11.0
Did not get prescription drugs due to cost	10.8	15.6	13.0	4.2	21.5	18.4	7.7
Did not get dental care due to cost	17.1	20.7	21.6	8.7	30.4	29.2	12.2

Actual Access

Utilization

Type of Use: Use of Selected Services (CDC 2011d; NCHS 2012)

Percentage having had procedures or contact by race/ethnicity or income

	Race					Poverty Status[2]		
	White	Black	Hispanic	Asian	Two or More Races	Poor	Near Poor	Not Poor
Began prenatal care first trimester (2008)	72.2	59.1	64.7	77.4	—	—	—	—
Vaccinations, children (19–35 months) (2011)								
One dose MMR	91.1	90.8	92.4	93.9	91.1	—	—	—
Four doses DTaP	85.0	81.3	84.1	92.0	87.1	—	—	—
Three doses polio	93.9	93.9	93.8	96.5	93.5	—	—	—
Saw dentist, past year (age 2+ years) (2010)	65.6	58.8	56.5	66.5	65.2	50.6	51.6	71.4

Women who received a mammogram in past two years (age 40+) (2010)	67.4	67.9	64.2	62.4	51.4	51.4	53.8	72.2
Women who received a Pap smear in past three years (age 18+) (2010)	72.8	77.9	73.6	68.0	70.8	65.1	64.3	77.2

Self-Assessed Health Status (NCHS 2012)

	Race					Poverty Status[2]		
	White	Black	Hispanic	Asian	Two or More Races	Poor	Near Poor	Not Poor
Percentage in fair or poor health (2010)	8.8	14.9	13.1	8.1	15.6	20.9	15.2	6.3
Percentage with at least one basic actions difficulty (2010)	31.2	32.3	24.7	17.5	36.3	40.6	38.7	27.1

Volume of Use (NCHS 2012)

		Race					Poverty Status[2]		
	White	Black	Hispanic	Asian	Two or More Races	Poor	Near Poor	Not Poor
Percentage with healthcare visit to doctor's office, emergency department, or home visit during the past year (2010)	84.7	84.3	76.5	79.6	86.1	79.6	79.1	86.8

Percentage with 1–3, 4–9, or 10+ healthcare visits to doctor's office, emergency department, or home visit during the past year (2010)

	White	Black	Hispanic	Asian	Two or More Races	Poor	Near Poor	Not Poor
1–3	44.9	47.2	43.2	49.9	42.3	37.5	42.1	47.9
4–9	26.1	24.7	22.6	22.1	25.2	25.1	23.1	26.5
10+	13.7	12.4	10.7	7.6	18.6	17.0	13.9	12.4

Unmet Need (Sondik, Madans, and Gentleman 2011)

Percentage of people not receiving needed medical care in the past year due to cost by race, income, insurance status, and current health status (2011)[4]

Race		
White	6.2	
Black	8.4	
Hispanic	8.0	
Asian	3.9	
Two or more races	9.8	
Poverty status[2]		
Poor	13.6	
Near poor	12.6	
Not poor	3.7	

Insurance (under age 65)	Private	2.9
	Medicaid	6.6
	Other	7.4
	Uninsured	21.9
Insurance (aged 65 or over)	Private	1.4
	Medicare and Medicaid	3.3
	Medicare only	4.1
	Other coverage	1.2
	Uninsured	19.0
Health status	Excellent or very good	3.9
	Good	8.8
	Fair or poor	17.8

Satisfaction							
General: Public Opinion (Schoen et al. 2010)							
Citizens' overall views of their healthcare system (2010)							
	Australia	Canada	New Zealand	Switzerland	United Kingdom	United States
Percentage who reported:							
Only minor changes needed	24	38	37	46	62	29
Fundamental changes needed	55	51	51	44	34	41
Rebuild completely	20	10	11	8	3	27
Citizens' views of access to and cost of care							
Access to doctor or nurse when sick or needed care	65	45	78	93	70	57
Percentage who reported wait times of two months or more for specialist appointment	28	41	22	5	19	9
Confident will receive most effective treatment if sick	76	76	84	89	92	70
Confident will be able to afford needed care	64	68	75	78	90	58

Did not fill a prescription due to cost	12	10	7	4	2	21
Did not get medical care due to cost	13	4	9	6	2	22
Did not get test, treatment, or follow-up care due to cost	14	5	8	4	3	22
Problems paying medical bills	8	6	6	6	2	20

Notes

1. Changes to definitional and reporting procedures affect the comparability of data across the years.

2. Poverty status is based on family income and family size as defined by the US Census Bureau's poverty thresholds for the previous calendar year. *Poor persons* are defined as individuals below the poverty threshold. *Near-poor persons* have incomes of 100 percent to less than 200 percent of the poverty threshold. *Not poor persons* have incomes that are 200 percent of the poverty threshold or greater. Because of the different income questions used in 2007 and beyond, poverty ratio estimates may not be comparable with those from earlier years.

3. N/A = not available. Estimates with a relative standard error greater than 50 percent are not shown.

4. Health insurance status for persons under age 65.

APPLYING HEALTH SERVICES RESEARCH IN POLICY ANALYSIS

Chapter Highlights

1. The objectives of health policy analysis are to produce and translate information for policymakers about the nature and causes of health-related problems and opportunities and to evaluate the consequences of actions taken to address them.
2. Different types of information and analysis are needed for the different types of decisions faced by policymakers in different stages of policymaking.
3. The HSR perspectives of effectiveness, efficiency, and equity offer theoretical frameworks, normative criteria, research methods, and measures that may be applied in policy analysis.
4. Researchers can enhance the application of HSR in the policy process by understanding the needs of policymakers and the role of research and analysis in the policy process.

Overview

This chapter links the major perspectives of HSR to policy analysis and shows how they can be applied to policy questions. An overview of the policymaking process and factors that tend to drive the process are described in the first section, followed by a discussion of the role of policy analysis in the policy process and a description of how the effectiveness, efficiency, and equity perspectives of HSR relate to the objectives and standards of policy analysis. The final section discusses the limitations of HSR as a resource for policy analysis.

The Policymaking Process

Public policies reflect the objectives of government and the strategies and resources for their achievement. Forms of public policy include laws and ordinances passed by Congress and by state and local legislative entities;

rules, regulations, and budgetary and operating decisions of government agencies; and decisions of the judicial courts (Longest Jr. 2009). The process of policy development is complex and multifaceted but can be divided into three broad stages: (1) formulation, which involves deciding which social conditions/issues to put on the policy agenda, which alternatives to consider to address them, and what action to take; (2) implementation, which includes the administration of rules, regulations, budgets, facilities, and human resources used in policy action; and (3) modification, which involves deciding if past policies have met intended goals and determining if change is needed (Exhibit 8.1).

In each stage of the process, demanders (e.g., employers, insurers/payers, providers of health services, consumers) attempt to influence policy, and suppliers (including elected officials and staff in the executive branch of government) produce policy in an environment of power struggles and shifts, technological change, national and international events, and evolving beliefs and values. The development of policy from one stage to the next is often iterative, moving backward and forward as policies are formulated, refined, implemented, and replaced in the context of changing circumstances (Longest Jr. 2009).

Demanders attempt to influence policy through their ability to shape the outcome of elections, their access to information, and their use of financial and other resources to shape public opinion and lobby policymakers. Suppliers introduce and pass legislation, promulgate rules and regulations, and deliver legal judgments. Their influence is derived from their position (i.e., legal authority) but also their political popularity, technical competency, and other factors.

In a classic study of the policy process, John Kingdon (2010) described three streams of activity that drive the policy process: (1) the problem stream, typically led by government and legislative staff involved in assessing the performance of past policies and elected officials interested in establishing new agendas and the need for change; (2) the solution stream, often led by analysts and researchers with expertise in a policy area and ideas about how to address a social problem; and (3) the political stream, led by elected officials and appointees involved in determining the general public's support for change and willingness to act. Each stream is driven by different factors, but—according to Kingdon's model—their convergence on a particular problem/policy combination creates the opportunity for significant change. Some of the features of the model are reflected in the ACA, which was brought on by a convergence of three factors: (1) the election of a new president who supports health reform, (2) widespread dissatisfaction with the US healthcare system, and (3) the existence of a reform strategy successfully implemented in a major state (the Massachusetts healthcare reform

Stages of Policymaking	Relevant Information	Type of Research/ Analysis
Formulation		
Define policy problems	Descriptive and analytic information on the scope, magnitude, importance, and causes of health and/or healthcare problems	Modeling, classification analysis, boundary analysis, and brainstorming
Identify alternatives	Projections of the consequences of alternatives	Extrapolative, theoretical, and judgmental forecasting
Evaluate alternatives	Comparisons of alternatives, considering multiple criteria and trade-offs	Outcomes research, cost-benefit analysis, and multi-attribute analysis
Implementation and Evaluation		
Describe consequences	Characteristics of interventions and populations served, health impacts, consumer satisfaction, and cost	Program evaluation research
Evaluate impacts	Adequacy, efficiency, and equity impacts of the policy	Outcomes research and cost-benefit analysis
Modification		
Determine if policy changes are needed	Policy performance, considering multiple criteria and trade-offs	Outcomes research, cost-benefit analysis, and multi-attribute analysis

EXHIBIT 8.1
Stages of Policymaking, Relevant Information, and Type of Research/ Analysis

law). Other aspects of the model are illustrated by the collapse of President Clinton's healthcare reform proposal in the early 1990s, when the critical mass of political will in Congress did not develop to support a well-developed (although complex) reform proposal that many thought had the potential to address the major problems of the US healthcare system.

Progress in the problem stream depends on agreement among the various actors about the scope and magnitude of unmet needs or opportunities and a sense of causation. Problem debates revolve around the definition of a social condition. For example, is the underuse of a given service for a certain condition a reflection of personal behavior, belief, or preference that is outside the purview of government, such as a religion-based preference for not using health services? Or is it a public concern—for example, the result of barriers to access imposed by market control by a large insurer or provider of health services (Munger 2000)? Driving factors include reaching agreement on the interpretation of social indicators of the condition (i.e., how widespread or severe the condition is) and finding evidence that links a condition to other problems (i.e., showing how rising healthcare costs contribute to government deficits or higher business expenses). Disagreement on scope, magnitude, and cause reduces the likelihood that a particular problem will be included on the policy agenda.

Policy solutions emerge from the solution stream if agreement is reached about the effectiveness of different alternatives for addressing a given problem or the alternatives' ability to achieve some specified value, such as effectiveness, efficiency, or equity. Agreement on policy solutions is difficult to reach when stakeholders have different opinions about the consequences of a given policy or the appropriate role of government. In these instances, debates tend to revolve more around different ideological views of policy than around pragmatic actions that could address a particular problem. In the policy stream, multiple possible actions tend to emerge for consideration. Projections are made and trade-offs among different valued outcomes are determined to identify a preferred alternative.

The political stream is the process by which citizens in a democracy decide whether they want to address a particular problem or adopt a particular policy. They may use direct democracy (referendum) or indirect democracy (elected representatives) to express their views. The political stream is important for determining who is in charge of the agenda, which values to prioritize, and the political will for action. The political stream reflects the mood of the general population, the influence of organized interest groups, election of new officials, and turnover of leadership in the branches of government. External factors, such as changing economic conditions and international conflicts, also may influence motivations for considering a particular problem/solution situation. For a particular strategy to emerge on the policy agenda and advance to the next stage of legislation, it must gain widespread political support. This process of determining political will is fluid, changes every day, and often leads to incompatible and inconsistent policies.

The Nature of Policy Analysis

The Role of Policy Analysis in the Policy Process

The role and influence of policy analysis depend on whether a particular policy process is aimed at comprehensive problem solving or incremental problem satisficing. In a problem-solving process, there is more agreement among policymakers on the role and goals of government, and policy debate is over the evidence, analysis, and cause–effect reasoning for policy change (Lasswell 1951). Indeed, early post–World War II views defined *policymaking* as primarily a problem-solving process, and *policy analysis* was thought of as the application of scientific theory and evidence to identify and solve society's problems. Analysts were initially employed by high-level government administrators for their technical understanding of the nature and causes of particular policy problems and their ability to identify and forecast the consequences of alternatives. Optimism about the availability of information, the capacity of analysts to reach definitive conclusions, and the motivation of policymakers to solve problems contributed to the early view of the policy analyst as a technical problem solver (Radin 2000).

A more realistic view emerged over the years as analysts were asked to take on more complex social problems for which information and theory were often lacking and political disagreement over the broad values and goals of policy and the role of government became more recognized. Policy analysts' response was the recognition that the role of analysis and the type of analysis possible for a particular problem substantially depend on the context in which the analyst is working. For example, severe resource constraints, short timelines, or major political conflicts suggest more modest objectives of identifying some of the likely causes of certain aspects of a policy problem or opportunity and offering incremental improvements rather than comprehensive solutions (Hayes 2001; Lindblom 1959). The problem-solving model, aimed at comprehensively understanding and resolving problems, yielded to the incremental model of acquiring a more limited understanding of some of the aspects of problems and using trial and error to better understand them. The problem-solving view emphasized prospective policy analysis and the application of theory in formulating policy alternatives; the incremental approach places more importance on monitoring and evaluating past actions and reformulating policy alternatives on the basis of feedback.

The challenge of low enrollment in a state's Children's Health Insurance Program (CHIP) illustrates the difference. The problem-solving approach would involve an extensive review of existing theory and experimental research on social marketing, outreach, and educational strategies to formulate alternative courses of action. The solution would be based on assessments of the strategies' potential to achieve specified enrollment targets at the least cost. The incremental approach also draws from research and theory but emphasizes experimenting with small modifications to current enrollment practices and monitoring the adequacy of improvement. Proponents of the incremental model tend to believe that successive incremental changes and feedback lead to better policy and that a comprehensive, problem-solving approach is unrealistic in most instances (Dunn 2009; Lindblom 1959).

Policy analysis also needs to relate to the political context in which analyses are conducted. In a highly politicized environment involving differences of opinion among interest groups about policy objectives and uncertainty about the consequences of different strategies, the policymaking process revolves more around conflict resolution than problem solving. The integrity of the political process through which the values and preferences of competing interest groups are considered is more relevant than evidence of a policy's merit in addressing a problem (Stone 2001). In such an environment, the policy analyst often ends up serving one interest group or another that has already taken a position or made a policy choice, and the analyst is asked to produce evidence to support the choice or rebut the opposition (Dryzek 1993; Habermas 1989). The goals of the analyst shift from technical proficiency in research and analysis to acquiring skills in public opinion assessment and consensus formation (Durning 1999; Fischer and Forester 1993; Forester 1993; Friedmann 1987; Munger 2000). The question is how to reconcile competing goals and satisfy multiple constraints in the pursuit of policy solutions.

Recognizing the political nature of policy processes, the policy analyst must have both the technical skills for rigorous analysis when problem solving is possible and the political skills for stakeholder assessment and consensus gathering when compromises need to be made. Technical skills are needed to understand scientific research principles and practices for high-quality analyses, and political skills are needed for the translation of research in an environment of political opportunity or political constraints (Heineman et al. 1990). While emphasizing the importance of producing objective information and analysis, the analyst also must consider political circumstances and client restrictions that may fundamentally change the set of actions implied by the research or the way a policy is framed. Analysts' ability to be objective depends on their sensitivity to and skills in the intervening political context.

Policy Analysis and the Stages of Policymaking

Policy analysis seeks to correctly formulate policy problems and identify, evaluate, and recommend solutions. As shown in Exhibit 8.1, the objectives of policy analysis, the type of information needed to support those objectives, and the various types of research required to produce that information are derived from the stages of the policy process (Bardach 2009; Dunn 2009;

MacRae and Whittington 1997; Munger 2000; Weimer and Vining 1999). Research and analysis at one stage are inappropriate and ineffective at the next because the questions are different at each stage.

At the policy formulation stage, analysts need factual information to document the scope and magnitude of social conditions and trends (e.g., a decrease in the number of uninsured, an increase in the costs of health services). Problem analysis involves clarifying the problem or opportunity, why it exists, whom it affects, and its possible causes. Most problems initially appear as vaguely defined concerns or signs of stress expressed by affected individuals or advocates. Analysts' first challenge is to describe the various representations or frames of a problem. The second is to attempt to consolidate those representations into more general terms that capture all important aspects of the problem. For example, analysts may decide whether low rates of mammography screening among the uninsured are due to the unavailability of low-cost healthcare providers in the area or to a lack of awareness of existing providers (Dunn 2009). Analysts need a model of causation to identify a problem and develop a solution.

The next step is to develop policy options that have the potential to correct, compensate for, or counteract the problem and to identify the potential consequences of implementing each alternative (e.g., forecast the number of people who would gain health insurance coverage under national healthcare reform). Policy options may derive from existing strategies or entirely new ideas. Methods for identifying new solutions range from brainstorming among stakeholders to analysis of the benefits of incremental modifications to—or adaptations of—existing solutions. A variety of systematic techniques may be employed to identify alternatives, from in-depth research and experimentation to quick surveys and literature reviews. The future consequences of alternatives should be projected in terms of the mix of goals and objectives that are to be used to evaluate the alternatives (Dunn 2009; Patton and Sawicki 1993).

Statistical models and simulation techniques may be used to generate projections. For example, during the 2009–2010 national healthcare reform debate, CMS used a variety of time series and behavioral modeling techniques to develop a ten-year projection of healthcare coverage and spending by population group (Foster 2010). More commonly, analysts must rely on simpler extrapolation techniques, such as linear projections, theoretical inference, or subjective opinion of experts, to generate forecasts (Bardach 2009).

In addition to forecasting, this step involves selecting criteria as bases for determining potential solutions and choosing among them. Another objective is to compare alternatives and recommend whether a particular one should be judged more beneficial than the others. For example, in addition to requesting factual information about the populations that would be covered under alternative health insurance reform proposals, the policymaker may ask the analyst to recommend on the basis of cost the preferred alternative for achieving a particular equity objective, such as equal coverage across income groups.

The introduction of criteria for judging policy requires the analyst to obtain normative information. Such information is always debatable and sometimes conflicting, and the analyst may be asked to identify the trade-offs among different criteria of various interest groups involved in the policy process (Dunn 2009). MacRae and Whittington (1997) provide practical guidance for selecting criteria: The criteria should focus on ends more than means, be quantitatively measurable, be comparable with other criteria and amenable to trade-off, and encompass the major concerns of stakeholders and the different aspects of the problem. The selection and application of criteria by the policy analyst represent a normative framework that should be justified with principled and logical argument.

The analyst may rely on the relevant policymaking body or affected stakeholders to define criteria. Criteria may be based on the preferences of elected officials; surveys of the general public; the analyst's own professional standards; interest group preferences; or analysis of past decisions, legislation, or testimony (MacRae and Whittington 1997; Patton and Sawicki 1993). For some cases, expert panels define criteria for policy analysis. For instance, the AHRQ clinical guidelines described in Chapter 3 offer criteria for identifying a problem in breast cancer policy: lack of access to mammography screening and cancer treatment—effective procedures shown to reduce mortality in women aged 40 to 70—among uninsured populations. On some occasions, government officials have defined normative standards in specific terms, such as the *Healthy People* 2020 objectives of the US Public Health Service (Office of Disease Prevention and Health Promotion 2012).

When choosing among alternatives, the analyst produces prescriptive information based on the application of criteria in comparative analysis. The availability of projected consequences is required for a policy alternative to be considered for action (Kingdon 2010). For example, after providing information about the potential of a Medicare prescription drug benefit proposal for achieving an effectiveness objective, a policy analyst may be asked to produce evidence of that proposal's cost-effectiveness relative to that of other proposals (i.e., different health impacts of alternative patient copayment options). Aids for developing prescriptive information include cost-benefit and cost-effectiveness analyses.

As the stage shifts from formulation to implementation and evaluation, the focus of policy analysis changes to assessing whether a policy was implemented as intended and had its anticipated effects. When assessing implementation, the analyst asks if standards are being followed and resources used as intended. Specific measures of inputs (e.g., personnel, facilities, equipment, supplies), processes (e.g., administrative, organizational, clinical, behavioral, political, attitudinal), and outputs (i.e., the goods and services provided) are obtained. When measuring effects, the analyst determines whether a change has occurred—for example, in the behavior, attitudes, or health status of targeted individuals, groups, organizations, or communities—and, if so, whether the change is attributable to the policy.

Approaches to evaluating past actions range from social indicator analysis, in which the analyst monitors overall changes in health status or some other indicator of targeted groups (e.g., infant mortality rates) over time and attempts to relate the changes to past policies (e.g., prenatal care access interventions), to studies of policy experiments or demonstrations, in which the analyst systematically isolates the effects of a policy from other factors (e.g., by separating the policy effects from an overall downward trend in infant mortality) (Dunn 2009). The menu of analytic tasks and methods used for the evaluation of alternatives in the policy formulation stage is also relevant to this stage (Exhibit 8.1), but the focus is on evaluating actual rather than potential consequences. To evaluate performance, the analyst must define policy objectives, operationalize them as specific criteria that can be used for evaluation, and evaluate the consequences of a policy or program on the basis of those criteria.

Analysts charged with meeting these informational needs (1) produce or interpret descriptive, normative, or prescriptive information about social conditions and past or future alternatives for improving them and (2) develop arguments translating such information into claims for action (Dunn 2009). Findings from the first objective are used to develop or influence the arguments in the second objective that identify a specific problem or recommend a policy action. The second objective involves critically assessing information by examining the validity of the data brought forth, the values applied to their interpretation, the internal logic of the argument, and the acceptability and uncertainty of the underlying assumptions. All these elements are relevant to supporting a policy claim.

HSR in Policy Analysis

The HSR perspectives of effectiveness, efficiency, and equity offer frameworks, methods, and measures for identifying policy problems and evaluating alternatives. The methods and measures of HSR are useful as indicators of the scope and magnitude of policy problems, and the frameworks provide criteria for judging the importance of problems and evaluating the consequences of policy alternatives. The HSR literature also provides valuable information about the possible causes of policy problems and suggests strategies for addressing them.

Criteria and Methods for Defining Problems

Effectiveness

As indicated in Chapter 2, the HSR literature defines problems with effectiveness from two perspectives: (1) the population perspective, which focuses broadly on the effectiveness of personal and community-based health services in determining the health of populations, and (2) the clinical perspective, which focuses narrowly on the benefits of health services for individual users or user groups (see Exhibit 8.2).

From the population perspective, effectiveness problems can be conceptualized in terms of detriments to population health associated with social, behavioral, environmental, or healthcare-related circumstances (Exhibit 8.3). The health effects associated with poverty, inadequate housing, smoking, or drug abuse might be contrasted with those resulting from poor access to health services in a given population. Explicit analyses of the relative health

EXHIBIT 8.2
Criteria for
Assessing
Health Policies
in Terms of
Effectiveness,
Efficiency, and
Equity

Dimensions	Criteria
Effectiveness	
Population perspective	Maximize population health
Clinical perspective	Maximize the health benefits of individuals receiving health services
Efficiency	
Allocative efficiency	Ensure a mix of health services and other health-related investments that maximizes population health and consumer satisfaction at the least cost
Production efficiency	Produce health services that maximize effectiveness at the least cost
Equity	
Distributive justice	Minimize disparities in the delivery of health services
Social justice	Minimize disparities in health and health risks
Deliberative justice	Minimize disparities in the participation of affected parties in the policy process

Dimensions	Analyses
Effectiveness	
Population perspective	Compare the relative contributions of health services and other population-oriented factors to the quality and quantity of life
Clinical perspective	Compare the actual and potential health benefits of individuals or groups receiving health services
Efficiency	
Allocative efficiency	Identify services, systems, organizational arrangements, and financial mechanisms that are not cost-beneficial
Production efficiency	Identify services and systems (with similar objectives) that are not cost-effective
Equity	
Distributive justice	Apply the equity-of-access model to estimate disparities in health services and systems
Social justice	Estimate disparities in health and health risks
Deliberative justice	Estimate the lack of participation of affected parties in policy development

EXHIBIT 8.3
Problem Analyses in Terms of Effectiveness, Efficiency, and Equity

effects of policies aimed at patient behavior and environmental conditions as well as access to health services are consistent with this perspective. For example, high breast cancer mortality rates among African-American women from different socioeconomic groups may be used as evidence of an access, a behavioral, or possibly a physiological problem.

Policy analysis aimed at improving clinical effectiveness draws on the framework proposed by Donabedian (2003, 1966) to evaluate quality and outcomes of health services. As discussed in Chapter 2, the clinical effectiveness framework can be divided into structure, process, and outcomes. *Structure* refers to factors associated with the receipt of services, such as affordability of insurance coverage and availability of healthcare providers.

Process refers to the quality and quantity of services being utilized. Both structure and process factors lead to *outcomes*.

The clinical perspective is helpful for identifying problems with the delivery of health services to individuals or groups under conditions of actual practice. From the clinical perspective, the standard for evaluating effectiveness is comparison of the actual benefits realized from healthcare delivery to the maximum benefits achievable. In the case of breast cancer, for example, evidence of a problem may be presented in terms of the lower survival rates among African-American women with cancer due to a lack of follow-up care after surgery.

Efficiency

Policy problems from the perspective of efficiency may be defined at the population level by evidence of a misallocation of health services and other health-related investments in social, environmental, or educational factors that negatively influences health (i.e., allocative inefficiency) or at the clinical level by a particular mix of inputs and production methods that fails to maximize benefits for individual patients at minimum cost (i.e., production inefficiency). Criteria for analysis in both cases include production and cost standards deduced from economic theories of efficiency in allocation of resources and production as well as measures derived from applying cost-effectiveness or cost-benefit analysis (Exhibit 8.2).

At the clinical level, the microeconomic model of healthcare provider performance analyzes the relationship between different levels and mixes of inputs, input prices, and technology that minimize the cost of service delivery (Exhibit 8.3). This model can be used in policy analysis when the concern is production of a specific service or mix of services. For example, each type of health services setting (e.g., community health center, hospital, nursing home) uses a particular combination of health personnel, supported by other inputs, to produce services. The microeconomic model suggests criteria that can be used to empirically identify the policy that produces the most efficient combination of personnel, supplies, and other inputs for a particular level of health services.

The cost-effectiveness framework, on the other hand, may be used when the concern is comparison of the relative efficiency of policies or programs that try to improve health through alternative methods of production. A cost-effectiveness ratio (e.g., cost per encounter, per case found, per quality-adjusted life year) is computed for each alternative and compared to that of other alternatives. For production to be efficient, services must be effective; a technical appraisal of effectiveness must precede an analysis of efficiency. Once a policy or program is shown to be effective, either in clinical or population-oriented terms, cost-effectiveness analysis compares its effectiveness and costs to those of other effective options. For example, one might determine whether the effectiveness of a case management program to increase surgery follow-up rates among African-American women with breast cancer is high enough to justify the cost of the intervention.

The broader goal of allocative efficiency can be applied in policy analysis using the cost-benefit framework. The analyst calculates and compares the costs and benefits of a policy, program, or service to determine if it contributes to social welfare—that is, if the social benefits exceed the social costs. All relevant social costs—including future cost savings that could be achieved by utilizing prevention services—and benefits should be identified and measured in dollars, if possible, so that comparisons can be made across possible actions. Future costs and benefits should be discounted to reflect their present value. Subtracting costs from benefits yields net benefits, the criterion indicating increased social welfare. Allocative inefficiencies are indicated when the aggregate costs of a policy or program exceed its aggregate benefits.

Equity

Equity criteria from the HSR literature relate to the distribution of health, health services, and health risks (Exhibit 8.2). Factors that affect equity in terms of the distributive justice paradigm include the characteristics of the healthcare delivery system (e.g., the availability and distribution of services), the characteristics of the population (e.g., ethnicity, gender, insurance coverage, access to a regular source of care), the use of services, and satisfaction with services (see Chapter 6, Exhibit 6.4). Equity problems are defined as healthcare disparities between advantaged and disadvantaged social groups (e.g., white and minority individuals), men and women, the insured and uninsured, people with and without disabilities, rural and urban residents, and people with high versus low education, all of whom have comparable need for health services (Exhibit 8.3). From the perspective of the socio-behavioral model of health services access (Andersen 1995), these disparities may be related to predisposing, enabling, or need factors that affect access to and use of health services. These factors include resources that affect access to services, such as income, health insurance coverage, knowledge about the healthcare system, transportation, and language proficiency. Professional and patient perceptions of need are another important set of predictors of health services use and outcomes. Need factors influence patients' and providers' choices independently and in connection with predisposing and enabling factors. Distributional equity problems may be evaluated at the institutional, system, or population level by applying these criteria, models, and measures.

Equity problems in health are defined on the basis of the social justice paradigm as disparities in health between social groups due to behavioral, environmental, or healthcare-related factors (see Exhibit 8.3) (Andersen 1995; Andersen and Aday 1978; Shi and Stevens 2005). Problems may include the availability of resources and training and practice styles, which may vary among providers or over time. Environmental problems may be due to social inequality, few community resources, or poor air and water quality. Personal factors include patients' age, gender, race/ethnicity, marital status, education, occupation, and health attitudes and beliefs, which may affect their healthcare-seeking or risk behavior independently or in conjunction with environmental and need factors.

Criteria and Methods for Identifying and Evaluating Policy Alternatives

Effectiveness

The structure/process/outcome framework developed by Donabedian (2003, 1966) offers a conceptual guide for the analytic tasks of identifying and evaluating policy alternatives (see Exhibit 8.4). This framework can be applied to patients at the system, institution, or individual level to improve the effectiveness of health services. Evidence linking the elements of the framework to outcomes suggests targets for policy interventions. For example, the structure/process/outcome framework suggests that the quality of nursing home care is influenced by structural factors such as the education, certification, and tenure of the nursing home administrator. Quality, in turn, has an influence on patient outcomes, including mortality, morbidity, functional status, and client satisfaction. Research on the role of this structural factor can inform the focus and content of a policy designed to improve the effectiveness of nursing home care (Bhaloo 2011).

Efficiency

Research concerned with allocative and production efficiency helps policymakers identify policy alternatives that are likely to deliver effective services at the lowest cost (Exhibit 8.4). Numerous empirical studies, for example, indicate that patients in fully capitated HMOs have lower admission rates to hospitals and shorter lengths of stay than do fee-for-service patients, with no corresponding reduction in the effectiveness of care (Miller and Luft 2002, 1997, 1994; Rosenthal and Newhouse 2002); that cost sharing reduces the use and cost of medical care with little or no decline in health status for the average patient, although it may lead some patients to curtail needed care (Newhouse et al. 1987); and that Medicaid coverage improves the quality of life of low-income populations (Baicker and Finkelstein 2011). Pushing for comparative effectiveness studies under healthcare reform, policymakers are asking researchers to provide better information on the efficiency of a variety of specific medical care services aimed at common medical problems and on the resources, organizational arrangements, and financing mechanisms involved in their provision.

Dimensions	Analyses
Effectiveness	
Population perspective	Apply the structure/process/outcome framework to identify policies associated with health improvements
Clinical perspective	Apply the structure/process/outcome framework to identify policies associated with improvements in health services and systems
Efficiency	
Allocative efficiency	Cost-benefit analysis of proposed medical and nonmedical services, organizational arrangements, and financing mechanisms
Production efficiency	Cost-effectiveness analysis of proposed services, organizational arrangements, and financing mechanisms
Equity	
Distributive justice	Apply the equity-of-access model to evaluate the impact of proposed health services and systems
Social justice	Analyze the impact of health services on disparities in health and health risks
Deliberative justice	Analyze the participation of affected parties in determining the need for health services

EXHIBIT 8.4
Solution Analyses in Terms of Effectiveness, Efficiency, and Equity

Solutions to efficiency problems may also be identified and evaluated through analysis of healthcare market conditions (see Chapter 4). Microeconomic theory identifies market conditions that lead to inefficient production or allocation if not corrected. Many of these conditions have been shown to be present in healthcare markets. For example, the uncertain consequences of some types of medical care make it difficult for patients to judge whether such care is in their best interest. The gap of knowledge between patients and providers leaves patients vulnerable to inappropriate care or care they would not choose for themselves if they were well informed. The external benefits and costs of some types of medical care (e.g., immunization to prevent infectious disease, which benefits populations as well as individuals) and investments in education, housing, and the environment may not be appropriately valued by private markets, leading to inefficient allocation of services. Documenting the presence of adverse conditions—in which markets are not suitable for achieving efficiencies—is another method used by analysts to suggest government interventions designed to improve production and allocational efficiency.

Applying the competitive economic model to enhance efficiency in health services assumes that maximizing satisfaction of consumer preferences is an appropriate policy goal, but its appropriateness is a value judgment that should be clearly stated when the model is applied. The goal of a needs-based model, such as maximizing the population's health status, may be substituted for consumer satisfaction in efficiency analysis, although the criteria for judging the determinants of allocative efficiency in the needs-based model are not as well developed as those in the competitive economic model. Both models are discussed in Chapter 4.

Equity

The two primary policy strategies for enhancing equity are lodged in the distributive and social justice paradigms and involve reducing disparities in (1) health services and (2) health (see Exhibit 8.4). Policies that address the various factors presumed to influence whether or not people receive care, experience social and behavioral risk factors, and suffer from poor health have the potential to enhance equity. Access indicators may be used to identify the content of possible solutions to equity problems, such as extension of insurance coverage and establishment of medical homes. The access model developed by Aday and Andersen (1974) is frequently used to examine if a policy has improved access to appropriate health services. Access is improved when need variables account for most of the variance in use among patient or population groups. Inequitable access results when demographic (e.g., sex, age), social (e.g., race/ethnicity), and enabling factors (e.g., income, insurance coverage) determine who receives appropriate health services.

Like efficiency analysis, equity analysis is ultimately concerned with identifying and evaluating medical and nonmedical services that are effective from both clinical and population perspectives—that is, for improving health and access to health services and reducing health and health services disparities. Evaluative criteria incorporating distributive justice norms regarding the distribution of health services can help policymakers identify desirable solutions from the equity perspective (Gelberg, Andersen, and Leake 2000). Criteria incorporating social justice norms regarding the distribution of health and health risks related to both health services and non-service factors (e.g., social-structural, cultural, environmental) can help policymakers identify equity solutions from the population perspective.

Along with its historical focus on delivery and outcomes of care, policy analysis of health services equity is increasingly focusing on equity in allocation of research resources. In recent decades, federal funding of HSR has become contingent on meeting various requirements aimed at achieving equity in HSR and in the subsequent development of health services programs and policies, such as the requirement to include women and minorities in clinical trials.

Criteria and Methods for Evaluating and Modifying Past Actions

Effectiveness

One of the major roles of HSR is to inform policymakers about what does and does not work. Effectiveness research supplies a conceptual framework, methods, and evidence to describe and evaluate the technical effectiveness of existing health policies. Structural factors—the quantity and efficacy of health services and other health-related inputs—can be linked to health outcomes to assess the impact of a particular intervention on desired policy outcomes. In the same way, studies on the effects of process—the quantity, quality, and appropriateness of services delivered or of investments made—on health outcomes guide evaluations of the success of actions taken to change the process of health services and social services delivery. For example, analysts might use this information to evaluate whether investments in public housing have lessened health disparities and thereby contributed to achieving the policy objective of improving the health of the population.

Efficiency

The concepts, definitions, and methods health economists have developed to examine the allocative and production efficiency of health services are important resources for describing and assessing the consequences of policy actions. Numerous studies of production efficiency (outlined in Chapters 4 and 5) are available to guide evaluations of the organization and production of health services. The RAND Health Insurance Experiment (discussed in Chapter 5), with its rigorous, large-scale design, is a good example of this kind of research. The Oregon Medicaid study (discussed in Chapter 4) is a more recent example. Findings indicated the costs and effects of alternative insurance strategies ranging from first-dollar coverage to catastrophic plans. Estimates were made of the excess spending that occurred under first-dollar coverage given the low marginal value of the added medical care services consumed. Studies of the efficiency of integrated HMO systems are another important example. Many well-conducted cost-effectiveness studies have provided useful information on the relative efficiency of alternative services and technologies (see Chapter 5).

Equity

Both analytic and evaluative research are relevant to the task of describing and evaluating the equity consequences of health policy and programs. Analytic research suggesting the causes of equity problems that are likely to be altered by government interventions provides criteria for evaluating the content and focus of policies. Empirical measurement of the specific effects of past actions (e.g., improving social support of high-risk mothers) is the primary basis for evaluating the equity consequences of alternative policies (e.g., investment in more prenatal care resources versus case management services using community health workers). Evaluative research on access (reviewed in Chapter 7) informs policy analysts of the success of specific programs or policies (e.g., the World Health Organization's Healthy Cities project and the Federally Qualified Health Centers program, both aimed at improving community health among underserved populations) for enhancing equity in distributional and social justice terms.

Challenges in Applying HSR in Policy Analysis

To the extent that the conceptual frameworks of effectiveness, efficiency, and equity are not well developed or research methods and empirical evidence are lacking, the HSR literature is limited as a source of information and argument in policy analysis. The previous sections in this chapter reviewed the potential contributions of HSR to policy analysis, and the discussion that follows highlights some of its limitations.

Effectiveness

No policy or professional consensus exists on how much emphasis should be placed on the population versus clinical perspectives in defining effectiveness in healthcare policy. The clinical perspective does not consider environmental and social factors that contribute to the health of populations. The population perspective requires that HSR address the health impact of factors (e.g., education, housing, quality of neighborhoods) for which causal information is limited. As indicated in Chapter 2, the clinical perspective has become more prominent of late in the United States, given the emphasis on comparative effectiveness research for evaluating the outcomes of specific clinical practices. Related to the debate over perspectives is the question of defining policy objectives in health. The population perspective emphasizes community health indicators, whereas the clinical perspective emphasizes individual patient health status.

The imprecision of measures of effectiveness is a critical weakness of effectiveness analysis at both clinical and population levels. Only rough estimates can be made of the direction and strength of the relationships between structure and outcomes and between processes and outcomes of care. Studies of variations in practice indicate that there is an extremely wide range of acceptable practice patterns (Brook 1994; Kane 1997; Wennberg et al. 2008). However, efforts by the federal government to invest in this type of research notwithstanding, it is difficult to determine precisely how much of the variation can be attributed to the provision of ineffective services.

Another limitation is that the extensive research on the medical and nonmedical determinants of health has not often been well linked across the levels of analysis defined in Chapter 2. Approaches that appear to be beneficial at one level may not be effective at the next level of analysis. For example, policies aimed at improving the quality of care of individual patients may not be effective at the community level because of the limited potency of healthcare interventions in general. When deciding how to invest societal resources to improve the health of the population, policymakers must take into account not only what works for the individual patient but also how these resources are best utilized for the population as a whole. Without information across levels of analysis, policymakers may make ineffective decisions.

Efficiency

Efficiency research provides useful but limited information on the optimal allocation of resources and optimal production methods. The effects of health services and other important medical and nonmedical investments on health and well-being are only beginning to be understood. Without this information, policymakers cannot determine the social value of resource allocation decisions with precision. The relative efficiency of different organizational models and resource mixes for producing cost-effective medical care is not clear despite the extensive research that has been done in some areas—for example, comparing managed care and consumer choice models of financing as policy strategies for improving allocational and production efficiency or comparing the costs and effectiveness of hospital inpatient and outpatient provision of various procedures and services (Altman and Levitt 2002). A conceptual difficulty in applying allocative efficiency criteria to the evaluation of policy alternatives is the inability to realistically assess the distributional consequences of alternatives (i.e., some win and some lose as a result of each alternative). Pareto-optimum criteria—that a policy is desirable for a community if the beneficiaries could use their winnings to adequately compensate those who paid for the policy and still be better off—can be used (see Chapter 4), but these criteria may not be acceptable from an equity perspective if they would prompt a substantial redistribution of income. The lack of distributional considerations in efficiency analysis implicitly accepts the current distribution of income and wealth.

The ability to compare projects also is limited because researchers apply different methods to their studies of efficiency (i.e., cost-effectiveness, cost-benefit, cost-utility, and cost-of-illness analyses). Guidelines have been developed, however, for researchers to follow (Gold et al. 1996). Furthermore, macro-international comparisons of efficiency are problematic due to the lack of a standard, international definition of health services; differences among nations' accounting practices; and currency differences (Edejer et al. 2003).

Equity

The focus of equity research would be enhanced if there were greater clarity and consensus on equity objectives. Chapter 6 proposes multiple paradigms as bases for alternative principles, criteria, and indicators of equity. Applying one framework (e.g., social justice) may lead to conflicts with another (e.g., distributive justice). A conceptual framework of equity that integrates these criteria and considers procedural and substantive equity and their interrelationship is presented in Chapter 6. Nevertheless, the relationships between indicators of procedural and substantive equity have not been thoroughly and uniformly documented. The challenge in HSR and policy analysis is to more accurately and fully document the contribution of medical and nonmedical factors to reducing health and health services inequalities—the ultimate criterion of distributive and social equity—across social and economic groups.

Summary and Conclusions

This chapter describes the policy process and the role of policy analysis, the objectives and standards of policy analysis, and the strengths and weaknesses of HSR as a resource for policy analysis. The linkages between the stages of policymaking and the tasks of policy analysis help policy analysts and health services researchers identify the types of information most relevant for policymakers in a given context. Because of the political nature of the policy process, the tasks of the rational model of policy analysis have been augmented by adding an awareness and sensitivity to political opportunity and feasibility.

HSR that meets the standards of scientific integrity—and is concerned broadly with both medical and nonmedical determinants of health—offers policy analysts perspectives and values useful for framing and clarifying problems, criteria and measures for identifying and evaluating policy options, and information about the likely performance of policy strategies for achieving specified goals. Despite their conceptual and empirical limitations, the effectiveness, efficiency, and equity perspectives of HSR provide a rich resource for policy development and assessment.

HEALTH DISPARITIES CASE STUDY

Chapter Highlights

1. This chapter applies the three HSR perspectives to a case study to evaluate a real-world policy question.
2. To set the context for the case, the chapter presents a brief history of health disparities in breast cancer screening, diagnosis, and treatment along with an overview of US policy addressing the problem.
3. Recent changes to the policy are described, and implementation of the changes is discussed.
4. Relevant criteria, measures, and data are identified and analyzed to evaluate the policy changes.

Overview

The case presented in this chapter focuses on the National Breast and Cervical Cancer Early Detection Program (NBCCEDP) created by federal legislation in 1990 to address disparities in breast and cervical cancer screening among low-income, uninsured, and underinsured women. The primary provisions of the NBCCEDP are described, as is the Texas Breast and Cervical Cancer Services (BCCS) Program created in 1991 to implement the NBCCEDP at the state level. We present the major features of recent policy changes that extended Medicaid coverage to women diagnosed with breast or cervical cancer through the program, and we evaluate this policy change by applying the effectiveness, efficiency, and equity perspectives of HSR.

Background

Breast cancer is the most common type of cancer affecting US women and the second leading cause of cancer-related death. Mammography screening for breast cancer saves lives by identifying disease at an early stage. Although consensus has not yet been reached on the age at which regular screening ought to begin, regular screening increases the chance of early detection among women developing breast cancer. Earlier detection enables earlier treatment, raising the likelihood of treatment effectiveness and longer survival. Several randomized clinical trials have found that regular screening by women aged 40 to 69 reduces mortality from breast cancer (Coldman and Phillips 2011; Feig 2002; Moss et al. 2006). The US Preventive Services Task Force (2009) recommends biennial mammograms for women aged 50 to 74 years. The American Cancer Society (2012) recommends yearly mammograms starting at age 40 and continuing for as long as a woman is in good health. A clinical breast exam (CBE) about every three years is recommended for women in their 20s and 30s and every year for women aged 40 or over. Those with abnormal screening should obtain a final diagnosis within 60 days, and diagnosed cases should obtain appropriate treatment within 60 days of the date of the diagnosis.

Low-income, uninsured women are less likely than the general population to meet these guidelines. They are less likely to participate in mammography screening (Breen et al. 2007) and less likely to have timely and complete follow-up after an abnormal screening result (Chang et al. 1996; Yabroff et al. 2004). They are also more likely to be diagnosed and treated at a later stage of breast cancer (Lantz et al. 2006; Li 2005; Smigal et al. 2006) and more likely to receive suboptimal treatment (Griggs et al. 2007, 2003; Richardson et al. 2006; Voti et al. 2006). Many programs and interventions in the United States have been implemented or are being proposed at the community level to increase breast cancer detection and follow-up among this population (Fernandez et al. 2009; Fernandez, Palmer, and Leong-Wu 2005; Komen Foundation 2012; Williams-Piehota et al. 2005).

The NBCCEDP was created in 1990 to address disparities in breast and cervical cancer screening among low-income, uninsured, and underinsured women at the national level. It was the first—and remains the largest—public health program in chronic disease prevention and control in the United States. In all 50 states, the District of Columbia, 12 tribes and tribal organizations, and five US territories, the program provides free or discounted mammograms, CBEs, and Pap tests to women who qualify. Federal funds from the CDC are granted to states to pay for the development of screening and diagnosis capacity, the delivery of screening and diagnostic services, education, quality assurance, and surveillance. Total appropriations of $30 million were distributed to eight states in 1992, growing to $192 million for all states; Washington, DC; the territories; and tribes by 2002 and reaching $215 million in 2010 (American Cancer Society 2010). States must fund $1 to the program for every $3 of federal funding.

When created, the NBCCEDP prohibited the use of program funds for treatment of breast and cervical cancer while requiring that contractors establish networks of providers willing to treat cases through charity care, for a reduced fee, or by another payment strategy (Lantz, Weisman, and Itani 2003). In 2000, Congress passed legislation enabling the states to offer Medicaid coverage for treatment of women diagnosed with breast or cervical cancer through the program (Lantz and Soliman 2009). The extension of Medicaid coverage for treatment increased the potential for this program to reduce the screening, diagnosis, and treatment gaps between low-income women and other populations.

Under an NBCCEDP agreement with the CDC, the Texas BCCS Program was created in 1991 to receive federal funds to provide free or discounted screening and diagnostic services to uninsured women with incomes up to 200 percent of the federal poverty level (FPL).[1] The Texas BCCS Program contracts with 47 local healthcare providers to screen women for breast and cervical cancer, notify them of screening results, track those needing diagnostic follow-up, provide diagnostic services, and ensure initiation of treatment of women with cancer. BCCS contractors must adhere to performance standards for screening, diagnostic follow-up of abnormal screening results, and treatment follow-up after a cancer diagnosis. Contractors are required to collect data on screening and diagnostic results and completion and timeliness of follow-up for all women who receive services. To be eligible for BCCS screening and diagnostic services, a woman must be at or below 200 percent of the FPL, uninsured or underinsured, and aged 40 or older. Symptomatic women under age 40 may be eligible for diagnostic services.

In response to the Medicaid policy change at the national level, in 2002 Texas began enrolling women in the Medicaid for Breast and Cervical Cancer Program (MBCCP). To qualify for MBCCP coverage, a woman must have received a diagnosis of breast or cervical cancer through the program and have family income at or below 200 percent of the FPL. She also must be uninsured, under age 65, a Texas resident, and a US citizen or eligible immigrant. In 2007, the Texas Legislature extended Medicaid coverage to eligible women diagnosed with breast or cervical cancer who are low-income and uninsured, regardless of their provider. Women potentially eligible after being diagnosed have to apply for Medicaid through a BCCS site. This policy evaluation focuses on the addition of Medicaid coverage in Texas for women diagnosed through the BCCS Program after 2002 and the extension in 2007 to women diagnosed outside the program.

Before the policy change in 2002, breast cancer was not a criterion for Medicaid eligibility. Women with cancer could qualify for Texas Medicaid coverage on the basis of their family status (e.g., a mother, pregnant, elderly) or a severe physical or mental disability and established income and asset eligibility thresholds (which are relatively low for adults in Texas—at

21 percent of the FPL—unless a person is severely disabled). Until 2003, women with incomes above the thresholds also could qualify if they had catastrophic healthcare expenses and became medically "needy." However, the medically needy program for adults was eliminated in Texas in 2003. The MBCCP establishes a pathway for more low-income women with breast and cervical cancer to obtain Medicaid coverage for treatment because the income thresholds are well above those required for enrollment in the regular Medicaid program, there are no asset or family categorical requirements, and recertification for as long as treatment is required is easier to obtain than enrollment in regular Medicaid.

Policy Evaluation Question and Tasks

For purposes of advising policymakers on the need for policy change, one role of policy analysis is to examine whether current policy is meeting performance objectives (MacRae and Whittington 1997). In this case, the policy question is whether the availability of Medicaid coverage increased the performance of the BCCS Program. Addressing this question involves a process of defining objectives for the program, developing specific criteria and measures that reflect the objectives, developing an evaluation design to determine the impact of the policy change, and gathering and analyzing data to evaluate the impact of the policy change in terms of valued outcomes. As discussed in previous chapters, the HSR perspectives of effectiveness, efficiency, and equity provide conceptual frameworks and analytic tools for policy evaluation.

In this illustrative case study, we identify hypothetical objectives of the Medicaid coverage policy, develop criteria and measures from each of the three HSR perspectives, make inferences and projections based on existing literature and available data, analyze the results, and offer recommendations. From the multi-perspective framework of HSR, we assess effectiveness in terms of changes in measures of program performance since the policy change. We assess efficiency by identifying incremental costs associated with the policy change and relating those costs to the associated change in performance. We evaluate equity by determining whether the policy change has the potential to significantly reduce disparities in treatment among different populations. Finally, we describe the specific tasks, measures, data sources, and analyses used to perform the evaluation.

Identifying Objectives
A simple logic model illustrating the potential impact of the availability of Medicaid coverage (Exhibit 9.1) suggests there is potential for more

low-income, uninsured women to access the screening program and for those with cancer to access treatment more quickly. The improvement in access and timeliness of treatment could occur if women are able to obtain treatment from any licensed Medicaid provider in the state. Offsetting this possible benefit is the potential for delayed treatment due to the additional time needed to complete the Medicaid eligibility process and locate a Medicaid provider. The eligibility process includes six steps. First, the breast cancer patient processes an MBCCP application at a BCCS clinic. Second, the BCCS clinic faxes the MBCCP application to the state BCCS office. Third, a BCCS nurse at the state office reviews the application for completeness and a qualifying diagnosis. Fourth, the completed application is faxed to the Medicaid eligibility contractor. Fifth, the eligibility contractor inputs the application and notifies the MBCCP eligibility department. Finally, the MBCCP eligibility department processes the MBCCP application and notifies the applicant of denial or acceptance into the MBCCP via mail.

The availability of Medicaid coverage also creates the potential for low-income women with cancer to obtain better-quality treatment. Improvements in the quality of care could occur if more women have financial access to surgical and nonsurgical services for the duration of their treatment. Together, the potential for improved access to timely, quality treatment (i.e., effectiveness and equity) could lead to increased survival rates. The achievement of these performance objectives must be compared to the additional cost to the state of paying for Medicaid case management and treatment (to assess efficiency).

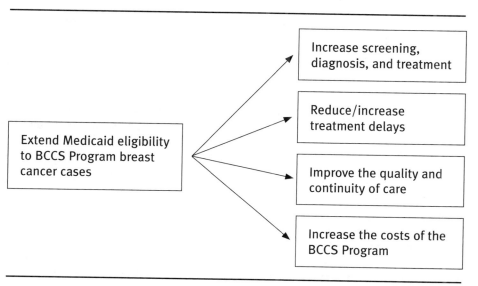

EXHIBIT 9.1
Logic Model of Impact

Increase screening, diagnosis, and treatment

Reduce/increase treatment delays

Extend Medicaid eligibility to BCCS Program breast cancer cases

Improve the quality and continuity of care

Increase the costs of the BCCS Program

Defining Criteria and Measures for Evaluation

Effectiveness

Criteria for evaluating the effectiveness of the policy change are based on the framework of Donabedian (2003, 1966) delineated in Chapter 2 (see Exhibits 2.2 and 2.3). The framework identifies structure, process, and outcome elements that determine the effectiveness of health services and system changes. In this case, the focus is on system structure, the policy change being the addition of Medicaid coverage. The process is the quality and timeliness of screening, diagnostic, and treatment services delivered by the program, and the process evaluation of the policy change assesses the degree to which Medicaid coverage might have improved the process of service delivery. Due to the short length of time that has elapsed since the policy change, our evaluation of effectiveness focuses on two process measures that suggest ultimate impact: (1) the timeliness of treatment follow-up of women following diagnosis of cancer and (2) the increase in the number of women diagnosed with cancer through the program (see Exhibit 9.2). To provide a preliminary assessment of effectiveness, we obtained pre- and post-change data on these measures and compared them.

　　　The first measure evaluates the extent to which the structural change in the program from introducing Medicaid coverage increased the number of women with breast cancer who received timely treatment services. The basis for this objective was the expectation that less time and effort on the part

EXHIBIT 9.2
Measures for
Analysis of
Effectiveness

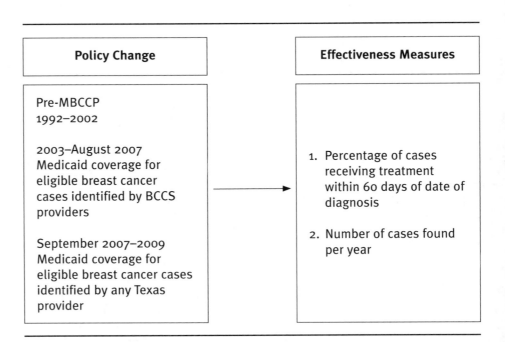

of BCCS staff and patients would need to be expended to find providers of free or discounted treatment. Offsetting this desirable effect is a confounding concern that the increased number of women applying for Medicaid and the time required to process Medicaid applications might actually delay treatment. This issue became particularly relevant after 2007, when the program began to allow women diagnosed by non-BCCS providers to apply for Medicaid but required that they do so through BCCS clinic staff (Lantz and Soliman 2009).

The timeliness measure was defined in terms of the program's performance benchmark:

- Benchmark: an interval of 60 days or less between diagnosis and initiation of treatment for breast cancer for a minimum of 80 percent of women needing treatment
- Measure: the percentage of women receiving treatment within 60 days of diagnosis

We estimated the effect of the policy change on timeliness of treatment by examining trends in the timeliness measure over three periods: the pre-Medicaid period between 1992 and 2002, the initial Medicaid period between 2003 and August 2007, and the period after Medicaid extension from September 2007 through 2009. We obtained BCCS Program data on the dates of screening, diagnosis, and initial treatment of women with breast cancer who were served by the BCCS Program, and then we calculated the percentage of women in each period who initiated treatment within 60 days of diagnosis.

Another expectation was that the availability of Medicaid coverage would increase the number of low-income women with breast cancer who obtain coverage for treatment. Because of the availability of Medicaid, more high-risk, low-income women might self-select the program or be referred to the program, increasing the effectiveness of the BCCS Program for providing high-quality care to more low-income women with cancer. To examine the impact of the policy change on the number of women diagnosed by the program, we tracked trends in the number of cancer cases receiving diagnoses through the Texas BCCS Program during the pre-Medicaid period (1992 to 2002), the initial Medicaid period (2003 to August 2007), and the period after Medicaid extension (September 2007 through 2009). The number in the post-extension period included women who were diagnosed outside the program (by non-BCCS providers) and received Medicaid assistance through the program (from BCCS providers).

The basis for using this measure to evaluate policy impact was the enabling role of Medicaid coverage, which encourages women to seek screening and diagnostic services and encourages providers to offer such services. Adams and colleagues (2009) and Chien and Adams (2010) showed that the availability of Medicaid through Georgia's BCCS Program increased the rate of Medicaid enrollment by women with cancer almost threefold and reduced disenrollment, both of which increase the potential for women with cancer to receive high-quality care. It also decreased the time gap between diagnosis and eventual Medicaid enrollment by about eight months. Research from the NBCCEDP in Washington found that 33.5 percent of cancer patients who were diagnosed between 1997 and 2002 (before Medicaid coverage was available through the program)—and who enrolled in Medicaid—disenrolled within one year of their diagnosis (Ramsey et al. 2008). Adams and colleagues (2009) assessed the effect of the introduction of Medicaid in the Georgia MBCCP on Medicaid disenrollment patterns of women with breast and cervical cancer. In a pre-/post-analysis, they found that, when Medicaid was made available through the program, the disenrollment rate declined 50 percent for women with breast and cervical cancer.

Efficiency
To assess efficiency, we calculated a cost-effectiveness ratio. The BCCS Program pays for Medicaid application processing, screening, and diagnostic workups, so we assessed cost-effectiveness from the program's perspective. The denominator reflected the incremental gain in health (or an intermediate outcome, such as timely receipt of treatment), and the numerator reflected the additional cost of the extended program over the status quo. Economic assessment models differ in terms of the measures used to express the benefits of any health-related screening or treatment service (Drummond et al. 2005; Gold et al. 1996). For a screening program, cost analyses usually consider the cost of the screening plus the cost of follow-up diagnostic services less cost savings from earlier treatment. Ideally, effects are measured in terms of quality-adjusted life-years saved. To do estimates, we need data or assumptions and models to measure and link screening, diagnosis, treatment, length of life, and quality of life, and then we project these factors to the end of life for treatment and comparison groups. We can simplify this analysis by focusing on intermediate outcomes, if those outcomes have been clearly linked by prior research to final health outcomes. Thus, in this case we focused on the relative efficiency of alternative strategies for getting women screened, diagnosed, and treated in a timely manner. Studies have shown that early breast cancer detection and treatment save lives well within the conventional efficiency norm of $50,000 per year of life saved. As long as the intervention to increase early screening and treatment is not too costly, intermediate outcome analysis can inform the selection of efficient policy (Chirikos et al. 2004).

In this case, the intermediate effect on timely treatment following diagnostic confirmation was expressed as the increase in the percentage of cases treated within 60 days of diagnosis compared to the cost of the program extension. The cost-effectiveness ratio was used to evaluate the program extension against the status quo option in terms of the incremental cost of the program extension divided by the percentage gain in the cases treated within 60 days of diagnosis.

Application of the cost-effectiveness framework can be facilitated by decision tree modeling of Medicaid coverage and possible subsequent treatment events. In this case, a simple decision tree model (Exhibit 9.3) is used to assess efficiency. The perspective of the model is a point-in-time choice between the BCCS Program with Medicaid and the BCCS Program without Medicaid. The model focuses only on women who are screened through participation in the program and assumes the number of women screened does not change with the introduction of Medicaid coverage.

Starting from the decision node on the left (indicated by a square box), the branches of the decision tree (Exhibit 9.3) indicate the alternatives, the subsequent possible events of the screen results, and diagnostic follow-up. The purpose of using the tree is to estimate the cost-effectiveness of Medicaid coverage in terms of expenditures on additional persons diagnosed with cancer who obtain treatment within 60 days of initial screening. To derive the net cost of Medicaid coverage per additional person receiving treatment within 60 days of screening, we use BCCS data to determine the difference between (1) the number of persons with Medicaid coverage who are expected to obtain treatment within 60 days of screening and (2) the number of persons without Medicaid coverage who are expected to obtain treatment within 60 days of screening, and then we divide this figure by the

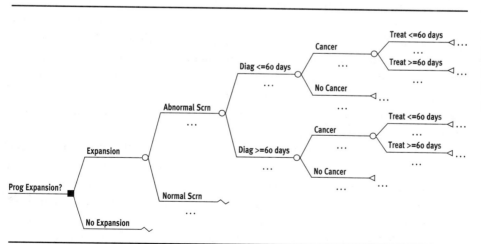

EXHIBIT 9.3

Framework for Analysis of Efficiency—Decision Tree Model

difference between the average cost of the BCCS Program with Medicaid and the cost of the status quo.

The upper branch of the decision tree leads to the Medicaid option and then to a chance node (indicated by a circle); at that node, the possibilities are that the participating woman would have either an abnormal or a normal screening test result. Abnormal screening results are defined as "a suspicious abnormality in need of biopsy," "a highly suggestive malignancy," or "an incomplete screen/additional imaging needs." To estimate the proportion of those screened who will have an abnormal result and the proportion of those screened who will have a normal result, we use the screening results from the BCCS Program before and after the introduction of Medicaid coverage. The estimated percentage of women included in each branch is based on the estimated percentage of women included in the preceding branch.

Following the second chance node, the tree branches into two groups: women with an abnormal screen result who received a diagnostic exam within 60 days of screening and women who received a diagnostic exam more than 60 days past the date of screening. The diagnostic procedures after abnormal screen may include diagnostic mammogram, ultrasound, fine needle/cyst aspiration, non-excisional biopsy, excisional biopsy, surgical consult, and pathology. A facility fee was added when a biopsy was involved. Only women who followed up through the program were considered for the chance node. The great majority of women do not receive a diagnostic exam because they do not have breast cancer and so do not have abnormal screen results, outside of the small proportion with false-positive screen results.

The diagnosis $\leq$ 60 days branch and the diagnosis > 60 days branch each lead to a chance node. Each of these nodes branches into two groups: women diagnosed with cancer on the basis of their workup results and women not diagnosed with cancer on the basis of their workup results. Finally, the "cancer" branch at the top of this section of the tree divides into two groups: women receiving treatment within 60 days of diagnosis and women receiving treatment more than 60 days after diagnosis. The "no cancer" branch positioned second from the top does not divide further but extends to indicate the group of women who do not initiate treatment, which includes all women not diagnosed with cancer.

In summary, determining whether the addition of Medicaid coverage to the BCCS Program improves efficiency involved estimation based on a decision tree model. We applied the normative value of clinical efficiency to evaluate whether the Medicaid-prompted increase in the proportion of women receiving treatment within 60 days of screening was large enough to justify the additional costs (i.e., for screening, diagnostic workup, and case management services) to the BCCS Program. We calculated an average cost-effectiveness ratio for all women to compare the BCCS Program with Medicaid to the BCCS Program without Medicaid:

$$\text{Incremental cost-effectiveness ratio} = \frac{(\textit{Cost of Medicaid} - \textit{Cost of status quo})}{\begin{array}{c}[\,(\textit{Percentage women treated} \leq 60 \textit{ days after screening} \\ \textit{under Medicaid}) - (\textit{Percentage of women treated} \\ \leq 60 \textit{ days after screening under status quo})\,].\end{array}}$$

Cost of adding Medicaid coverage = *Eligibility assessment cost + Screening cost + Diagnostic follow-up cost.*

Cost of status quo = *Screening cost + Diagnostic follow-up cost.*

Equity

Substantial barriers impede the availability of breast cancer screening and related treatment services to low-income, uninsured women and this population's use of these services. These barriers cause disparities in early diagnosis, treatment, and survival relative to other populations. Mammography screening facilities are less available in rural and inner-city areas, which generally have a disproportionate number of older and minority women. The availability and promotion of recommended screening also vary across healthcare plans and provider settings. Although private and public insurers may cover mammography screening, other factors—eligibility disruptions, deductibles, copayments, and resulting treatment costs—are burdensome to many (especially low-income) women (Feresu et al. 2008; Lee-Feldstein et al. 2000; Lin et al. 2005; McAlearney et al. 2007; O'Malley, Forrest, and Mandelblatt 2002; Perkins et al. 2001; Trivedi, Rakowski, and Ayanian 2008). The extension of Medicaid eligibility and the introduction of premium subsidies in the individual and small-group insurance markets under the provisions of the ACA may help alleviate the financial barriers for many people, especially when combined with programs that are explicitly directed at helping eligible women diagnosed with breast or cervical cancer enroll in Medicaid (e.g., the Texas BCCS Program).

Exhibit 7.1 (see Chapter 7) provides a summary of broad criteria for assessing the equity of health policies and illustrative examples of the application of these criteria in breast cancer screening and treatment decisions. The cost-effectiveness norm focuses on enhancing access to prevention and treatment benefits and services that are most likely to be cost-effective. Mammography screening has been documented to be the most effective technology to date for detecting early-stage breast cancer (Feig 2002; Humphrey et al. 2002; National Cancer Institute 2011a; Smith et al. 2010). Although the rates of mammography use and adherence have increased over the past decade, they remain short of the *Healthy People* 2010 objectives, especially among Hispanic, multiracial, and low-income women (see Appendix 7.1).

The similar-treatment norm argues for minimizing disparities in access to benefits and services across subgroups, particularly among those most at risk. The predisposing, enabling, and need dimensions of the equity framework (Chapter 7, Exhibit 7.1) provide guidance for identifying potential equity issues related to the similar-treatment norm. Equitable access is defined to exist when predisposing factors, such as need, account for most of the variation in use. Inequitable access occurs when healthcare system factors and predisposing social characteristics, such as age, race/ethnicity, and geographic location, determine who receives care (Andersen 1995; Andersen and Davidson 2001). Variation in the rate of health insurance coverage is a sentinel indicator of likely problems with the equity of healthcare services use.

The similar-treatment norm and related evidence regarding subgroup variations in breast cancer screening rates, cancer detection, and referral to a care source are central to evaluating the mammography screening policy for low-income, uninsured women presented in this chapter. Death rates and rates of late-stage diagnosis are higher among elderly, black, low-income, and uninsured women. Nonetheless, mammography utilization and adherence rates decline with age; are lower among minority, low-income, and uninsured women; and are lower among women in rural areas. Having a regular source of care enhances mammography screening rates, although other barriers—such as lack of transportation and limited access to screening services—may influence screening rates, especially among women most at risk (Amey, Miller, and Albrecht 1997; Bloom et al. 2001; Coughlin et al. 2002; Harper et al. 2009; Hirschman, Whitman, and Ansell 2007; Khan et al. 2010; Kim and Jang 2008; Legler et al. 2002; Lorant et al. 2002; Miller and Champion 1997; Qureshi et al. 2000; Selvin and Brett 2003).

As noted earlier in the chapter in the section on effectiveness, one of the potential impacts of the program was an increase in the number of low-income, uninsured women diagnosed with breast cancer and enrolled in Medicaid after the implementation of Medicaid eligibility in 2003. To assess the contribution of Medicaid coverage in the BCCS Program toward increasing equity in breast cancer screening, diagnosis, and treatment access, we obtained data on the number of cases identified by the program before and after the 2003 and 2007 program changes and compared the number of cases identified by the program to the estimated total number of low-income, uninsured women diagnosed with breast cancer in Texas. This comparison provides evidence that the policy change may be helping the program assist a greater number of low-income, uninsured women diagnosed with breast cancer.

In addition to evaluating effectiveness, efficiency, and equity, we examined breast cancer detection and Medicaid referral by age, Hispanic versus non-Hispanic ethnicity, and geographic location (residing in a metropolitan or nonmetropolitan area) before and after the 2003 and 2007 program changes. We then compared the estimates for each period to determine any change in the characteristics of low-income women with breast cancer who were reached by the program.

Analyzing the Results

Effectiveness

To evaluate the effectiveness of the policy change, we obtained BCCS Program data on service delivery to women aged 40 to 64 from 1992 through 2009. Over the period between 1992 and 2002 (pre-MBCCP), 14,295 BCCS-paid screens were done per year, on average. Over the period between 2003 and August 2007 (the initial MBCCP), the number of screens declined slightly to 13,207 per year. Over the period from September 2007 through 2009 (the extended MBCCP), the number of screens was slightly greater than that over the previous four years, at 13,601 per year, but lower than that in the pre-MBCCP period (see Exhibit 9.4). Most of the women screened received both mammograms and CBEs, paid for by the program as part of the screen, but some received one and not the other.

	1992–2002 (11 years)		2003–August 2007 (4.67 years)		September 2007– 2009 (2.33 years)	
	Total	*Per Year*	*Total*	*Per Year*	*Total*	*Per Year*
Number of screens (mammogram and CBE)	157,245	14,295	61,679	13,207	31,691	13,601
Mammogram only	6,281	571	2,064	442	2,992	1,284
CBE only	3,888	353	2,149	460	2,855	1,225
Mammogram and CBE	147,076	13,371	57,466	12,305	25,844	11,092
Number of abnormal screens	16,132	1,467	7,535	1,613	3,710	1,592
Number of diagnosed cases	933	85	1,009	216	550	236

EXHIBIT 9.4
Number of Screens by Type of Screen

The number of abnormal screens per year was 1,467 pre-MBCCP (1992 to 2002), 1,613 per year during the initial Medicaid period (2003 to August 2007), and 1,592 per year during the period after Medicaid extension (September 2007 through 2009) (see Exhibit 9.4). The number of cases diagnosed by BCCS providers over the entire study period totaled 2,492, increasing from 85 per year pre-MBCCP to 216 in the initial Medicaid period to 236 per year in the post-extension period.

The timeliness of follow-up treatment is summarized in Exhibit 9.5. The proportion of women receiving treatment within 60 days increased from 85.9 percent in the pre-MBCCP period to 90.4 percent in the initial Medicaid period and then declined slightly to 88.7 percent in the period after the Medicaid extension.

Further analysis is needed to determine if the introduction of Medicaid was associated with a significant change in the timeliness of treatment initiation (net of the underlying trends taking place over the period of the study) and whether benchmarks were reached. A logistic regression model could be used to determine if there was a change in the likelihood of receiving a follow-up diagnosis, receiving a diagnosis within 60 days of an abnormal mammogram, receiving appropriate treatment, and receiving treatment within 60 days of diagnosis. We could control for such covariates as age, race/ethnicity, presence of self-reported breast symptoms, receipt of a previous mammogram, positive CBE before the mammogram, CBE and other diagnostics paid by the Texas BCCS Program, and year of first mammogram. While analyzing treatment provision, we also could control for stage of diagnosis.

The second measure of effectiveness of the Medicaid change, the number of women whose cancers were detected through the program,

EXHIBIT 9.5
Percentage of Women with a Diagnosis Who Initiated Treatment Through the Program

	1992–2002 (11 years)		2003–August 2007 (4.67 years)		September 2007–2009 (2.33 years)	
	Total	*Per Year*	*Total*	*Per Year*	*Total*	*Per Year*
Number of diagnosed cases	933	85	1,009	216	550	236
Number of initiated treatments	918	83	981	210	496	213
Percentage with treatment initiated within 60 days		85.9		90.4		88.7

	1992–2002 (11 years)		2003–August 2007 (4.67 years)		September 2007–2009 (2.33 years)	
	Total	*Per Year*	*Total*	*Per Year*	*Total*	*Per Year*
BCCS	933	85	1,009	216	550	236
MBCCP	0	0	0	0	1,568	673
Total	933	85	1,009	216	2,118	909

EXHIBIT 9.6
Number of Cases Detected Through the BCCS/MBCCP

increased from an average of 85 cases per year pre-MBCCP to 216 in the initial extension period to 236 per year in the post-2007 extension period (Exhibit 9.6). If we add the MBCCP cases who were diagnosed outside the program but enrolled in Medicaid through the program, the number of cases per year increases to 909. Clearly, the number cases found through this program increased as a result of the Medicaid extension.

In summary, the analysis of the effectiveness measures indicates that the performance of the BCCS Program improved in terms of timeliness of treatment and number of cases found. More low-income, uninsured women with cancer—particularly those whose cancers were detected by other providers—have received Medicaid coverage and timely treatment since the Medicaid extension was introduced.

Efficiency

The probability values necessary for computing cost and early treatment outcomes as reflected in the decision tree are summarized in Exhibit 9.7. The values were derived from the BCCS Program data for the pre- and post-MBCCP periods. Data included normal and abnormal screening rates, timeliness of diagnostic follow-up, breast cancer rates, and timeliness of treatment following diagnostic follow-up.

We estimated the unit cost of screening by multiplying the number of screening office visits and screening exams (for new and established patients) by the 2010 Texas reimbursement CPT (Current Procedural Terminology) unit cost values (see Exhibit 9.8). Office visits included visits for CBEs, mammograms, and re-screenings. We divided the sum of the weighted costs for office visits and screening services by the number of women served during the period to arrive at an average screening cost of $236 before program extension and $288 after program extension. We used the screening cost before extension for both pre- and post-extension events to eliminate any influence the cost of screening might have had on the results of our analysis.

EXHIBIT 9.7
Decision
Tree Values:
Mammography
Screening
Program
Extension

Variables	Pre-Medicaid Percentages	Post-Medicaid Percentages
Screening		
Abnormal	16.64	17.94
Normal	83.36	82.06
Timeliness of diagnostic follow-up (Dx)		
Abnormal screen		
Dx ≤ 60 days	77.80	85.71
Dx > 60 days	22.20	14.29
Normal screen (false negatives)*		
Dx ≤ 60 days	79.40	93.63
Dx > 60 days	20.60	6.37
Breast cancer rate		
Abnormal screen and Dx ≤ 60 days		
Cancer	5.21	10.35
No cancer	94.79	89.65
Abnormal screen and Dx > 60 days		
Cancer	4.20	7.99
No cancer	95.80	92.01
Normal screen and Dx ≤ 60 days (false negatives)		
Cancer	0.54	1.05
No cancer	99.46	98.95
Normal screen and Dx > 60 days (false negatives)		
Cancer	1.13	3.70
No cancer	98.87	96.30
Timeliness of treatment initiated (Tx)		
Abnormal screen and Dx ≤ 60 days and cancer		
Tx ≤ 60 days	86.68	90.42
Tx > 60 days	13.32	9.58
Abnormal screen and Dx > 60 days and cancer		
Tx ≤ 60 days	78.84	79.34
Tx > 60 days	21.17	20.66
Normal screen and Dx ≤ 60 days and cancer (false negatives)		
Tx ≤ 60 days	100.00	87.50
Tx > 60 days	0	12.50
Normal screen and Dx > 60 days and cancer (false negatives)		
Tx ≤ 60 days	83.33	100.00
Tx > 60 days	16.67	0

*False negatives refer to a small number of cases in which cancer is found subsequent to a normal screen (via a rescreen or another procedure).

Source: CDC (2010).

Screening Procedures	CPT Code	Cost Per Procedure
Mammogram: new screening	77057	$85.37
Mammogram: re-screening	77057	$85.37
Office visit: new patient	99203	$93.10
Office visit: established patient	99213	$59.07
Diagnostic Procedures	**CPT Code**	**Cost Per Procedure**
Diagnostic mammogram	77056	$101.92
Ultrasound	76645	$74.05
Fine needle/cyst aspiration	10021+88173	$266.75
Non-excisional biopsy	19101	$299.06
Excisional biopsy	19120	$411.73
Surgical consult	99242	$89.73
Pathology	88305	$101.83
Facility fee	101FX 120FX	$478.00

EXHIBIT 9.8
Reimbursement Rates for Screening and Diagnostic Services, Fiscal Year 2010

Source: Texas Department of State Health Services (2010).

For diagnostic workups following an abnormal screen, we estimated the number of abnormal results from a mammogram or CBE and multiplied this number by the percentage of cases who underwent each diagnostic procedure following an abnormal screen (see Exhibit 9.9). We multiplied the estimated number for each diagnostic procedure by the respective CPT unit cost value (see Exhibit 9.8) and then divided the weighted sum of the expected cost by the number of women served in each period to estimate the average diagnostic workup cost. The estimated costs were $305 pre-Medicaid and $380 after introduction of Medicaid. Again, for purposes of the analysis, we used the pre-Medicaid diagnostic cost for both program periods.

For processing the Medicaid applications of women diagnosed with cancer, BCCS providers are reimbursed $100 per case (Texas Department of State Health Services 2012, 2010). We determined the total cost of processing patients' Medicaid applications in the period after MBCCP extension by multiplying the number of women diagnosed with breast cancer by $100, assuming that all women diagnosed with breast cancer submitted the

EXHIBIT 9.9
Estimated Rate
of Diagnostic
Procedures
Following an
Abnormal
Screen

	Abnormal Mammogram	Abnormal CBE
Diagnostic mammogram	46.7%	6.7%
Ultrasound	73.2%	73.1%
Fine needle/cyst aspiration	3.4%	1.6%
Non-excisional biopsy	8.9%	1.8%
Excisional biopsy	17.9%	3.5%
Surgical consult	32.2%	50.3%
Pathology	30.2%	6.9%

Source: Texas Department of State Health Services (2010).

MBCCP application for the initiation of treatment. This cost was not applied to any women diagnosed with cancer in the pre-extension period because no financial support for treatment was available for women diagnosed with cancer before 2003.

The pre/post results of the efficiency analysis indicate that the introduction of Medicaid coverage in the BCCS Program may have increased the percentage of women who were diagnosed with cancer and received treatment within 60 days of their diagnosis. It also may have increased the diagnostic and case management costs of the program. The rate increase implies that out of a population of 10,000 women participating in screening, about 122 would have received timely treatment for cancer in the pre-Medicaid period and about 250 would have received timely treatment in the period after introduction of Medicaid (see Exhibit 9.10).

EXHIBIT 9.10
Cost-
Effectiveness
Analysis

Strategy	Cost per Screen ($)	Incremental Increase in Cost ($)	% Treated ≤ 60 Days of Diagnosis	Incremental % Increase in Timeliness of Treatment	Incremental Cost-Effectiveness Ratio ($)
Pre-Medicaid	503.579	—	1.224	—	—
After introduction of Medicaid	543.796	40.217	2.501	1.277	3,149

The marginal cost of screening, including the CBE, mammography, and diagnostic workup was approximately $544 in the period after introduction of Medicaid and approximately $503 in the pre-Medicaid period. Thus, for women participating in screening, the cost-effectiveness of the Medicaid strategy—the incremental cost-effectiveness ratio (ICER)—versus no Medicaid was $3,149 per additional woman who received timely treatment for breast cancer ($40.217/0.0127).

These results are not sensitive to the assumption that the abnormal screening rate did not change between the pre- and post-extension periods. Under this assumption, the ICER would be $3,511. The results are sensitive to the cost of the diagnostic workup but are not affected by increases in the cost of mammography screening. When the cost of the diagnostic workup was hypothetically increased from $305 to $1,021 in the model, the ICER increased from $3,149 to $10,034.

Equity

As noted earlier in the results for effectiveness, the number of low-income, uninsured women diagnosed with breast cancer through the BCCS Program increased from 85 per year in the pre-Medicaid period to 216 per year in the initial Medicaid period and to more than 900 per year under extended Medicaid. We roughly estimated the percentage of low-income, uninsured women diagnosed with breast cancer in Texas in 2009 by multiplying the number of uninsured Texans in 2009 (6.1 million) by the percentage of uninsured Texans below 200 percent of the FPL (59 percent); then by the percentage of adults in that uninsured, low-income group (73 percent), and then finally by the percentage of females in that uninsured, low-income, adult group (47 percent). We multiplied the resulting estimate of low-income, uninsured women (6.1 million × 0.59 × 0.73 × 0.47 ≈ 1,234,817) by the breast cancer incidence for 2009 (0.001155 per 1,000), arriving at an estimate of 1,426 low-income, uninsured women diagnosed with breast cancer in 2009, or 9.9 percent of all women diagnosed with breast cancer in Texas in that year (see Exhibit 9.11). Applying that percentage to the number of women diagnosed with breast cancer in 2002 (12,600) yielded a rough estimate of 1,245 low-income, uninsured women with breast cancer in 2002. We compared these two estimates to the number of women identified through the BCCS/MBCCP in those years to assess the change in the proportion of low-income, uninsured women with breast cancer reached by the program.

The percentage increase in women identified through the BCCS/MBCCP is remarkable: from 7.9 percent of low-income, uninsured cases in 2002 to 63.7 percent in 2009. This substantial increase suggests that these programs have the potential to reduce disparities in the process of care between low-income, uninsured women with breast cancer in Texas and those with coverage and higher income.

	2002	2009
New female BC cases	12,600	14,428
Uninsured, low-income cases*	1,245	1,426
BCCS/MBCCP cases	98	909
Percentage	7.9	63.7

*6.1 million uninsured Texans (2009) $\times$ 0.59 (< 200% FPL) $\times$ 0.73 (adults) $\times$ 0.47 (female) $\times$ 0.001155 (2009 breast cancer incidence rate) = 1,426. Therefore, 1,426 ÷ 14,428 $\times$ 12,600 = 1,245.

The addition of Medicaid eligibility for BCCS Program participants in 2003 and the inclusion of community-identified cancer cases in 2007 increased the number of women with breast cancer who gained eligibility for Medicaid. We examined the distribution of cases across five age categories, ethnicity (Hispanic versus non-Hispanic), and urban versus rural status to see if programmatic changes in 2003 and 2007 modified the patterns of women diagnosed with cancer through the BCCS/MBCCP (see Exhibits 9.12–9.14). All comparisons were based on the average number of women identified per year. The distribution of women across the five age groups was remarkably flat from the introduction of the BCCS Program in 1995 through the introduction of the MBCCP in 2007 (see Exhibit 9.12). None of the program expansions prompted statistically significant (at the $p \leq 0.05$ confidence level) age differences in the women identified with cancer. The same was true of the distribution between Hispanic and non-Hispanic women (see Exhibit 9.13). There was, however, a significant shift in urban versus rural representation after the 2007 extension (see Exhibit 9.14). Women in rural counties comprised 26.54 percent of the women identified by the BCCS Program before the 2003 extension. This percentage declined slightly, although not by a statistically significant amount, to 22 percent after the introduction of Medicaid in 2003. After the 2007 program extension, however, rural representation declined to 11.82 percent among BCCS Program participants and 10.91 percent among MBCCP participants (11.1 percent combined; $\chi^2 = 30.3$, df = 2, $p \leq 0.0001$).

Conclusion and Recommendations

Given current disparities and preliminary evidence that mammography screening and treatment services increase health benefits and may be cost-effective, a policy of extending Medicaid coverage to low-income, uninsured

EXHIBIT 9.12
Age Distribution of Women Identified with Cancer Across Program Eras

	Age	1995–2002 (8 years)			2003–August 2007 (4.67 years)			September 2007–2009 (2.33 years)		
		Total	Per Year	%	Total	Per Year	%	Total	Per Year	%
BCCS Program	40–44	107	13	13.68	171	37	16.91	66	28	11.98
	45–49	122	15	15.60	205	44	20.28	115	49	20.87
	50–54	205	26	26.21	229	49	22.65	138	59	25.05
	55–59	161	20	20.59	218	47	21.56	125	54	22.69
	60–64	187	23	23.91	188	40	18.60	107	46	19.42
	Total	782	98	100.00	1,011	216	100.00	551	236	100.00
MBCCP	40–44							277	119	17.67
	45–49							343	147	21.88
	50–54							314	135	20.03
	55–59							315	135	20.09
	60–64							319	137	20.34
	Total							1,568	673	100.00

EXHIBIT 9.13
Ethnicity
Distribution
of Women
Identified with
Cancer Across
Program Eras

	Ethnicity	1995–2002 (8 years)			2003–August 2007 (4.67 years)			September 2007–2009 (2.33 years)		
		Total	Per Year	%	Total	Per Year	%	Total	Per Year	%
BCCS Program (in-situ/invasive)	Hispanic	396	50	50.77	446	96	44.20	234	100	42.55
	Non-Hispanic	384	48	49.23	548	117	54.31	315	135	57.27
	Unknown	0	0	0.00	15	3	1.49	1	0	0.18
	Total	780	98	100.00	1,009	216	100.00	550	236	100.00
MBCCP (applications submitted)	Hispanic							592	254	37.76
	Non-Hispanic							975	418	62.18
	Unknown							1	0	0.06
	Total							1,568	673	100.00

EXHIBIT 9.14
Urban/Rural
Distribution
of Women
Identified with
Cancer Across
Program Eras

		1995–2002 (8 years)			2003–August 2007 (4.67 years)			September 2007–2009 (2.33 years)		
		Total	Per Year	%	Total	Per Year	%	Total	Per Year	%
BCCS (in-situ/ invasive)	Urban	573	72	73.46	787	169	78.00	485	208	88.18
	Rural	207	26	26.54	222	48	22.00	65	28	11.82
	Total	780	98	100.00	1,009	216	100.00	550	236	100.00
MBCCP (applications submitted)	Urban							1,397	600	89.09
	Rural							171	73	10.91
	Total							1,568	673	100.00

women and shifting costs from the private to the public sector could be a good investment.

The effectiveness analysis shows that the use of BCCS staff to process Medicaid applications for women diagnosed with breast cancer increased the percentage of women receiving timely follow-up care and the number of low-income women with breast cancer served by the program. Additional analysis is needed to verify the trends while controlling for year-to-year changes related to program experiences and other confounders that might have influenced the results. Ultimately, an outcomes study linking BCCS Program and Texas Cancer Registry (TCR) data needs to be done to compare the outcomes (e.g., stage at diagnosis, survival) of breast cancer cases diagnosed through the BCCS Program to comparable cancer cases diagnosed outside the program.

The efficiency analysis, which compared the additional BCCS diagnostic and case management costs associated with the introduction of Medicaid to the increase in the number of cases receiving timely treatment, suggests that the Medicaid policy may be cost-effective for low-income women from the perspective of state government. After the introduction of Medicaid coverage, there was an increase in the number of women who were diagnosed through the BCCS Program and received timely breast cancer treatment, at a cost of $3,149 per additional woman. Whether this investment is worthwhile depends on whether this improvement leads to treatment of more breast cancer cases at an earlier stage and higher survival rates.

Equity analysis indicates that the extension of Medicaid eligibility may have significantly increased the percentage of low-income women with cancer diagnosed through the program and enrolled in Medicaid. The age and Hispanic ethnicity distributions of the women served did not change, but there was a significant increase in the proportion of program participants residing in urban areas after the introduction of the MBCCP in 2007. Interestingly, the shift from rural to urban distribution was noted among program participants identified by BCCS Program contractors as well as those referred by community providers. Clearly, further work is needed to determine whether the shift resulted from program characteristics or from factors outside the BCCS Program. The magnitude of the increase in public insurance coverage depends on how many women who were uninsured prior to the 2003 BCCS Program expansion ultimately gained this coverage. This information could be obtained through a merger of TCR data and data from Medicaid enrollment files. Our example is limited by the roughness of our estimate of the overall number of low-income, uninsured women diagnosed with breast cancer in Texas. While a more precise estimate would give us greater confidence in our results, it is nonetheless clear from the data that the BCCS/MBCCP expansion substantially increased the number of women identified through the program and that a potentially commensurate number gained access to public insurance coverage.

These rudimentary analyses of the effectiveness, efficiency, and equity of screening demonstrate how HSR can inform goal-oriented, evidence-based policy decision making. The discussion in this and previous chapters examines the conceptual, descriptive, and prescriptive information that can be produced by applying the effectiveness, efficiency, and equity perspectives of HSR to policy issues. It analyzes the balances and trade-offs that influence policies and programs designed to realize these objectives. It reviews the methods used to measure the extent to which each of these goals has been achieved. And it encourages dialogue among health services researchers, policy analysts, policymakers, and administrators who study, recommend, formulate, and implement health policy. To design a healthcare system that optimizes the policy ideals of effectiveness, efficiency, and equity, we must critically examine the meaning of these goals and systematically apply the criteria presented in this book to gain a better understanding of existing problems and unrealized opportunities.

Note

1. The case study is limited to the breast cancer component of the Texas BCCS Program.

REFERENCES

Aaron, H. J. 2003. "The Costs of Health Care Administration in the United States and Canada—Questionable Answers to a Questionable Question." *New England Journal of Medicine* 349 (8): 801–803.

Aaron, H. J., and P. B. Ginsburg. 2009. "Is Health Spending Excessive? If So, What Can We Do About It?" *Health Affairs* 28 (5): 1260–75.

Abbaszadeh, A., A. A. Haghdoost, M. Taebi, and S. Kohan. 2007. "The Relationship Between Women's Health Beliefs and Their Participation in Screening Mammography." *Asian Pacific Journal of Cancer Prevention* 8 (4): 471–75.

Abelson, J., P. G. Forest, J. Eyles, P. Smith, E. Martin, and F. P. Gauvin. 2003. "Deliberations About Deliberative Methods: Issues in the Design and Evaluation of Public Participation Processes." *Social Science & Medicine* 57 (2): 239–51.

Abelson, R., and G. Harris. 2010. "Critics Question Study Cited in Health Debate." *New York Times* (June 2).

Achman, L., and M. Gold. 2002. "Medicare+Choice 1999–2001: An Analysis of Managed Care Plan Withdrawals and Trends in Benefits and Premiums." New York: The Commonwealth Fund.

Adams, E. K., L. N. Chien, C. S. Florence, and C. Raskind-Hood. 2009. "The Breast and Cervical Cancer Prevention and Treatment Act in Georgia: Effects on Time to Medicaid Enrollment." *Cancer* 115 (6): 1300–309.

Adams, P. F., K. M. Heyman, and J. L. Vickerie. 2009. "Summary Health Statistics for the U.S. Population: National Health Interview Survey, 2008." *Vital Health Statistics. Series 10* (243): 1–104.

Aday, L. A. 2005. *Reinventing Public Health: Policies and Practices for a Healthy Nation.* San Francisco: Jossey-Bass.

———. 2001. *At Risk in America: The Health and Health Care Needs of Vulnerable Populations in the United States,* second edition. San Francisco: Jossey-Bass.

———. 1996. *Designing and Conducting Health Surveys: A Comprehensive Guide.* San Francisco: Jossey-Bass.

Aday, L. A., and R. M. Andersen. 1981. "Equity of Access to Medical Care: A Conceptual and Empirical Overview." *Medical Care* 19 (12): 4–27.

———. 1974. "A Framework for the Study of Access to Medical Care." *Health Services Research* 9 (3): 208–20.

Aday, L. A., R. Andersen, and G. V. Fleming. 1980. *Health Care in the U.S.: Equitable for Whom?* Beverly Hills, CA: Sage Publications.

Aday, L. A., and W. C. Awe. 1997. "Health Services Utilization Models." In *Handbook of Health Behavior Research I: Personal and Social Determinants*, edited by D. S. Gochman, 153–72. New York: Plenum Press.

Aday, L. A., C. E. Begley, D. R. Lairson, and C. H. Slater. 1993. *Evaluating the Medical Care System: Effectiveness, Efficiency, and Equity.* Chicago: Health Administration Press.

Aday, L. A., C. E. Begley, D. R. Lairson, C. H. Slater, A. J. Richard, and I. D. Montoya. 1999. "A Framework for Assessing the Effectiveness, Efficiency, and Equity of Behavioral Healthcare." *American Journal of Managed Care* 5 Spec No: SP25–44.

Aday, L. A., and L. J. Cornelius. 2006. *Designing and Conducting Health Surveys: A Comprehensive Guide.* San Fransisco: Jossey-Bass.

Adler, N. E., W. T. Boyce, M. A. Chesney, S. Folkman, and S. L. Syme. 1993. "Socioeconomic Inequalities in Health. No Easy Solution." *Journal of the American Medical Association* 269 (24): 3140–45.

Agabiti, N., M. Pirani, P. Schifano, G. Cesaroni, M. Davoli, L. Bisanti, N. Caranci, G. Costa, F. Forastiere, C. Marinacci, A. Russo, T. Spadea, and C. A. Perucci. 2009. "Income Level and Chronic Ambulatory Care Sensitive Conditions in Adults: A Multicity Population-Based Study in Italy." *BMC Public Health* 9: 457.

Agency for Healthcare Research and Quality (AHRQ). 2013. "Medical Expenditure Panel Survey (MEPS)." www.meps.ahrq.gov/mepsweb.

———. 2012a. "Consumer Assessment of Healthcare Providers and Systems (CAHPS)." US Department of Health & Human Services. www.cahps.ahrq.gov/default.asp.

———. 2012b. "Data Sources Available from AHRQ." www.ahrq.gov/data/data resources.htm.

———. 2011. "AHRQ Home." US Department of Health & Human Services. www.ahrq.gov.

———. 2009. "The Guide to Clinical Preventive Services 2009: Recommendations of the U.S. Preventive Services Task Force." US Department of Health & Human Services.

Albrecht, G., S. Freeman, and N. Higginbotham. 1998. "Complexity and Human Health: The Case for a Transdisciplinary Paradigm." *Culture Medicine and Psychiatry* 22 (1): 55–92.

Alliance for Health Policy and Systems Research. 2011. *Annual Report 2010: Building and Strengthening Partnerships.* Geneva, Switzerland: WHO Press. www.who.int/alliance-hpsr/resources/alliancehpsr_annualreport2010.pdf.

Al Snih, S., K. S. Markides, L. A. Ray, J. L. Freeman, G. V. Ostir, and J. S. Goodwin. 2006. "Predictors of Healthcare Utilization Among Older Mexican Americans." *Ethnicity & Disease* 16 (3): 640–46.

Altman, D. E., and L. Levitt. 2002. "The Sad History of Health Care Cost Containment as Told in One Chart." *Health Affairs (Millwood)* 21 (Suppl. Web Exclusives): W83–84.

Altman, S. H., and U. E. Reinhardt, eds. 1996. *Strategic Choices for a Changing Health Care System*. Chicago: Health Administration Press.

American Cancer Society. 2012. "Cancer Facts & Figures 2012." www.cancer.org /acs/groups/content/@epidemiologysurveilance/documents/document /acspc-031941.pdf.

———. 2010. "Decades of Detection: Progress and Challenges of the National Breast and Cervical Cancer Screening and Treatment Programs." www.acscan.org/pdf /breastcancer/dod-report.pdf.

American College of Osteopathic Family Physicians. 2010. "ACO/Medical Home." www.acofp.org/Practice_Management/ACO/Medical_Home.

American College of Physicians. 2008. "Improved Availability of Comparative Effectiveness Information: An Essential Feature for a High-Quality and Efficient United States Healthcare System." Position paper. Philadelphia, PA: American College of Physicians.

American Hospital Association (AHA). 2010. *Hospital Statistics*. Chicago: American Hospital Association.

———. 2009. *TrendWatch Chartbook 2009: Trends Affecting Hospitals and Health Systems*. Chicago: American Hospital Association.

Amey, C. H., M. K. Miller, and S. L. Albrecht. 1997. "The Role of Race and Residence in Determining Stage at Diagnosis of Breast Cancer." *Journal of Rural Health* 13 (2): 99–108.

Andersen, R. M. 1995. "Revisiting the Behavioral Model and Access to Medical Care: Does It Matter?" *Journal of Health & Social Behavior* 36 (1): 1–10.

Andersen, R. M., and L. A. Aday. 1978. "Access to Medical Care in the U.S.: Realized and Potential." *Medical Care* 16 (7): 533–46.

Andersen, R. M., L. A. Aday, C. S. Lyttle, L. J. Cornelius, and M. Chen. 1987. *Ambulatory Care and Insurance Coverage in an Era of Constraint*. Chicago: Pluribus Press, Inc.

Andersen, R. M., and P. L. Davidson. 2001. "Improving Access to Care in America: Individual and Contextual Indicators." In *Changing the U.S. Health Care System: Key Issues in Health Services, Policy, and Management*, edited by R. M. Andersen, T. H. Rice, and G. F. Kominski, 3–30. San Francisco: Jossey-Bass.

Anderson, G. F., U. E. Relnhardt, P. S. Hussey, and V. Petrosyan. 2003. "It's the Prices, Stupid: Why the United States Is So Different from Other Countries." *Health Affairs (Millwood)* 22 (3): 89–105.

Anderson, G. F., and D. A. Squires. 2010. "Measuring the U.S. Health Care System: A Cross-National Comparison." Published June 29. New York: The Commonwealth Fund.

Anderson, G. M., R. Brook, and A. Williams. 1991. "A Comparison of Cost-Sharing Versus Free Care in Children: Effects on the Demand for Office-Based Medical Care." *Medical Care* 29 (9): 890–98.

Anderson, J. M., P. Rodney, S. Reimer-Kirkham, A. J. Browne, K. B. Khan, and M. J. Lynam. 2009. "Inequities in Health and Healthcare Viewed Through the Ethical Lens of Critical Social Justice: Contextual Knowledge for the Global Priorities Ahead." *Advances in Nursing Science* 32 (4): 282–94.

Anderson, O. W. 1991. *The Evolution of Health Services Research: Personal Reflections on Applied Social Science.* San Francisco: Jossey-Bass.

———. 1989. *The Health Services Continuum in Democratic States: An Inquiry into Solvable Problems.* Chicago: Health Administration Press.

Andrulis, D., L. Duchon, C. Pryor, and N. Goodman. 2003. "Paying for Health Care When You're Uninsured: How Much Support Does the Safety Net Offer?" Boston: The Access Project.

Angelelli, J., D. Gifford, O. Intrator, P. Gozalo, L. Laliberte, and V. Mor. 2002. "Access to Postacute Nursing Home Care Before and After the BBA: Balanced Budget Act." *Health Affairs (Millwood)* 21 (5): 254–64.

Anglin, M. K. 1998. "Dismantling the Master's House: Cancer Activists, Discourses of Prevention, and Environmental Justice." *Identities* 5 (2): 183–217.

Anthony, D. 2003. "Changing the Nature of Physician Referral Relationships in the US: The Impact of Managed Care." *Social Science & Medicine* 56 (10): 2033–44.

Arnstein, S. 1969. "A Ladder of Citizen Participation." *Journal of the American Institute of Planners* 35 (July): 216–24.

Aronson, R. E., A. B. Wallis, P. J. O'Campo, and P. Schafer. 2007. "Neighborhood Mapping and Evaluation: A Methodology for Participatory Community Health Initiatives." *Maternal and Child Health Journal* 11 (4): 373–83.

Arrow, K. J. 1963. "Uncertainty and the Welfare Economics of Medical Care." *American Economic Review* 53 (5): 941–73.

Audit Commission. 2011. "Paying GPs to Improve Quality: Auditing Payments Under the Quality and Outcomes Framework." Health briefing, published in February. London: Audit Commission Publishing Team.

Baicker, K., and A. Finkelstein. 2011. "The Effects of Medicaid Coverage—Learning from the Oregon Experiment." *New England Journal of Medicine* 365 (8): 683–85.

Bailey, J. E., and D. Gibson. 2005. "Public Reporting Needed to Improve the Health of Tennesseans." *Tennessee Medicine* 98 (11): 539–40, 545.

Bailit Health Purchasing, LLC. 2002. "Ensuring Quality Providers: A Purchaser's Toolkit for Using Incentives." Published in May. Washington, DC: National Health Care Purchasing Institute.

Bailit Health Purchasing, LLC, and Sixth Man Consulting, Inc. 2001. "The Growing Case for Using Physician Incentives to Improve Health Care Quality." Published in December. Washington, DC: National Health Care Purchasing Institute.

Baker, L. C. 2001. "Managed Care and Technology Adoption in Health Care: Evidence from Magnetic Resonance Imaging." *Journal of Health Economics* 20 (3): 395–421.

Baker, L. C., and C. S. Phibbs. 2002. "Managed Care, Technology Adoption, and Health Care: The Adoption of Neonatal Intensive Care." *RAND Journal of Economics* 33 (3): 524–48.

Ball, R. M. 1995. "What Medicare's Architects Had in Mind." *Health Affairs (Millwood)* 14 (4): 62–72.

Balance, D., D. Kornegay, and P. Evans. 2009. "Factors That Influence Physicians to Practice in Rural Locations: A Review and Commentary." *Journal of Rural Health* 25 (3): 276–81.

Banerjee, M., J. George, C. Yee, W. Hryniuk, and K. Schwartz. 2007. "Disentangling the Effects of Race on Breast Cancer Treatment." *Cancer* 110 (10): 2169–77.

Bardach, E. 2009. *A Practical Guide for Policy Analysis: The Eightfold Path to More Effective Problem Solving.* Washington, DC: CQ Press.

Bartholomew, L. K., G. S. Parcel, G. Kok, N. H. Gottlieb, and M. E. Fernandez. 2011. *Planning Health Promotion Programs: An Intervention Mapping Approach.* San Francisco: Jossey-Bass.

Basu, R., L. Franzini, P. M. Krueger, and D. R. Lairson. 2010. "Gender Disparities in Medical Expenditures Attributable to Hypertension in the United States." *Women's Health Issues* 20 (2): 114–25.

Bazzoli, G. J., S. M. Shortell, N. Dubbs, C. Chan, and P. Kralovec. 1999. "A Taxonomy of Health Networks and Systems: Bringing Order Out of Chaos." *Health Services Research* 33 (6): 1683–717.

Beauchamp, D. E. 1998. "Public Health, Privatization, and Market Populism: A Cautionary Note." In *Managed Care & Public Health*, edited by P. K. Halverson, A. D. Kaluzny, and C. P. McLaughlin, 339–49. Gaithersburg, MD: Aspen Publishers, Inc.

———. 1988. *The Health of the Republic: Epidemics, Medicine, and Moralism as Challenges to Democracy.* Philadelphia, PA: Temple University Press.

———. 1985. "Community: The Neglected Tradition of Public Health." *Hastings Center Report* 15 (6): 28–36.

———. 1976. "Public Health as Social Justice." *Inquiry* 13 (1): 3–14.

Beauchamp, D. E., and B. Steinbock. 1999. *New Ethics for the Public's Health.* New York: Oxford University Press.

Beck, A. H. 2004. "The Flexner Report and the Standardization of American Medical Education." *Journal of the American Medical Association* 291 (17): 2139–40.

Begg, C., M. Cho, S. Eastwood, R. Horton, D. Moher, I. Olkin, R. Pitkin, D. Rennie, K. F. Schulz, D. Simel, and D. F. Stroup. 1996. "Improving the Quality of Reporting of Randomized Controlled Trials. The CONSORT Statement." *Journal of the American Medical Association* 276 (8): 637–39.

Begley, C. E., L. A. Aday, D. R. Lairson, and C. H. Slater. 2002. "Expanding the Scope of Health Reform: Application in the United States." *Social Science & Medicine* 55 (7): 1213–29.

Bentley, T. G., R. M. Effros, K. Palar, and E. B. Keeler. 2008. "Waste in the U.S. Health Care System: A Conceptual Framework." *Milbank Quarterly* 86 (4): 629–59.

Berk, M. L., C. L. Schur, and J. C. Cantor. 1995. "Ability to Obtain Health Care: Recent Estimates from the Robert Wood Johnson Foundation National Access to Care Survey." *Health Affairs (Millwood)* 14 (3): 139–46.

Berki, S. 1972. *Hospital Economics.* Lexington, MA: Lexington Books.

Berkman, L. F. 2000. "Social Support, Social Networks, Social Cohesion and Health." *Social Work in Health Care* 31 (2): 3–14.

Berlowitz, D. R., A. S. Ash, E. C. Hickey, R. H. Friedman, M. Glickman, B. Kader, and M. A. Moskowitz. 1998. "Inadequate Management of Blood Pressure in a Hypertensive Population." *New England Journal of Medicine* 339 (27): 1957–63.

Bernstein, J. 2009. "Changes in Health Care Financing & Organization: Impact of the Economy on Health Care." Robert Wood Johnson Foundation, issue brief, published in August. www.rwjf.org/content/dam/farm/reports /issue_briefs/2009/rwjf44843.

Bhaloo, T. 2011. "The Role of a Nursing Home Administrator's Education in Influencing Quality of Care in US Nursing Homes." Texas Medical Center Dissertations (via ProQuest), Paper AAI3459835. http://digitalcommons .library.tmc.edu/dissertations/AAI3459835.

Bibb, S. C. 2001. "The Relationship Between Access and Stage at Diagnosis of Breast Cancer in African American and Caucasian Women." *Oncology Nursing Forum* 28 (4): 711–19.

Biello, K. B., J. Rawlings, A. Carroll-Scott, R. Browne, and J. R. Ickovics. 2010. "Racial Disparities in Age at Preventable Hospitalization Among U.S. Adults." *American Journal of Preventive Medicine* 38 (1): 54–60.

Biles, B., J. Pozen, and S. Guterman. 2009. "The Continuing Cost of Privatization: Extra Payments to Medicare Advantage Plans Jump to $11.4 Billion in 2009." Issue brief, published May 4. New York: The Commonwealth Fund.

Billings, J., G. M. Anderson, and L. S. Newman. 1996. "Recent Findings on Preventable Hospitalizations." *Health Affairs (Project Hope)* 15 (3): 239–49.

Bindman, A. B., and M. R. Gold. 1998. "Measuring Access to Care Through Population-Based Surveys in a Managed Care Environment: A Special Supplement to HSR." *Health Services Research* 33 (3 Pt. 2): entire issue.

Bindman, A. B., K. Grumbach, D. Osmond, M. Komaromy, K. Vranizan, N. Lurie, J. Billings, and A. Stewart. 1995. "Preventable Hospitalizations and Access to Health Care." *Journal of the American Medical Association* 274 (4): 305–11.

Blacksher, E., and G. S. Lovasi. 2012. "Place-Focused Physical Activity Research, Human Agency, and Social Justice in Public Health: Taking Agency Seriously in Studies of the Built Environment." *Health & Place* 18 (2): 172–79.

Blackwell, D. L., M. E. Martinez, J. F. Gentleman, C. Sanmartin, and J. M. Berthelot. 2009. "Socioeconomic Status and Utilization of Health Care Services in Canada and the United States: Findings from a Binational Health Survey." *Medical Care* 47 (11): 1136–46.

Blackwell, D. L., and L. Tonthat. 2003. "Summary Health Statistics for the U.S. Population: National Health Interview Survey, 1999." *Vital and Health Statistics* 10 (211): 1–94.

Blendon, R. J., C. Schoen, C. M. DesRoches, R. Osborn, K. L. Scoles, and K. Zapert. 2002. "Inequities in Health Care: A Five-Country Survey." *Health Affairs (Millwood)* 21 (3): 182–91.

Bloom, B., R. A. Cohen, and G. Freeman. 2011. "Summary Health Statistics for U.S. Children: National Health Interview Survey, 2010." National Center for Health Statistics. *Vital and Health Statistics* 10 (250).

Bloom, J. R., S. L. Stewart, J. Koo, and R. A. Hiatt. 2001. "Cancer Screening in Public Health Clinics: The Importance of Clinic Utilization." *Medical Care* 39 (12): 1345–51.

Blumenschein, K., and M. Johannesson. 1996. "Economic Evaluation in Healthcare: A Brief History and Future Directions." *Pharmacoeconomics* 10 (2): 114–22.

Blumenthal, D. S. 1985. *Introduction to Environmental Health.* New York: Springer Publishing Company.

Blumenthal, D., and A. M. Epstein. 1996. "Quality of Health Care. Part 6: The Role of Physicians in the Future of Quality Management." *New England Journal of Medicine* 335 (17): 1328–31.

Bodenheimer, T. S. 1969. "Regional Medical Programs: No Road to Regionalization." *Medical Care Review* 26: 1125–66.

Bodenheimer, T., and H. H. Pham. 2010. "Primary Care: Current Problems and Proposed Solutions." *Health Affairs (Millwood)* 29 (5): 799–805.

Boucher, A., S. Bowman, C. Piselli, and R. Scichilone. 2006. "The Evolution of DRGs." *Journal of AHIMA* 77 (7): 68A–68C.

Boudreaux, E. D., B. L. Cruz, and B. M. Baumann. 2006. "The Use of Performance Improvement Methods to Enhance Emergency Department Patient Satisfaction in the United States: A Critical Review of the Literature and Suggestions for Future Research." *Academic Emergency Medicine* 13 (7): 795–802.

Boudreaux, E. D., and E. L. O'Hea. 2004. "Patient Satisfaction in the Emergency Department: A Review of the Literature and Implications for Practice." *Journal of Emergency Medicine* 26 (1): 13–26.

Boukus, E., A. Cassil, and A. O'Malley. 2009. "A Snapshot of U.S. Physicians: Key Findings from the 2008 Health Tracking Physician Survey." *Data Bulletin (Center for Studying Health System Change)* 35: 1–11.

Boyce, W. F. 2001. "Disadvantaged Persons' Participation in Health Promotion Projects: Some Structural Dimensions." *Social Science & Medicine* 52 (10): 1551–64.

Bradley, E. H., L. A. Curry, and K. J. Devers. 2007. "Qualitative Data Analysis for Health Services Research: Developing Taxonomy, Themes, and Theory." *Health Services Research* 42 (4): 1758–72.

Bradley, E. H., S. A. McGraw, L. Curry, A. Buckser, K. L. King, S. V. Kasl, and R. Andersen. 2002. "Expanding the Andersen Model: The Role of Psychosocial Factors in Long-Term Care Use." *Health Services Research* 37 (5): 1221–42.

Braybrooke, D. 1998. *Moral Objectives, Rules, and the Forms of Social Change.* Toronto, Canada: University of Toronto Press.

———. 1987. *Meeting Needs.* Princeton, NJ: Princeton University Press.

Breen, N., A. Cronin, H. I. Meissner, S. H. Taplin, F. K. Tangka, J. A. Tiro, and T. S. McNeel. 2007. "Reported Drop in Mammography: Is This Cause for Concern?" *Cancer* 109 (12): 2405–409.

Brereton, L., and V. Vasoodaven. 2010. "The Impact of the NHS Market: An Overview of the Literature." Published March 1. London: Civitas: Institute for the Study of Civil Society.

Brook, R. H. 1994. "Appropriateness: The Next Frontier." *BMJ* 308 (6923): 218–19.

Brook, R. H., and K. N. Lohr. 1985. "Efficacy, Effectiveness, Variations, and Quality. Boundary-Crossing Research." *Medical Care* 23 (5): 710–22.

Brown, C., J. Barner, T. Bohman, and K. Richards. 2009. "A Multivariate Test of an Expanded Andersen Health Care Utilization Model for Complementary and Alternative Medicine (CAM) Use in African Americans." *Journal of Alternative and Complementary Medicine* 15 (8): 911–19.

Brown, D. M. 1988. "Do Physicians Underutilize Aides?" *Journal of Human Resources* 23 (3): 342–55.

Brown, E. R., P. L. Davidson, H. Yu, R. Wyn, R. M. Andersen, L. Becerra, and N. Razack. 2004. "Effects of Community Factors on Access to Ambulatory Care for Lower-Income Adults in Large Urban Communities." *Inquiry* 41 (1): 39–56.

Brown, H. S. III. 2003. "Managed Care and Technical Efficiency." *Health Economics* 12 (2): 149–58.

Brown, L. D. 1991. "Knowledge and Power: Health Services Research as a Political Resource." In *Health Services Research: Key to Health Policy*, edited by E. Ginzberg, 20–45. Cambridge, MA: Harvard University Press.

Brown, P. 1995. "Race, Class, and Environmental Health: A Review and Systematization of the Literature." *Environmental Research* 69 (1): 15–30.

Brownson, R. C., C. Royer, R. Ewing, and T. D. McBride. 2006. "Researchers and Policymakers: Travelers in Parallel Universes." *American Journal of Preventive Medicine* 30 (2): 164–72.

Bryan, K. A., and L. Martinez. 2008. "On the Evolution of Income Inequality in the United States." *Economic Quarterly* 94 (2): 97–120.

Buerhaus, P. I. 2008. "Current and Future State of the US Nursing Workforce." *Journal of the American Medical Association* 300 (20): 2422–25.

Bullard, R. D. 2000. *Dumping in Dixie: Race, Class, and Environmental Quality.* Boulder, CO: Westview Press.

Bunker, J. P. 1970. "Surgical Manpower. A Comparison of Operations and Surgeons in the United States and in England and Wales." *New England Journal of Medicine* 282 (3): 135–44.

Bunker, J. P., H. S. Frazier, and F. Mosteller. 1994. "Improving Health: Measuring Effects of Medical Care." *Milbank Quarterly* 72 (2): 225–58.

Burns, L. R., G. J. Bazzoli, L. Dynan, and D. R. Wholey. 2000. "Impact of HMO Market Structure on Physician-Hospital Strategic Alliances." *Health Services Research* 35 (1 Pt. 1): 101–32.

Burtram, S. G. 1994. "A Critical Assessment of the National Institutes of Health Consensus Development Program Against the Eras Which Shaped It." PhD dissertation, University of Texas School of Public Health. http://digital commons.library.tmc.edu/dissertations/AAI9513520.

Callahan, D. 2001. *Promoting Healthy Behavior: How Much Freedom? Whose Responsibility?* Washington, DC: Georgetown University Press.

Canadian Agency for Drugs and Technologies in Health. 2006. *Guidelines for the Economic Evaluation of Health Technologies: Canada*, third edition. www.cadth .ca/media/pdf/186_EconomicGuidelines_e.pdf.

Canadian Institute for Health Information. 2009. *The Health Indicators Project. Report from the Third Consensus Conference on Health Indicators.* Ottawa, Canada: Canadian Institute for Health Information.

———. 2005. *The Health Indicators Project: The Next 5 Years. Report from the Second Consensus Conference on Population Health Indicators.* Ottawa, Canada: Canadian Institute for Health Information.

———. 1999. *Final Report: National Consensus Conference on Population Health Indicators.* Ottawa, Canada: Canadian Institute for Health Information.

Caplan, L. S., E. R. Schoenfeld, E. S. O'Leary, and M. C. Leske. 2000. "Breast Cancer and Electromagnetic Fields: A Review." *Annals of Epidemiology* 10 (1): 31–44.

Carrier, E., M. N. Gourevitch, and N. R. Shah. 2009. "Medical Homes: Challenges in Translating Theory into Practice." *Medical Care* 47 (7): 714–22.

Casale, A. S., R. A. Paulus, M. J. Selna, M. C. Doll, A. E. Bothe Jr., K. E. McKinley, S. A. Berry, D. E. Davis, R. J. Gilfillan, B. H. Hamory, and G. D. Steele Jr. 2007. "'ProvenCareSM': A Provider-Driven Pay-for-Performance Program for Acute Episodic Cardiac Surgical Care." *Annals of Surgery* 246 (4): 613–21.

Casalino, L., and J. C. Robinson. 2003. "Alternative Models of Hospital-Physician Affiliation as the United States Moves Away from Tight Managed Care." *Milbank Quarterly* 81 (2): 331–51.

Catlin, A., C. Cowan, M. Hartman, and S. Heffler; National Health Expenditure Accounts Team. 2008. "National Health Spending in 2006: A Year of Change for Prescription Drugs." *Health Affairs (Millwood)* 27 (1): 14–29.

Center for Studying Health System Change. 2003. "Tracking Health Care Costs: Trends Stabilize but Remain High in 2002." *Data Bulletin (Center for Studying Health System Change)* 25: 1–2.

Center for the Evaluation of Value and Risk in Health. "Cost-Effectiveness Analysis Registry." Institute for Clinical Research and Health Policy Studies, Tufts Medical Center. https://research.tufts-nemc.org/cear4/Home.aspx.

Centers for Disease Control and Prevention (CDC). 2011a. "CDC Health Disparities and Inequalities Report—United States, 2011." *Morbidity and Mortality Weekly Report* 60 (Suppl.); published January 14. www.cdc.gov/mmwr/pdf/other/su6001.pdf.

———. 2011b. "Data & Statistics." www.cdc.gov/DataStatistics.

———. 2011c. "DATA2010 . . . the Healthy People 2010 Database." US Department of Health & Human Services. http://wonder.cdc.gov/data2010.

———. 2011d. "Vaccine-Specific Coverage Levels by Race/Ethnicity and Poverty Level." www.cdc.gov/vaccines/stats-surv/nis/data/tables_2011.htm.

———. 2010. "April 2010 Submission of NBCCEDP Minimum Data Elements (MDE)." Atlanta, GA: US Department of Health and Human Services.

———. 2006. "The Behavioral Risk Factor Surveillance System Operational and User's Guide, Version 3.0." Published December 12. ftp://ftp.cdc.gov/pub/Data/Brfss/userguide.pdf.

Centers for Medicare & Medicaid Services (CMS). 2013a. "Data Compendium." www.cms.gov/DataCompendium/14_2010_Data_Compendium.asp#TopOfPage.

———. 2013b. "Medicare Plan Finder." www.medicare.gov/find-a-plan/questions/home.aspx.

———. 2013c. "Nursing Home Compare." www.medicare.gov/NHCompare/Include/DataSection/Questions/SearchCriteriaNEW.asp?version=default&browser=IE|6|WinXP&language=English&defaultstatus=0&pagelist=Home&CookiesEnabledStatus=True.

———. 2013d. "Research, Statistics, Data & Systems." www.cms.gov/home/rsds.asp.

———. 2012a. "Medicare Current Beneficiary Survey (MCBS)." www.cms.gov/mcbs.

———. 2012b. "Medicare Physician Fee Schedule." www.cms.gov/apps/physician-fee-schedule.

———. 2011a. "Medicaid Managed Care Enrollment Report." US Department of Health & Human Services. www.medicaid.gov/Medicaid-CHIP-Program-Information/By-Topics/Data-and-Systems/Downloads/2011-Medicaid-MC-Enrollment-Report.pdf.

———. 2011b. "Medicare & Medicaid Statistical Supplement." www.cms.gov/Research-Statistics-Data-and-Systems/Statistics-Trends-and-Reports/MedicareMedicaidStatSupp/2011.html.

———. 2011c. "National Health Expenditure Data." www.cms.gov/NationalHealthExpendData.

———. 2010a. "Innovators' Guide to Navigating Medicare, Version 2.0." www.cms .gov/CouncilonTechInnov/Downloads/InnovatorsGuide5_10_10.pdf.

———. 2010b. "Medicare 'Accountable Care Organizations' Shared Savings Program—New Section 1899 of Title XVIII: Preliminary Questions & Answers." http://healthreformgps.org/wp-content/uploads/AccountableCare Organization1.pdf.

Chandra, A., J. Gruber, and R. McKnight. 2010. "Patient Cost-Sharing and Hospitalization Offsets in the Elderly." *American Economic Review* 100 (1): 193–213.

Chang, S. W., K. Kerlikowske, A. Nápoles-Springer, S. F. Posner, E. A. Sickles, and E. J. Pérez-Stable. 1996. "Racial Differences in Timeliness of Follow-Up After Abnormal Screening Mammography." *Cancer* 78 (7): 1395–402.

Chao, S., K. Anderson, and L. Hernandez. 2009. "Toward Health Equity and Patient-Centeredness: Integrating Health Literacy, Disparities Reduction, and Quality Improvement. Workshop Summary." Institute of Medicine. Washington, DC: National Academies Press.

Charles, C., and S. DeMaio. 1993. "Lay Participation in Health Care Decision Making: A Conceptual Framework." *Journal of Health Politics, Policy & Law* 18 (4): 881–904.

Chassin, M. R., R. H. Brook, R. E. Park, J. Keesey, A. Fink, J. Kosecoff, K. Kahn, N. Merrick, and D. H. Solomon. 1986. "Variations in the Use of Medical and Surgical Services by the Medicare Population." *New England Journal of Medicine* 314 (5): 285–90.

Cheadle, A., E. Wagner, M. Walls, P. Diehr, M. Bell, C. Anderman, C. McBride, R. F. Catalano, E. Pettigrew, R. Simmons, and H. Neckerman. 2001. "The Effect of Neighborhood-Based Community Organizing: Results from the Seattle Minority Youth Health Project." *Health Services Research* 36 (4): 671–89.

Chernew, M. E., R. A. Hirth, and D. M. Cutler. 2009. "Increased Spending on Health Care: Long-Term Implications for the Nation." *Health Affairs (Millwood)* 28 (5): 1253–55.

Chernew, M. E., I. A. Juster, M. Shah, A. Wegh, S. Rosenberg, A. B. Rosen, M. C. Sokol, K. Yu-Isenberg, and A. M. Fendrick. 2010. "Evidence That Value-Based Insurance Can Be Effective." *Health Affairs (Millwood)* 29 (3): 530–36.

Chernew, M. E., and J. P. Newhouse. 2008. "What Does the RAND Health Insurance Experiment Tell Us About the Impact of Patient Cost Sharing on Health Outcomes?" *American Journal of Managed Care* 14 (7): 412–14.

Chernew, M. E., L. M. Sabik, A. Chandra, T. B. Gibson, and J. P. Newhouse. 2010. "Geographic Correlation Between Large-Firm Commercial Spending and Medicare Spending." *American Journal of Managed Care* 16 (2): 131–38.

Chien, A. T., Z. Li, and M. B. Rosenthal. 2010. "Improving Timely Childhood Immunizations Through Pay for Performance in Medicaid-Managed Care." *Health Services Research* 45 (6 Pt. 2): 1934–47.

Chien, L. N., and E. K. Adams. 2010. "The Effect of the Breast and Cervical Cancer Prevention and Treatment Act on Medicaid Disenrollment." *Women's Health Issues* 20 (4): 266–71.

Chirikos, T. N., L. K. Christman, S. Hunter, and R. G. Roetzheim. 2004. "Cost-Effectiveness of an Intervention to Increase Cancer Screening in Primary Care Settings." *Preventive Medicine* 39 (2): 230–38.

Chlebowski, R. T. 2000. "Reducing the Risk of Breast Cancer." *New England Journal of Medicine* 343 (3): 191–98.

Choi, M., B. D. Sommers, and J. M. McWilliams. 2011. "Children's Health Insurance and Access to Care During and After the CHIP Expansion Period." *Journal of Health Care for the Poor and Underserved* 22 (2): 576–89.

Choi, T., and J. N. Greenberg. 1982. *Social Science Approaches to Health Services Research.* Chicago: Health Administration Press.

Chou, R., and M. Helfand. 2005. "Challenges in Systematic Reviews That Assess Treatment Harms." *Annals of Internal Medicine* 142 (12 Pt. 2): 1090–99.

Chou, S. Y., M. Grossman, and H. Saffer. 2004. "An Economic Analysis of Adult Obesity: Results from the Behavioral Risk Factor Surveillance System." *Journal of Health Economics* 23 (3): 565–87.

Christianson, J. B., and S. Trude. 2003. "Managing Costs, Managing Benefits: Employer Decisions in Local Health Care Markets." *Health Services Research* 38 (1 Pt. 2): 357–73.

Christianson, J. B., K. M. Volmar, J. Alexander, and D. P. Scanlon. 2010. "A Report Card on Provider Report Cards: Current Status of the Health Care Transparency Movement." *Journal of General Internal Medicine* 25 (11): 1235–41.

Chung, S., L. P. Palaniappan, L. M. Trujillo, H. R. Rubin, and H. S. Luft. 2010. "Effect of Physician-Specific Pay-for-Performance Incentives in a Large Group Practice." *American Journal of Managed Care* 16 (2): 35–42.

Cinnamon, J., N. Schuurman, and V. A. Crooks. 2008. "A Method to Determine Spatial Access to Specialized Palliative Care Services Using GIS." *BMC Health Services Research* 8: 140.

Claxton, G., B. DiJulio, H. Whitmore, J. D. Pickreign, M. McHugh, A. Osei-Anto, and B. Finder. 2010. "Health Benefits in 2010: Premiums Rise Modestly, Workers Pay More Toward Coverage." *Health Affairs (Millwood)* 29 (10): 1942–50.

Claxton, G., J. Feder, D. Shactman, and S. Altman. 1997. "Public Policy Issues in Nonprofit Conversions: An Overview." *Health Affairs (Millwood)* 16 (2): 9–28.

Cleverly, W. O. 1997. *Essentials of Health Care Finance.* Gaithersburg, MD: Aspen Publishers, Inc.

Coburn, D., K. Denny, E. Mykhalovskiy, P. McDonough, A. Robertson, and R. Love. 2003. "Population Health in Canada: A Brief Critique." *American Journal of Public Health* 93 (3): 392–96.

Cochrane, A. L. 1971. *Effectiveness and Efficiency*. London: Nuffield Provincial Hospitals Trust.

Cohen, J. 1994. "The Earth Is Round (p < .05)." *American Psychologist* 49 (12): 997–1003.

Cohen, J. W., A. C. Monheit, K. M. Beauregard, S. B. Cohen, D. C. Lefkowitz, D. E. Potter, J. P. Sommers, A. K. Taylor, and R. H. Arnett III. 1996. "The Medical Expenditure Panel Survey: A National Health Information Resource." *Inquiry* 33 (4): 373–89.

Cohen, S. B. 2005. "Medical Expenditure Panel Survey (MEPS)." In *Encyclopedia of Biostatistics*, second edition, edited by P. Armitage and T. Colton. Hoboken, NJ: John Wiley & Sons.

Colby, D. C., and L. C. Baker. 2009. "Health Services Research in 2020: An Assessment of the Field's Workforce Needs." *Health Services Research* 44 (6): 2193–97.

Colby, D. C., B. C. Quinn, C. H. Williams, L. T. Bilheimer, and S. Goodell. 2008. "Research Glut and Information Famine: Making Research Evidence More Useful for Policymakers." *Health Affairs (Millwood)* 27 (4): 1177–82.

Coldman, A., and N. Phillips. 2011. "Population Studies of the Effectiveness of Mammographic Screening." *Preventive Medicine* 53 (3): 115–17.

Coleman, R. 2011. "The Independent Medicare Advisory Committee: Death Panel or Smart Governing?" *Issues in Law & Medicine* 27 (2): 121–77.

Collins, S. R., K. Davis, M. M. Doty, and A. Ho. 2004. "Wages, Health Benefits, and Workers' Health." *Issue Brief (Commonwealth Fund)* 788: 1–16.

Colwill, J. M., J. M. Cultice, and R. L. Kruse. 2008. "Will Generalist Physician Supply Meet Demands of an Increasing and Aging Population?" *Health Affairs (Millwood)* 27 (3): w232–41.

Comber, A. J., C. Brunsdon, and R. Radburn. 2011. "A Spatial Analysis of Variations in Health Access: Linking Geography, Socio-Economic Status and Access Perceptions." *International Journal of Health Geographics* 10: 44.

Committee for Economic Development Research and Policy Committee. 2007. "Quality, Affordable Health Care for All: Moving Beyond the Employer-Based Health-Insurance System." Published October 15. Washington, DC: Committee for Economic Development.

Commonwealth Fund. 2010. "2010 Commonwealth Fund International Health Policy Survey." www.commonwealthfund.org/Content/Surveys/2010/Nov/2010-International-Survey.aspx.

Community Care Coordination Learning Network. 2010. *Connecting Those at Risk to Care: A Guide to Building a Community "HUB" to Promote a System of Collaboration, Accountability, and Improved Outcomes*. Rockville, MD: Agency for Healthcare Research and Quality.

Cook, B. L. 2007. "Effect of Medicaid Managed Care on Racial Disparities in Health Care Access." *Health Services Research* 42 (1 Pt. 1): 124–45.

Cooper, M. H. 1994. "Jumping on the Spot: Health Reform New Zealand Style." *Health Economics* 3 (2): 69–72.

Copeland, V. C., S. H. Scholle, and J. A. Binko. 2003. "Patient Satisfaction: African American Women's Views of the Patient-Doctor Relationship." *Journal of Health & Social Policy* 17 (2): 35–48.

Corso, L. C., L. B. Landrum, D. Lenaway, R. Brooks, and P. K. Halverson. 2007. "Building a Bridge to Accreditation—The Role of the National Public Health Performance Standards Program." *Journal of Public Health Management and Practice* 13 (4): 374–77.

Coughlin, S. S., T. D. Thompson, H. I. Hall, P. Logan, and R. J. Uhler. 2002. "Breast and Cervical Carcinoma Screening Practices Among Women in Rural and Nonrural Areas of the United States, 1998–1999." *Cancer* 94 (11): 2801–12.

Council on Health Care Technology. 1990. *Improving Consensus Development for Health Technology Assessment: An International Perspective.* Washington, DC: National Academies Press.

Cowan, C. A., P. A. McDonnell, K. R. Levit, and M. A. Zezza. 2002. "Burden of Health Care Costs: Businesses, Households, and Governments, 1987–2000." *Health Care Financing Review* 23 (3): 131–59.

Cowing, T. G., A. G. Holtmann, and S. Powers. 1983. "Hospital Cost Analysis: A Survey and Evaluation of Recent Studies." *Advances in Health Economics and Health Services Research* 4: 257–303.

Cram, P., G. E. Rosenthal, and M. S. Vaughan-Sarrazin. 2005. "Cardiac Revascularization in Specialty and General Hospitals." *New England Journal of Medicine* 352 (14): 1454–62.

Cram, P., M. S. Vaughan-Sarrazin, B. Wolf, J. N. Katz, and G. E. Rosenthal. 2007. "A Comparison of Total Hip and Knee Replacement in Specialty and General Hospitals." *Journal of Bone and Joint Surgery. American Volume* 89 (8): 1675–84.

Crawford, M. J., D. Rutter, C. Manley, T. Weaver, K. Bhui, N. Fulop, and P. Tyrer. 2002. "Systematic Review of Involving Patients in the Planning and Development of Health Care." *British Medical Journal* 325 (7375): 1263–65.

Cromwell, J., M. Trisolini, G. Pope, J. Mitchell, and L. Greenwald. 2011. *Pay for Performance in Health Care: Methods and Approaches.* Research Triangle Park, NC: RTI Press.

Cuellar, A. E., and P. J. Gertler. 2005. "How the Expansion of Hospital Systems Has Affected Consumers." *Health Affairs (Millwood)* 24 (1): 213–19.

Culyer, A. J. 1992. "The Morality of Efficiency in Health Care: Some Uncomfortable Implications." *Health Economics* 1 (1): 7–18.

Cunningham, P. J. 2002. "Mounting Pressures: Physicians Serving Medicaid Patients and the Uninsured, 1997–2001." *Tracking Report (Center for Studying Health System Change)* 6 (6): 1–4.

Cunningham, P. J., J. Hadley, G. Kenney, and A. J. Davidoff. 2007. "Identifying Affordable Sources of Medical Care Among Uninsured Persons." *Health Services Research* 42 (1 Pt. 1): 265–85.

Currie, J., and E. Moretti. 2003. "Mother's Education and the Intergenerational Transmission of Human Capital: Evidence from College Openings." *Quarterly Journal of Economics* 118 (4): 1495–1532.

Cutler, D. M. 2006. "The Economics of Health System Payment." *De Economist* 154 (1): 1–18.

———. 2002. "Equality, Efficiency, and Market Fundamentals: The Dynamics of International Medical-Care Reform." *Journal of Economic Literature* 40 (3): 881–906.

Cutler, D. M., and A. Lleras-Muney. 2010. "Understanding Differences in Health Behaviors by Education." *Journal of Health Economics* 29 (1): 1–28.

Cutler, D. M., A. Lleras-Muney, and T. Vogl. 2008. "Socioeconomic Status and Health: Dimensions and Mechanisms." NBER Working Paper No. 14333. Published in September. Cambridge, MA: National Bureau of Economic Research.

Cutler, D. M., and M. McClellan. 2001a. "Is Technological Change in Medicine Worth It?" *Health Affairs (Millwood)* 20 (5): 11–29.

———. 2001b. "Productivity Change in Health Care." *American Economic Review* 91 (2): 281–86.

Dal Maso, L., A. Zucchetto, R. Talamini, D. Serraino, C. F. Stocco, M. Vercelli, F. Falcini, and S. Franceschi. 2008. "Effect of Obesity and Other Lifestyle Factors on Mortality in Women with Breast Cancer." *International Journal of Cancer* 123 (9): 2188–94.

Daly, M. 1994. *Communitarianism: A New Public Ethics*. Belmont, CA: Wadsworth Publishing Company.

Daniels, N. 2011. "Reflective Equilibrium." In *The Stanford Encyclopedia of Philosophy (Spring 2011 Edition)*, edited by E. N. Zalta. http://plato.stanford.edu /archives/spr2011/entries/reflective-equilibrium.

———. 2009. "Just Health: Replies and Further Thoughts." *Journal of Medical Ethics* 35 (1): 36–41.

———. 2008. *Just Health: Meeting Health Needs Fairly*. New York: Cambridge University Press.

———. 2006. "Equity and Population Health: Toward a Broader Bioethics Agenda." *Hastings Center Report* 36 (4): 22–35.

———. 2001. "Justice, Health, and Healthcare." *American Journal of Bioethics* 1 (2): 2–16.

———. 1998. "Appendix D: Distributive Justice and the Use of Summary Measures of Population Health Status." In *Summarizing Population Health: Directions for the Development and Application of Population Metrics*, edited by M. J. Field and M. R. Gold, 58–71. Washington, DC: National Academies Press.

———. 1996. "Justice, Fair Procedures, and the Goals of Medicine." *Hastings Center Report* 26 (6): 10–12.

———. 1985. *Just Health Care.* Cambridge, UK: Cambridge University Press.

Daniels, N., B. Kennedy, and I. Kawachi. 2000. *Is Inequality Bad for Our Health?* Boston: Beacon Press.

Daniels, N., and J. E. Sabin. 2002. *Setting Limits Fairly: Can We Learn to Share Medical Resources?* New York: Oxford University Press.

Daniels, N., B. Saloner, and A. H. Gelpi. 2009. "Access, Cost, and Financing: Achieving an Ethical Health Reform." *Health Affairs (Millwood)* 28 (5): w909–16.

Dartmouth Atlas of Healthcare. 2013. "Understanding of the Efficiency and Effectiveness of the Health Care System." www.dartmouthatlas.org.

Davidson, P. L., R. M. Andersen, R. Wyn, and E. R. Brown. 2004. "A Framework for Evaluating Safety-Net and Other Community-Level Factors on Access for Low-Income Populations." *Inquiry* 41 (1): 21–38.

Davies, G., and J. Burgess. 2004. "Challenging the 'View from Nowhere': Citizen Reflections on Specialist Expertise in a Deliberative Process." *Health Place* 10 (4): 349–61.

Davis, K., C. Schoen, and K. Stremikis. 2010. "Mirror, Mirror on the Wall: How the Performance of the U.S. Health Care System Compares Internationally, 2010 Update." Published June 23. New York: The Commonwealth Fund.

Davis, L. 2008. *Multi-Stakeholder Community Inventory Modules.* Rockville, MD: Agency for Healthcare Research and Quality. www.ahrq.gov/qual/value /cimodules.pdf.

Davis, M. V., M. M. Cannon, L. Corso, D. Lenaway, and E. L. Baker. 2009. "Incentives to Encourage Participation in the National Public Health Accreditation Model: A Systematic Investigation." *American Journal of Public Health* 99 (9): 1705–11.

Davis, R. M. 1997. "Healthcare Report Cards and Tobacco Measures." *Tobacco Control* 6 (Suppl. 1): S70–77.

Davis, S. K., Y. Liu, and G. H. Gibbons. 2003. "Disparities in Trends of Hospitalization for Potentially Preventable Chronic Conditions Among African Americans During the 1990s: Implications and Benchmarks." *American Journal of Public Health* 93 (3): 447–55.

Deaton, A. 2002. "Policy Implications of the Gradient of Health and Wealth." *Health Affairs (Project Hope)* 21 (2): 13–30.

Deb, P., and A. M. Holmes. 1998. "The Formal Mental Health Care Burden Among Recently Deinstitutionalized Patients." *Journal of Behavioral Health Services & Research* 25 (3): 346–56.

DeFriese, G. H., T. C. Ricketts III, and J. Stein. 1989. *Methodological Advances in Health Services Research.* Chicago: Health Administration Press.

De Koning, H. J. 2000. "Breast Cancer Screening: Cost-Effective in Practice?" *European Journal of Radiology* 33 (1): 32–37.

DeNavas-Walt, C., B. D. Proctor, and J. C. Smith. 2010. *Income, Poverty, and Health Insurance Coverage in the United States: 2009.* US Census Bureau, Current Population Reports, P60-238. Washington, DC: US Government Printing Office.

Devers, K. J. 2011. "Qualitative Methods in Health Services and Management Research: Pockets of Excellence and Progress, but Still a Long Way to Go." *Medical Care Research and Review* 68 (1): 41–48.

Devers, K. J., L. R. Brewster, and P. B. Ginsburg. 2003. "Specialty Hospitals: Focused Factories or Cream Skimmers?" *Issue Brief (Center for Studying Health System Change)* 62: 1–4.

DeVoe, J. E., G. E. Fryer, R. Phillips, and L. Green. 2003. "Receipt of Preventive Care Among Adults: Insurance Status and Usual Source of Care." *American Journal of Public Health* 93 (5): 786–91.

DeVoe, J. E., C. J. Tillotson, S. E. Lesko, L. S. Wallace, and H. Angier. 2011. "The Case for Synergy Between a Usual Source of Care and Health Insurance Coverage." *Journal of General Internal Medicine* 26 (9): 1059–66.

De Vries, R., A. Stanczyk, I. F. Wall, R. Uhlmann, L. J. Damschroder, and S. Y. Kim. 2010. "Assessing the Quality of Democratic Deliberation: A Case Study of Public Deliberation on the Ethics of Surrogate Consent for Research." *Social Science & Medicine* 70 (12): 1896–903.

Deyo, R. A. 1995. "Promises and Limitations of the Patient Outcome Research Teams: the Low-Back Pain Example." *Proceedings of the Association of American Physicians* 107 (3): 324–28.

D'Intignano, B. 1990. "Incentives in Health Care Management." Second World Congress on Health Economics, University of Zurich, Switzerland, September 10–14.

Docteur, E. R., D. C. Colby, and M. Gold. 1996. "Shifting the Paradigm: Monitoring Access in Medicare Managed Care." *Health Care Financing Review* 17 (4): 5–21.

Donabedian, A. 2005. "Evaluating the Quality of Medical Care." *Milbank Quarterly* 83 (4): 691–729.

———. 2003. *An Introduction to Quality Assurance in Health Care.* New York: Oxford University Press.

———. 1990. "The Seven Pillars of Quality." *Archives of Pathology & Laboratory Medicine* 114 (11): 1115–18.

———. 1982. *Explorations in Quality Assessment and Monitoring. Volume II—The Criteria and Standards of Quality.* Chicago: Health Administration Press.

———. 1980. *Explorations in Quality Assessment and Monitoring. Volume I—The Definition of Quality and Approaches to Its Assessment.* Chicago: Health Administration Press.

———. 1973. *Aspects of Medical Care Administration: Specifying Requirements for Health Care.* Cambridge, MA: Harvard University Press.

————. 1966. "Evaluating the Quality of Medical Care." *Milbank Memorial Fund Quarterly* 44 (3 Suppl.): 166–206.

Donelan, K., J. R. Mailhot, D. Dutwin, K. Barnicle, S. A. Oo, K. Hobrecker, S. Percac-Lima, and B. A. Chabner. 2011. "Patient Perspectives of Clinical Care and Patient Navigation in Follow-Up of Abnormal Mammography." *Journal of General Internal Medicine* 26 (2): 116–22.

Doran, T., and M. Roland. 2010. "Lessons from Major Initiatives to Improve Primary Care in the United Kingdom." *Health Affairs (Millwood)* 29 (5): 1023–29.

d'Oronzio, J. C. 2001. "A Human Right to Healthcare Access: Returning to the Origins of the Patients' Rights Movement." *Cambridge Quarterly of Healthcare Ethics* 10 (3): 285–98.

Dowling, W. L. 1974. "Prospective Reimbursement of Hospitals." *Inquiry* 11 (3): 163–80.

Dranove, D., and W. D. White. 1998. "Medicaid-Dependent Hospitals and Their Patients: How Have They Fared?" *Health Services Research* 33 (2 Pt. 1): 163–85.

Draper, D. A., R. E. Hurley, C. S. Lesser, and B. C. Strunk. 2002. "The Changing Face of Managed Care." *Health Affairs (Millwood)* 21 (1): 11–23.

Drummond, M. F., M. J. Sculpher, G. W. Torrance, B. J. O'Brien, and G. L. Stoddart. 2005. *Methods for the Economic Evaluation of Health Care Programmes*, third edition. New York: Oxford University Press, USA.

Dryzek, J. S. 1993. "Policy Analysis and Planning: From Science to Argument." In *The Argumentative Turn in Policy Analysis and Planning*, edited by F. Fischer and J. Forester, 213–32. Durham, NC: Duke University Press.

Dunet, D. O., P. B. Sparling, J. Hersey, P. Williams-Piehota, M. D. Hill, M. Reyes, C. Hanssen, and F. Lawrenz. 2008. "Peer Reviewed: A New Evaluation Tool to Obtain Practice-Based Evidence of Worksite Health Promotion Programs." *Preventing Chronic Disease* 5 (4): A118.

Dunn, W. N. 2009. *Public Policy Analysis: An Introduction*, fourth edition. Upper Saddle River, NJ: Pearson Prentice Hall.

DuPlessis, H. M., M. Inkelas, and N. Halfon. 1998. "Assessing the Performance of Community Systems for Children." *Health Services Research* 33 (4 Pt. 2): 1111–42.

Durairaj, L., J. C. Torner, E. A. Chrischilles, M. S. Vaughan-Sarrazin, J. Yankey, and G. E. Rosenthal. 2005. "Hospital Volume-Outcome Relationships Among Medical Admissions to ICUs." *Chest* 128 (3): 1682–89.

Durning, D. 1999. "The Transition from Traditional to Postpositivist Policy Analysis: A Role for Q-Methodology." *Journal of Policy Analysis and Management* 18 (3): 389–410.

Eddy, D. M. 2005. "Evidence-Based Medicine: A Unified Approach." *Health Affairs (Millwood)* 24 (1): 9–17.

————. 1991. "Clinical Decision Making: From Theory to Practice. What's Going On in Oregon?" *Journal of the American Medical Association* 266 (3): 417–20.

————. 1980. *Screening for Cancer: Theory, Analysis, and Design*. Englewood Cliffs, NJ: Prentice-Hall.

Edejer, T. T., R. Baltussen, T. Adam, R. Hutubessy, A. Acharya, D. B. Evans, and C. J. L. Murray, eds. 2003. "Making Choices in Health: WHO Guide to Cost-Effectiveness Analysis." Geneva, Switzerland: World Health Organization. www.who.int/choice/publications/p_2003_generalised_cea.pdf.

Eibner, C., P. S. Hussey, and F. Girosi. 2010. "The Effects of the Affordable Care Act on Workers' Health Insurance Coverage." *New England Journal of Medicine* 363 (15): 1393–95.

Eng, P. M., E. B. Rimm, G. Fitzmaurice, and I. Kawachi. 2002. "Social Ties and Change in Social Ties in Relation to Subsequent Total and Cause-Specific Mortality and Coronary Heart Disease Incidence in Men." *American Journal of Epidemiology* 155 (8): 700–709.

Enthoven, A. 2010. "Curing Fragmentation with Integrated Delivery Systems: What They Do, What Has Blocked Them, Why We Need Them, and How to Get There from Here." In *The Fragmentation of U.S. Health Care: Causes and Solutions*, edited by E. Elhauge. New York: Oxford University Press.

————. 1990. "What Can Europeans Learn from Americans?" In *Health Care Systems in Transition: The Search for Efficiency*, 51–71. Paris, France: Organisation for Economic Co-operation and Development.

Epstein, A. 1995. "Performance Reports on Quality: Prototypes, Problems, and Prospects." *New England Journal of Medicine* 333 (1): 57–61.

Epstein, A. J. 2001. "The Role of Public Clinics in Preventable Hospitalizations Among Vulnerable Populations." *Health Services Research* 36 (2): 405–20.

Epstein, A. M., and D. Blumenthal. 1993. "Physician Payment Reform: Past and Future." *Milbank Quarterly* 71 (2): 193–215.

Epstein, R. M., K. Fiscella, C. S. Lesser, and K. C. Stange. 2010. "Why the Nation Needs a Policy Push on Patient-Centered Health Care." *Health Affairs (Millwood)* 29 (8): 1489–95.

Escarce, J. J., and S. Goodell. 2007. "Racial and Ethinic Disparities in Access to and Quality of Health Care." Published September 1. www.rwjf.org/pr/product.jsp?id=20651.

Estabrooks, C. A., D. S. Thompson, J. J. Lovely, and A. Hofmeyer. 2006. "A Guide to Knowledge Translation Theory." *Journal of Continuing Education in the Health Professions* 26 (1): 25–36.

Ettner, S. L. 1996. "The Timing of Preventive Services for Women and Children: The Effect of Having a Usual Source of Care." *American Journal of Public Health* 86 (12): 1748–54.

Etzioni, A. 2003a. *My Brother's Keeper: A Memoir and a Message*. Lanham, MD: Rowman & Littlefield Publishers, Inc.

———. 2003b. *The Monochrome Society*. Princeton, NJ: Princeton University Press.

———. 2000a. *Next: The Road to the Good Society*. New York: Basic Books.

———. 2000b. *The New Golden Rule: Community and Morality in a Democratic Society*. New York: Basic Books.

———. 1999. *Civic Repentance*. Lanham, MD: Rowman & Littlefield Publishers, Inc.

———. 1998. *The Essential Communitarian Reader*. Lanham, MD: Rowman & Littlefield Publishers, Inc.

European Observatory on Health Care Systems. 2002. *Health Care Systems in Eight Countries: Trends and Challenges*. London: London School of Economics & Political Science.

European Science Foundation. 2008. *Shared Responsibilities in Sharing Research Data: Policies and Partnerships*. Report of an ESF–DFG workshop, September 21, 2007.

Evans, G. W., and E. Kantrowitz. 2002. "Socioeconomic Status and Health: The Potential Role of Environmental Risk Exposure." *Annual Review of Public Health* 23: 303–31.

Evans, R. G., M. Barer, and T. R. Marmor, eds. 1994. *Why Are Some People Healthy and Others Not? The Determinants of Health of Populations*. Hawthorne, NY: Aldine De Gruyter.

Evans, R. G., and G. L. Stoddart. 2003. "Consuming Research, Producing Policy?" *American Journal of Public Health* 93 (3): 371–79.

Feig, S. A. 2002. "Current Status of Screening Mammography." *Obstetrics & Gynecology Clinics of North America* 29 (1): 123–36.

Feldstein, P. J. 1998. *Health Care Economics*. Albany, NY: Delmar Publishers.

Felland, L. E., J. M. Grossman, and H. T. Tu. 2011. "Key Findings from HSC's 2010 Site Visits: Health Care Markets Weather Economic Downturn, Brace for Health Reform." *Issue Brief (Center for Studying Health System Change)* 135: 1–8.

Felt-Lisk, S., M. McHugh, and E. Howell. 2002. "Monitoring Local Safety-Net Providers: Do They Have Adequate Capacity?" *Health Affairs (Millwood)* 21 (5): 277–83.

Feresu, S. A., W. Zhang, S. E. Puumala, F. Ullrich, and J. R. Anderson. 2008. "Breast and Cervical Cancer Screening Among Low-Income Women in Nebraska: Findings from the Every Woman Matters Program, 1993–2004." *Journal of Health Care for the Poor and Underserved* 19 (3): 797–813.

Fernandez, M. E., A. Gonzales, G. Tortolero-Luna, J. Williams, M. Saavedra-Embesi, W. Chan, and S. W. Vernon. 2009. "Effectiveness of Cultivando la Salud: A Breast and Cervical Cancer Screening Promotion Program for Low-Income Hispanic Women." *American Journal of Public Health* 99 (5): 936–43.

Fernandez, M. E., R. C. Palmer, and C. A. Leong-Wu. 2005. "Repeat Mammography Screening Among Low-Income and Minority Women: A Qualitative Study." *Cancer Control* 12 (Suppl. 2): 77–83.

Ferrante, J. M., D. C. Fyffe, M. L. Vega, A. K. Piasecki, P. A. Ohman-Strickland, and B. F. Crabtree. 2010. "Family Physicians' Barriers to Cancer Screening in Extremely Obese Patients." *Obesity (Silver Spring)* 18 (6): 1153–59.

Fields, D., E. Leshen, and K. Patel. 2010. "Analysis & Commentary. Driving Quality Gains and Cost Savings Through Adoption of Medical Homes." *Health Affairs (Millwood)* 29 (5): 819–26.

Fineberg, H. V. 2009. "Health Reform Beyond Health Insurance." President's Address, Institute of Medicine Annual Meeting. Published October 12. www.iom.edu /About-IOM/~/media/Files/About%20the%20IOM/PresAddress%20 2009.pdf.

Finkelstein, A., S. Taubman, B. Wright, M. Bernstein, J. Gruber, J. P. Newhouse, H. Allen, K. Baicker, and the Oregon Health Study Group. 2011. "The Oregon Health Insurance Experiment: Evidence from the First Year." NBER Working Paper No. 17190, published in July. Cambridge, MA: National Bureau of Economic Research.

Finks, J. F., N. H. Osborne, and J. D. Birkmeyer. 2011. "Trends in Hospital Volume and Operative Mortality for High-Risk Surgery." *New England Journal of Medicine* 364 (22): 2128–37.

Fiscella, K., P. Franks, M. P. Doescher, and B. G. Saver. 2002. "Disparities in Health Care by Race, Ethnicity, and Language Among the Insured: Findings from a National Sample." *Medical Care* 40 (1): 52–59.

Fischer, F., and J. Forester. 1993. *The Argumentative Turn in Policy Analysis and Planning.* Durham, NC: Duke University Press.

Fisher, E. S., M. B. McClellan, J. Bertko, S. M. Lieberman, J. J. Lee, J. L. Lewis, and J. S. Skinner. 2009. "Fostering Accountable Health Care: Moving Forward in Medicare." *Health Affairs (Millwood)* 28 (2): w219–31.

Fisher, E. S., and S. M. Shortell. 2010. "Accountable Care Organizations: Accountable for What, to Whom, and How." *Journal of the American Medical Association* 304 (15): 1715–16.

Fishman, P., S. Taplin, D. Meyer, and W. Barlow. 2000. "Cost-Effectiveness of Strategies to Enhance Mammography Use." *Effective Clinical Practice* 3 (5): 213–20.

Flexner, A. 1910. *Medical Education in the United States and Canada: A Report to the Carnegie Foundation for the Advancement of Teaching.* Boston: Merrymount Press.

Flobbe, K., A. M. Bosch, A. G. Kessels, G. L. Beets, P. J. Nelemans, M. F. von Meyenfeldt, and J. M. van Engelshoven. 2003. "The Additional Diagnostic Value of Ultrasonography in the Diagnosis of Breast Cancer." *Archives of Internal Medicine* 163 (10): 1194–99.

Flook, E. E., and P. J. Sanazaro. 1973. *Health Services Research and R & D in Perspective.* Chicago: Health Administration Press.

Folland, S., A. C. Goodman, and M. Stano. 2010. *The Economics of Health and Health Care,* sixth edition. Upper Saddle River, NJ: Pearson Prentice Hall.

Ford, E. S., and S. Capewell. 2011. "Proportion of the Decline in Cardiovascular Mortality Disease Due to Prevention Versus Treatment: Public Health Versus Clinical Care." *Annual Review of Public Health* 32: 5–22.

Forester, J. 1993. *Critical Theory, Public Policy and Planning Practice: Toward a Critical Pragmatism.* Albany, NY: State University of New York Press.

Forrest, C. B., J. P. Weiner, J. Fowles, C. Vogeli, K. D. Frick, K. W. Lemke, and B. Starfield. 2001. "Self-Referral in Point-of-Service Health Plans." *Journal of the American Medical Association* 285 (17): 2223–31.

Foster, R. S. 2010. "Estimated Financial Effect of the 'Patient Protection and Affordable Care Act,' as Amended." Published April 22. www.cms.gov/Actuarial Studies/downloads/PPACA_2010-04-22.pdf.

Fottler, M. D., D. J. Slovensky, and S. J. Rogers. 1988. "HCFA Release of Hospital Specific Death Rates: Where Are We and Where Are We Going?" *Journal of the American Medical Records Association* 59 (9): 25–29.

Fournier, G. M., and J. M. Mitchell. 1992. "Hospital Costs and Competition for Services: A Multiproduct Analysis." *Review of Economics and Statistics* 74 (4): 627–34.

Foxall, M. J., C. R. Barron, and J. F. Houfek. 2001. "Ethnic Influences on Body Awareness, Trait Anxiety, Perceived Risk, and Breast and Gynecologic Cancer Screening Practices." *Oncology Nursing Forum* 28 (4): 727–38.

Francis, D. P., P. R. Baker, J. Doyle, B. J. Hall, and E. Waters. 2011. "Reviewing Interventions Delivered to Whole Communities: Learnings and Recommendations for Application to Policy, Practice and Evidence Development." *Journal of Public Health (Oxford, England)* 33 (2): 322–25.

Franzini, L. 2008. "Self-Rated Health and Trust in Low-Income Mexican-Origin Individuals in Texas." *Social Science & Medicine* 67 (12): 1959–69.

Franzini, L., M. Caughy, W. Spears, and M. E. Fernandez-Esquer. 2005. "Neighborhood Economic Conditions, Social Processes, and Self-Rated Health in Low-Income Neighborhoods in Texas: A Multilevel Latent Variables Model." *Social Science & Medicine* 61 (6): 1135–50.

Franzini, L., M. N. Elliott, P. Cuccaro, M. Schuster, M. J. Gilliland, J. A. Grunbaum, F. Franklin, and S. R. Tortolero. 2009. "Influences of Physical and Social Neighborhood Environments on Children's Physical Activity and Obesity." *American Journal of Public Health* 99 (2): 271–78.

Franzini, L., and M. E. Fernandez-Esquer. 2004. "Socioeconomic, Cultural, and Personal Influences on Health Outcomes in Low Income Mexican-Origin Individuals in Texas." *Social Science & Medicine* 59 (8): 1629–46.

Franzini, L., O. I. Mikhail, and J. S. Skinner. 2010. "McAllen and El Paso Revisited: Medicare Variations Not Always Reflected in the Under-Sixty-Five Population." *Health Affairs (Millwood)* 29 (12): 2302–309.

Franzini, L., W. Taylor, M. N. Elliott, P. Cuccaro, S. R. Tortolero, M. Janice Gilliland, J. Grunbaum, and M. A. Schuster. 2010. "Neighborhood Characteristics

Favorable to Outdoor Physical Activity: Disparities by Socioeconomic and Racial/Ethnic Composition." *Health Place* 16 (2): 267–74.

Fraser, I., W. Encinosa, and L. Baker. 2010. "Payment Reform. Introduction." *Health Services Research* 45 (6 Pt. 2): 1847–53.

Frech, H. E., and P. B. Ginsburg. 1974. "Optimal Scale in Medical Practice: A Survivor Analysis." *Journal of Business* 47 (1): 23–36.

Freire, P. 1995. *Pedagogy of Hope: Reliving Pedagogy of the Oppressed.* New York: Continuum International Publishing Group, Inc.

———. 1970. *Pedagogy of the Oppressed.* New York: Seabury Press.

Friedmann, J. 1987. *Planning in the Public Domain: From Knowledge to Action.* Princeton, NJ: Princeton University Press.

Freudenberg, N., D. Silver, J. M. Carmona, D. Kass, B. Lancaster, and M. Speers. 2000. "Health Promotion in the City: A Structured Review of the Literature on Interventions to Prevent Heart Disease, Substance Abuse, Violence and HIV Infection in US Metropolitan Areas, 1980–1995." *Journal of Urban Health* 77 (3): 443–57.

Frost, L., and S. Stone. 2009. "Community-Based Collaboration: A Philanthropic Model for Positive Social Change." *Foundation Review* 1 (1): 55–68.

Fuchs, V. R. 1974. *Who Shall Live? Health, Economics, and Social Choice.* New York: Basic Books.

———. 1972. "Health Care and the United States Economic System: An Essay in Abnormal Physiology." *Milbank Memorial Fund Quarterly* 50 (2): 211–44.

Fung, A. E., R. Palanki, S. J. Bakri, E. Depperschmidt, and A. Gibson. 2009. "Applying the CONSORT and STROBE Statements to Evaluate the Reporting Quality of Neovascular Age-Related Macular Degeneration Studies." *Ophthalmology* 116 (2): 286–96.

Fung, C. H., Y. W. Lim, S. Mattke, C. Damberg, and P. G. Shekelle. 2008. "Systematic Review: The Evidence That Publishing Patient Care Performance Data Improves Quality of Care." *Annals of Internal Medicine* 148 (2): 111–23.

Gabel, J., L. Levitt, E. Holve, J. Pickreign, H. Whitmore, K. Dhont, S. Hawkins, and D. Rowland. 2002. "Job-Based Health Benefits in 2002: Some Important Trends." *Health Affairs (Millwood)* 21 (5): 143–51.

Gabel, J. R., A. T. Lo Sasso, and T. Rice. 2002. "Consumer-Driven Health Plans: Are They More than Talk Now?" *Health Affairs (Millwood)* (Suppl. Web Exclusives): W395–407.

Gagnon, F., J. Turgeon, and C. Dallaire. 2007. "Healthy Public Policy: A Conceptual Cognitive Framework." *Health Policy* 81 (1): 42–55.

Galea, S., and M. Tracy. 2007. "Participation Rates in Epidemiologic Studies." *Annals of Epidemiology* 17 (9): 643–53.

Galewitz, P. 2011. "Medicare Advantage Premiums to Fall 4% Next Year." Kaiser Health News, September 15. www.kaiserhealthnews.org/stories/2011/september /15/medicare-advantage-premiums-fall-next-year.aspx.

Garber, A. M. 2001. "Evidence-Based Coverage Policy." *Health Affairs (Millwood)* 20 (5): 62–82.

Garcia, R., and C. Fenwick. 2009. "Social Science, Equal Justice, and Public Health Policy: Lessons from Los Angeles." *Journal of Public Health Policy* 30 (Suppl. 1): S26–32.

Gaskin, D. J., and J. Hadley. 1997. "The Impact of HMO Penetration on the Rate of Hospital Cost Inflation, 1985–1993." *Inquiry* 34 (3): 205–16.

Gaskin, D. J., J. Hadley, and V. G. Freeman. 2001. "Are Urban Safety-Net Hospitals Losing Low-Risk Medicaid Maternity Patients?" *Health Services Research* 36 (1 Pt. 1): 25–51.

Gaskin, D. J., and C. Hoffman. 2000. "Racial and Ethnic Differences in Preventable Hospitalizations Across 10 States." *Medical Care Research & Review* 57 (Suppl.): 85–107.

Gauthier, A. K., D. L. Rogal, N. L. Barrand, and A. B. Cohen. 1992. "Administrative Costs in the U.S. Health Care System: The Problem or the Solution?" *Inquiry* 29 (3): 308–20.

Gawande, A. 2009. "The Cost Conundrum: What a Texas Town Can Teach Us About Healthcare." *New Yorker* (June 1).

Gelberg, L., R. M. Andersen, and B. D. Leake. 2000. "The Behavioral Model for Vulnerable Populations: Application to Medical Care Use and Outcomes for Homeless People." *Health Services Research* 34 (6): 1273–302.

Gellad, W. F., H. A. Huskamp, A. Li, Y. Zhang, D. G. Safran, and J. M. Donohue. 2011. "Use of Prescription Drug Samples and Patient Assistance Programs, and the Role of Doctor-Patient Communication." *Journal of General Internal Medicine* 26 (12): 1458–64.

Gerdtham, U. G., M. Johannesson, L. Lundberg, and D. Isacson. 1999. "The Demand for Health: Results from New Measures of Hospital Capital." *European Journal of Political Economy* 15: 501–21.

Getzen, T. E. 2003. *Health Economics: Fundamentals and Flow of Funds*, second edition. Hoboken, NJ: John Wiley & Sons, Inc.

Getzen, T. E., and B. H. Allen. 2007. *Health Care Economics*. Hoboken, NJ: John Wiley & Sons.

Giacomini, M. K., and D. J. Cook. 2000a. "Users' Guides to the Medical Literature: XXIII. Qualitative Research in Health Care A. Are the Results of the Study Valid? Evidence-Based Medicine Working Group." *Journal of the American Medical Association* 284 (3): 357–62.

———. 2000b. "Users' Guides to the Medical Literature: XXIII. Qualitative Research in Health Care B. What Are the Results and How Do They Help Me Care for My Patients? Evidence-Based Medicine Working Group." *Journal of the American Medical Association* 284 (4): 478–82.

Gilbert, G. H., G. R. Shah, B. J. Shelton, M. W. Heft, E. H. Bradford Jr., and L. S. Chavers. 2002. "Racial Differences in Predictors of Dental Care Use." *Health Services Research* 37 (6): 1487–507.

Ginzberg, E. 1991. *Health Services Research: Key to Health Policy.* Cambridge, MA: Harvard University Press.

Given, R. S. 1996. "Economies of Scale and Scope as an Explanation of Merger and Output Diversification Activities in the Health Maintenance Organization Industry." *Journal of Health Economics* 15 (6): 685–713.

Glance, L. G., Y. Li, T. M. Osler, A. Dick, and D. B. Mukamel. 2006. "Impact of Patient Volume on the Mortality Rate of Adult Intensive Care Unit Patients." *Critical Care Medicine* 34 (7): 1925–34.

Glanz, K., F. M. Lewis, and B. Rimer. 2002. *Health Behavior and Health Education: Theory, Research, and Practice,* third edition. San Francisco: Jossey-Bass.

Glaser, B. G. 1965. "The Constant Comparative Method of Qualitative Analysis." *Social Problems* 12 (4): 436–45.

Glasgow, R. E., E. Lichtenstein, and A. C. Marcus. 2003. "Why Don't We See More Translation of Health Promotion Research to Practice? Rethinking the Efficacy-to-Effectiveness Transition." *American Journal of Public Health* 93 (8): 1261–67.

Glasgow, R. E., D. J. Magid, A. Beck, D. Ritzwoller, and P. A. Estabrooks. 2005. "Practical Clinical Trials for Translating Research to Practice: Design and Measurement Recommendations." *Medical Care* 43 (6): 551–57.

Glasgow, R. E., T. M. Vogt, and S. M. Boles. 1999. "Evaluating the Public Health Impact of Health Promotion Interventions: The RE-AIM Framework." *American Journal of Public Health* 89 (9): 1322–27.

Glennerster, H. 1995. "Internal Markets: Context and Structure." In *Health Care Reform Through Internal Markets,* edited by M. Jerome-Forget, J. White, and J. Wiener, 17–26. Washington, DC: The Brookings Institution.

Glied, S. 2003. "Health Care Costs: On the Rise Again." *Journal of Economic Perspectives* 17 (2): 125–48.

Glouberman, S., and J. Millar. 2003. "Evolution of the Determinants of Health, Health Policy, and Health Information Systems in Canada." *American Journal of Public Health* 93 (3): 388–92.

Glover, J. A. 1938. "The Incidence of Tonsillectomy in School Children." *Proceedings of the Royal Society of Medicine* 31 (10): 1219–36.

Gold, J. 2011. "Accountable Care Organizations, Explained." Published January 18. www.npr.org/2011/04/01/132937232/accountable-care-organizations-explained.

Gold, M. R., J. E. Siegel, L. B. Russell, and M. C. Weinstein. 1996. *Cost-Effectiveness in Health and Medicine.* New York: Oxford University Press.

Goldsmith, B., J. Dietrich, Q. Du, and R. S. Morrison. 2008. "Variability in Access to Hospital Palliative Care in the United States." *Journal of Palliative Medicine* 11 (8): 1094–102.

Gong, F., S. Baron, L. Ayala, L. Stock, S. McDevitt, and C. Heaney. 2009. "The Role for Community-Based Participatory Research in Formulating Policy Initiatives: Promoting Safety and Health for In-Home Care Workers and

Their Consumers." *American Journal of Public Health* 99 (Suppl. 3): S531–38.

Gonzalez, C. A., and E. Riboli. 2010. "Diet and Cancer Prevention: Contributions from the European Prospective Investigation into Cancer and Nutrition (EPIC) Study." *European Journal of Cancer* 46 (14): 2555–62.

Gosfield, A. G. 1997. "Who Is Holding Whom Accountable for Quality?" *Health Affairs (Millwood)* 16 (3): 26–40.

Goss, C., and C. Renzi. 2007. "Patient and Citizen Participation in Health Care Decisions in Italy." *German Journal for Quality in Health Care* 101 (4): 236–40.

Gould, E. 2009. "The Erosion of Employer-Sponsored Health Insurance: Declines Continue for the Seventh Year Running." *International Journal of Health Services* 39 (4): 669–97.

Graham, H. 2002. "Building an Inter-Disciplinary Science of Health Inequalities: The Example of Lifecourse Research." *Social Science & Medicine* 55 (11): 2005–16.

Grannemann, T. W., R. S. Brown, and M. V. Pauly. 1986. "Estimating Hospital Costs: A Multiple-Output Analysis." *Journal of Health Economics* 5 (2): 107–27.

Graves, B. A. 2008. "Integrative Literature Review: A Review of Literature Related to Geographical Information Systems, Healthcare Access and Health Outcomes." *Perspectives in Health Information Management* 5: 11.

Grayson, C. 2004. "Every Patient Deserves a Doctor: Improving Access to Care for Medicaid Patients in Georgia. An Argument for Improving Physician Medicaid Payments." *Journal of the Medical Association of Georgia* 2: 15–20.

Green, L. W., R. W. Wilson, and K. G. Bauer. 1983. "Data Requirements to Measure Progress on the Objectives for the Nation in Health Promotion and Disease Prevention." *American Journal of Public Health* 73 (1): 18–24.

Greene, J. J. 1976. "The Health Professions Educational Assistance Act of 1976: A New Prescription?" *Fordham Urban Law Journal* 5 (2): 279–302.

Greene, J., J. Blustein, and D. Remler. 2005. "The Impact of Medicaid Managed Care on Primary Care Physician Participation in Medicaid." *Medical Care* 43 (9): 911–20.

Greenfield, S., S. Kaplan, and J. E. Ware Jr. 1985. "Expanding Patient Involvement in Care. Effects on Patient Outcomes." *Annals of Internal Medicine* 102 (4): 520–28.

Grembowski, D. 2001. *The Practice of Health Program Evaluation*. Thousand Oaks, CA: Sage Publications, Inc.

Gresenz, C. R., J. Rogowski, and J. J. Escarce. 2009. "Community Demographics and Access to Health Care Among U.S. Hispanics." *Health Services Research* 44 (5 Pt. 1): 1542–62.

Griggs, J. J., E. Culakova, M. E. Sorbero, M. S. Poniewierski, D. A. Wolff, J. Crawford, D. C. Dale, and G. H. Lyman. 2007. "Social and Racial Differences in

Selection of Breast Cancer Adjuvant Chemotherapy Regimens." *Journal of Clinical Oncology* 25 (18): 2522–27.

Griggs, J. J., M. E. Sorbero, A. T. Stark, S. E. Heininger, and A. W. Dick. 2003. "Racial Disparity in the Dose and Dose Intensity of Breast Cancer Adjuvant Chemotherapy." *Breast Cancer Research and Treatment* 81 (1): 21–31.

Grimshaw, J. M., and I. T. Russell. 1993. "Effect of Clinical Guidelines on Medical Practice: A Systematic Review of Rigorous Evaluations." *Lancet* 342 (8883): 1317–22.

Gross, D. J., L. Alecxih, M. J. Gibson, J. Corea, C. Caplan, and N. Brangan. 1999. "Out-of-Pocket Health Spending by Poor and Near-Poor Elderly Medicare Beneficiaries." *Health Services Research* 34 (1 Pt. 2): 241–54.

Grosse, S. D., S. M. Teutsch, and A. C. Haddix. 2007. "Lessons from Cost-Effectiveness Research for United States Public Health Policy." *Annual Review of Public Health* 28: 365–91.

Grossman, M. 1972. *The Demand for Health: A Theoretical and Empirical Investigation.* New York: National Bureau of Economic Research.

Grumbach, K., K. Vranizan, and A. B. Bindman. 1997. "Physician Supply and Access to Care in Urban Communities." *Health Affairs (Millwood)* 16 (1): 71–86.

Grytten, J., and R. Sorensen. 2001. "Type of Contract and Supplier-Induced Demand for Primary Physicians in Norway." *Journal of Health Economics* 20 (3): 379–93.

Guadagnoli, E., and P. Ward. 1998. "Patient Participation in Decision-Making." *Social Science & Medicine* 47 (3): 329–39.

Gunning, T., and R. Sickles. 2011. "A Multi-Product Cost Function for Physician Private Practices." *Journal of Productivity Analysis* 35 (2): 119–28.

Guo, S., L. Wang, and R. Yan. 2002. "Health Service Needs of Women with Reproductive Tract Infections in Selected Areas of China." *Chinese Medical Journal* 115 (8): 1253–56.

Haas, J. S., K. A. Phillips, D. Sonneborn, C. E. McCulloch, and S. Y. Liang. 2002. "Effect of Managed Care Insurance on the Use of Preventive Care for Specific Ethnic Groups in the United States." *Medical Care* 40 (9): 743–51.

Habermas, J. 2002. *On the Pragmatics of Social Interaction: Preliminary Studies in the Theory of Communicative Action.* Cambridge, MA: MIT Press.

———. 1996. *Between Facts and Norms: Contributions to a Discourse Theory of Law and Democracy.* Cambridge, MA: MIT Press.

———. 1995. *Moral Consciousness and Communicative Action.* Cambridge, MA: MIT Press.

———. 1989. *The Structural Transformation of the Public Sphere: An Inquiry into a Category of Bourgeois Society.* Cambridge, MA: MIT Press.

Habermas, J., and B. Fultner. 2003. *Truth and Justification.* Cambridge, MA: MIT Press.

Hacker, J. 1996. *The Road to Nowhere: The Genesis of President Clinton's Plan for Health Security.* Princeton, NJ: Princeton University Press.

Haddix, A. C., S. M. Teutsch, and P. S. Corso. 2003. *Prevention Effectiveness: A Guide to Decision Analysis and Economic Evaluation.* New York: Oxford University Press.

Hadorn, D. C. 1991. "Setting Health Care Priorities in Oregon: Cost-Effectiveness Meets the Rule of Rescue." *Journal of the American Medical Association* 265 (17): 2218–25.

Hahn, J. 2010. "Medicare Physician Payment Updates and the Sustainable Growth Rate (SGR) System." Published August 6. Washington, DC: Congressional Research Service.

Halfon, N., and M. Hochstein. 2002. "Life Course Health Development: An Integrated Framework for Developing Health, Policy, and Research." *Milbank Quarterly* 80 (3): 433–79.

Halm, E. A., C. Lee, and M. R. Chassin. 2002. "Is Volume Related to Outcome in Health Care? A Systematic Review and Methodologic Critique of the Literature." *Annals of Internal Medicine* 137 (6): 511–20.

Hansen, K. K., and J. Zwanziger. 1996. "Marginal Costs in General Acute Care Hospitals: A Comparison Among California, New York and Canada." *Health Economics* 5 (3): 195–216.

Hanson, G. 2003. "Operation Medicaid: The War on Women." National Women's Health Network. http://nwhn.org/print/660.

Hanson, M. J., and D. Callahan. 2001. *The Goals of Medicine: The Forgotten Issue in Health Care Reform.* Washington, DC: Georgetown University Press.

Harden, V. A. 1986. *Inventing the NIH: Federal Biomedical Research Policy, 1887–1937.* Baltimore, MD: Johns Hopkins University Press.

Hargraves, J. L., P. J. Cunningham, and R. G. Hughes. 2001. "Racial and Ethnic Differences in Access to Medical Care in Managed Care Plans." *Health Services Research* 36 (5): 853–68.

Harper, S., J. Lynch, S. C. Meersman, N. Breen, W. W. Davis, and M. C. Reichman. 2009. "Trends in Area-Socioeconomic and Race-Ethnic Disparities in Breast Cancer Incidence, Stage at Diagnosis, Screening, Mortality, and Survival Among Women Ages 50 Years and Over (1987–2005)." *Cancer Epidemiology, Biomarkers & Prevention* 18 (1): 121–31.

Harris, E. N. 1987. "Syndrome of the Black Swan." *British Journal of Rheumatology* 26 (5): 324–26.

Harris, J., M. Westerby, T. Hill, T. Sellers, and A. Hutchinson. 2001. "User Satisfaction: Measurement and Interpretation." *Journal of Family Planning & Reproductive Health Care* 27 (1): 41–45.

Hartman, M., A. Martin, O. Nuccio, and A. Catlin; National Health Expenditure Accounts Team. 2010. "Health Spending Growth at a Historic Low in 2008." *Health Affairs (Millwood)* 29 (1): 147–55.

Havlicek, P. L. 1996. *Medical Groups in the US: A Survey of Practice Characteristics.* Chicago: American Medical Association.

Hawks, D. 1997. "The New Public Health: Nanny in a New Hat?" *Addiction* 92 (9): 1175–77.

Hayes, M. T. 2001. *The Limits of Policy Change: Incrementalism, Worldview, and the Rule of Law*. Washington, DC: Georgetown University Press.

Health Resources and Services Administration. 2011. "Area Resource File (ARF)." US Department of Health & Human Services. http://arf.hrsa.gov.

Heineman, R. A., W. T. Bluhm, S. A. Peterson, and E. N. Kearney. 1990. *The World of the Policy Analyst: Rationality, Values, and Politics*. Chatham, NJ: Chatham House Publishers.

Helmchen, L. A., and A. T. Lo Sasso. 2010. "How Sensitive Is Physician Performance to Alternative Compensation Schedules? Evidence from a Large Network of Primary Care Clinics." *Health Economics* 19 (11): 1300–17.

Hendryx, M. S., M. M. Ahern, N. P. Lovrich, and A. H. McCurdy. 2002. "Access to Health Care and Community Social Capital." *Health Services Research* 37 (1): 87–103.

Hensen, P., S. Beissert, L. Bruckner-Tuderman, T. A. Luger, N. Roeder, and M. L. Müller. 2008. "Introduction of Diagnosis-Related Groups in Germany: Evaluation of Impact on In-Patient Care in a Dermatological Setting." *European Journal of Public Health* 18 (1): 85–91.

Hiatt, M. D., and C. G. Stockton. 2003. "The Impact of the Flexner Report on the Fate of Medical Schools in North America After 1909." *Journal of American Physicians and Surgeons* 8 (2): 37–40.

Hill, A. B. 1965. "The Environment and Disease: Association or Causation?" *Proceedings of the Royal Society of Medicine* 58: 295–300.

Hillman, B. J., C. A. Joseph, M. R. Mabry, J. H. Sunshine, S. D. Kennedy, and M. Noether. 1990. "Frequency and Costs of Diagnostic Imaging in Office Practice: A Comparison of Self-Referring and Radiologist-Referring Physicians." *New England Journal of Medicine* 323 (23): 1604–608.

Hipp, J. R., and C. M. Lakon. 2010. "Social Disparities in Health: Disproportionate Toxicity Proximity in Minority Communities over a Decade." *Health Place* 16 (4): 674–83.

Hirschman, J., S. Whitman, and D. Ansell. 2007. "The Black:White Disparity in Breast Cancer Mortality: The Example of Chicago." *Cancer Causes & Control* 18 (3): 323–33.

Hixon, A. L., and L. E. Buenconsejo-Lum. 2010. "Developing the Rural Primary Care Workforce in Hawaii—A 10-Point Plan." *Hawaii Medical Journal* 69 (6 Suppl. 3): 53–55.

Hofer, A. N., J. M. Abraham, and I. Moscovice. 2011. "Expansion of Coverage Under the Patient Protection and Affordable Care Act and Primary Care Utilization." *Milbank Quarterly* 89 (1): 69–89.

Hoilette, L. K., S. J. Clark, A. Gebremariam, and M. M. Davis. 2009. "Usual Source of Care and Unmet Need Among Vulnerable Children: 1998–2006." *Pediatrics* 123 (2): e214–19.

Holahan, J., C. Hoffman, and M. Wang. 2003. "The New Middle-Class of Uninsured Americans: Is It Real?" Kaiser Commission on Medicaid and the

Uninsured; published in March. www.kff.org/uninsured/loader.cfm?url= /commonspot/security/getfile.cfm&PageID=14321.

Holahan, J., and A. Yemane. 2009. "Enrollment Is Driving Medicaid Costs—but Two Targets Can Yield Savings." *Health Affairs (Millwood)* 28 (5): 1453–65.

Holden, D. J., D. E. Jonas, D. S. Porterfield, D. Reuland, and R. Harris. 2010. "Systematic Review: Enhancing the Use and Quality of Colorectal Cancer Screening." *Annals of Internal Medicine* 152 (10): 668–76.

Hollingsworth, B. 2008. "The Measurement of Efficiency and Productivity of Health Care Delivery." *Health Economics* 17 (10): 1107–28.

Homer, J. B., and G. B. Hirsch. 2006. "System Dynamics Modeling for Public Health: Background and Opportunities." *American Journal of Public Health* 96 (3): 452–58.

Hsiao, W. C., P. Braun, D. Dunn, E. R. Becker, M. DeNicola, and T. R. Ketcham. 1988. "Results and Policy Implications of the Resource-Based Relative-Value Study." *New England Journal of Medicine* 319 (13): 881–88.

Hubbard, G., L. Kidd, E. Donaghy, C. McDonald, and N. Kearney. 2007. "A Review of Literature About Involving People Affected by Cancer in Research, Policy and Planning and Practice." *Patient Education and Counseling* 65 (1): 21–33.

Humphrey, L. L., M. Helfand, B. K. Chan, and S. H. Woolf. 2002. "Breast Cancer Screening: A Summary of the Evidence for the U.S. Preventive Services Task Force." *Annals of Internal Medicine* 137 (5 Pt. 1): 347–60.

Hurley, R. E., and M. J. McCue. 2000. *Partnership Pays: Making Medicaid Managed Care Work in a Turbulent Environment.* Princeton, NJ: Center for Health Care Strategies.

ICPSR and Robert Wood Johnson Foundation. 2011. "The Community Tracking Study." www.icpsr.umich.edu/icpsrweb/content/HMCA/community -tracking-study.html.

Iezzoni, L. I. 2003. *Risk Adjustment for Measuring Health Care Outcomes,* third edition. Chicago: Health Administration Press.

Iglehart, J. K. 2009a. "Finding Money for Health Care Reform—Rooting Out Waste, Fraud, and Abuse." *New England Journal of Medicine* 361 (3): 229–31.

———. 2009b. "Prioritizing Comparative-Effectiveness Research—IOM Recommendations." *New England Journal of Medicine* 361 (4): 325–28.

Institute of Medicine (IOM). 2012. "Crossing the Quality Chasm: The IOM Health Care Quality Initiative." www.iom.edu/Global/News%20Announcements /Crossing-the-Quality-Chasm-The-IOM-Health-Care-Quality-Initiative.aspx.

———. 2003. *Unequal Treatment: Confronting Racial and Ethnic Disparities in Health Care.* Washington, DC: National Academies Press.

———. 2002a. *The Future of the Public's Health in the 21st Century.* Washington, DC: National Academies Press.

———. 2002b. *Guidance for the National Health Disparities Report.* Washington, DC: National Academies Press.

———. 2001. *Crossing the Quality Chasm: A New Health System for the 21st Century.* Washington, DC: National Academies Press.

———. 2000. "Interpreting the Volume: Outcome Relationship in the Context of Health Care Quality: Workshop Summary." Washington, DC: National Academies Press.

———. 1998. "Summarizing Population Health: Directions for the Development and Application of Population Metrics." Washington, DC: National Academies Press.

———. 1995. *Health Services Research: Work Force and Educational Issues.* Washington, DC: National Academies Press.

———. 1993. *Access to Health Care in America.* Washington, DC: National Academies Press.

———. 1992. *Guidelines for Clinical Practice.* Washington, DC: National Academies Press.

———. 1991. *Improving Information Services for Health Services Researchers: A Report to the National Library of Medicine.* Washington, DC: National Academies Press.

———. 1988. *The Future of Public Health.* Washington, DC: National Academies Press.

———. 1979. *Report on Health Services Research.* Washington, DC: National Academies Press.

Institute of Medicine (IOM) Committee on Comparative Effectiveness Research Prioritization. 2009. *Initial National Priorities for Comparative Effectiveness Research.* Washington, DC: National Academies Press.

Israel, B. A., B. Checkoway, A. Schulz, and M. Zimmerman. 1994. "Health Education and Community Empowerment: Conceptualizing and Measuring Perceptions of Individual, Organizational, and Community Control." *Health Education Quarterly* 21 (2): 149–70.

Israel, B. A., C. M. Coombe, R. R. Cheezum, A. J. Schulz, R. J. McGranaghan, R. Lichtenstein, A. G. Reyes, J. Clement, and A. Burris. 2010. "Community-Based Participatory Research: A Capacity-Building Approach for Policy Advocacy Aimed at Eliminating Health Disparities." *American Journal of Public Health* 100 (11): 2094–102.

Israel, B. A., A. J. Schulz, E. A. Parker, and A. B. Becker. 1998. "Review of Community-Based Research: Assessing Partnership Approaches to Improve Public Health." *Annual Review of Public Health* 19: 173–202.

Iversen, M. D., R. K. Chhabriya, and N. Shadick. 2011. "Predictors of the Use of Physical Therapy Services Among Patients with Rheumatoid Arthritis." *Physical Therapy* 91 (1): 65–76.

Jacobs, P., J. Rapoport, and D. Edbrooke. 2004. "Economies of Scale in British Intensive Care Units and Combined Intensive Care/High Dependency Units." *Intensive Care Medicine* 30 (4): 660–64.

Jencks, S. F., T. Cuerdon, D. R. Burwen, B. Fleming, P. M. Houck, A. E. Kussmaul, D. S. Nilasena, D. L. Ordin, and D. R. Arday. 2000. "Quality of Medical Care Delivered to Medicare Beneficiaries: A Profile at State and National Levels." *Journal of the American Medical Association* 284 (13): 1670–76.

Jensen, G. A., M. A. Morrisey, S. Gaffney, and D. K. Liston. 1997. "The New Dominance of Managed Care: Insurance Trends in the 1990s." *Health Affairs (Millwood)* 16 (1): 125–36.

Jiang, H. J., R. Andrews, D. Stryer, and B. Friedman. 2005. "Racial/Ethnic Disparities in Potentially Preventable Readmissions: The Case of Diabetes." *American Journal of Public Health* 95 (9): 1561–67.

Johnson, A. D., and S. E. Wegner. 2007. "High-Deductible Health Plans and the New Risks of Consumer-Driven Health Insurance Products." *Pediatrics* 119 (3): 622–26.

Johnson, M. L., W. Crown, B. C. Martin, C. R. Dormuth, and U. Siebert. 2009. "Good Research Practices for Comparative Effectiveness Research: Analytic Methods to Improve Causal Inference from Nonrandomized Studies of Treatment Effects Using Secondary Data Sources: The ISPOR Good Research Practices for Retrospective Database Analysis Task Force Report—Part III." *Value in Health* 12 (8): 1062–73.

Johnson, T. D. 2011. "Accreditation Program for Health Departments Launches: Voluntary Program to Drive Improvement." *The Nation's Health* 41 (9): 1–14.

Johnson-Thompson, M. C., and J. Guthrie. 2000. "Ongoing Research to Identify Environmental Risk Factors in Breast Carcinoma." *Cancer* 88 (5 Suppl.): 1224–29.

Jones, D., C. Heflinger, and R. Saunders. 2007. "The Ecology of Adolescent Substance Abuse Service Utilization." *American Journal of Community Psychology* 40 (3): 345–58.

Jones, N. III, S. L. Jones, and N. A. Miller. 2004. "The Medicare Health Outcomes Survey Program: Overview, Context, and Near-Term Prospects." *Health and Quality of Life Outcomes* 2: 33.

Joumard, I., C. André, and C. Nicq. 2010. "Health Care Systems: Efficiency and Institutions." Economics Department Working Paper No. 769. Paris, France: Organisation for Economic Co-operation and Development.

Kahn, J. M., C. H. Goss, P. J. Heagerty, A. A. Kramer, C. R. O'Brien, and G. D. Rubenfeld. 2006. "Hospital Volume and the Outcomes of Mechanical Ventilation." *New England Journal of Medicine* 355 (1): 41–50.

Kahn, J. M., T. R. Ten Have, and T. J. Iwashyna. 2009. "The Relationship Between Hospital Volume and Mortality in Mechanical Ventilation: An Instrumental Variable Analysis." *Health Services Research* 44 (3): 862–79.

Kahn, K. L., E. B. Keeler, M. J. Sherwood, W. H. Rogers, D. Draper, S. S. Bentow, E. J. Reinisch, L. V. Rubenstein, J. Kosecoff, and R. H. Brook. 1990. "Comparing Outcomes of Care Before and After Implementation of the

DRG-Based Prospective Payment System." *Journal of the American Medical Association* 264 (15): 1984–88.

Kahn, M. G., and D. Ranade. 2010. "The Impact of Electronic Medical Records Data Sources on an Adverse Drug Event Quality Measure." *Journal of the American Medical Informatics Association* 17 (2): 185–91.

Kaiser Commission on Medicaid and the Uninsured. 2012. "Medicaid and Managed Care: Key Data, Trends, and Issues." Policy brief, published in February. Washington, DC: Kaiser Family Foundation.

———. 2010. "The Uninsured: A Primer. Key Facts About Americans Without Health Insurance." Published in December. www.kff.org/uninsured /upload/7451-06.pdf.

———. 2008. "The Medicaid Program at a Glance." Published in November. www .kff.org/medicaid/upload/7235_03-2.pdf.

———. 2002. "Underinsured in America: Is Health Coverage Adequate?" Published in July. www.kff.org/uninsured/loader.cfm?url=/commonspot/security /getfile.cfm&PageID=14136.

Kaiser Family Foundation. 2012. "Explaining Health Care Reform: Questions About Health Insurance Subsidies." Published in July. www.kff.org/healthreform /upload/7962-02.pdf.

———. 2011a. "Number of HMOs, July 2011." www.statehealthfacts.org/compare maptable.jsp?yr=270&typ=1&ind=347&cat=7&sub=85.

———. 2011b. "Registered Nurses per 100,000 Population, 2011." www.state healthfacts.org/comparemaptable.jsp?cat=8&ind=439.

———. 2010a. "Health Reform Implementation Timeline." www.kff.org/health reform/upload/8060.pdf.

———. 2010b. "Medicare: A Primer." Published in April. www.kff.org/medicare /upload/7615-03.pdf.

Kanaan, S. B. 2000. "The National Committee on Vital and Health Statistics 1949–1999: A History." US Department of Health & Human Services. http:// ncvhs.hhs.gov/50history.htm#top.

Kanavos, P., and E. Mossialos. 1999. "International Comparisons of Health Care Expenditures: What We Know and What We Do Not Know." *Journal of Health Services & Research Policy* 4 (2): 122–26.

Kane, C. K. 2011. "The Practice Arrangements of Patient Care Physicians, 2007–2008: An Analysis by Age Cohort and Gender." Chicago: American Medical Association.

Kane, R. L. 1997. *Understanding Health Care Outcomes Research*. Gaithersburg, MD: Aspen Publishers.

Kann, L., S. K. Telljohann, and S. F. Wooley. 2007. "Health Education: Results from the School Health Policies and Programs Study 2006." *Journal of School Health* 77 (8): 408–34.

Kanouse, D. E., R. H. Brook, J. D. Winkler, J. Kosecoff, S. H. Berry, G. M. Carter, J. P. Kahan, L. McCloskey, W. H. Rogers, C. M. Winslow, G. M. Anderson,

L. Brodsley, A. Fink, and L. S. Meredith. 1989. *Changing Medical Practice Through Technology Assessment: An Evaluation of the NIH Consensus Development Program.* Santa Monica, CA: RAND.

Kaplan, S. H., B. Gandek, S. Greenfield, W. Rogers, and J. E. Ware. 1995. "Patient and Visit Characteristics Related to Physicians' Participatory Decision-Making Style. Results from the Medical Outcomes Study." *Medical Care* 33 (12): 1176–87.

Katz, M. H. 2010. "Future of the Safety Net Under Health Reform." *Journal of the American Medical Association* 304 (6): 679–80.

Katz, M. H., and T. M. Brigham. 2011. "Transforming a Traditional Safety Net into a Coordinated Care System: Lessons from Healthy San Francisco." *Health Affairs (Millwood)* 30 (2): 237–45.

Katz, J. N., E. Losina, C. B. Phillips, N. N. Mahomed, R. A. Lew, W. H. Harris, R. Poss, J. A. Baron, A. H. Fossel, N. Maher, J. Barrett, and J. Tullar. 2002. "The Relationship of Surgical Volume to Quality of Care: Scientific Considerations and Policy Implications." *Journal of Bone and Joint Surgery. American Volume* 84A (8): 1483–85.

Katz, J. N., C. B. Phillips, J. A. Baron, A. H. Fossel, N. N. Mahomed, J. Barrett, E. A. Lingard, W. H. Harris, R. Poss, R. A. Lew, E. Guadagnoli, E. A. Wright, and E. Losina. 2003. "Association of Hospital and Surgeon Volume of Total Hip Replacement with Functional Status and Satisfaction Three Years Following Surgery." *Arthritis & Rheumatism* 48 (2): 560–68.

Kawachi, I., and L. F. Berkman. 2001. "Social Ties and Mental Health." *Journal of Urban Health* 78 (3): 458–67.

Kazdin, A. E. 2008. "Evidence-Based Treatment and Practice: New Opportunities to Bridge Clinical Research and Practice, Enhance the Knowledge Base, and Improve Patient Care." *American Psychologist* 63 (3): 146–59.

Keckley, P. H., S. Coughlin, S. Gupta, and C. Vasquez. 2011. "Comparative Effectiveness Research in the United States: Update and Implications." Issue brief. Washington, DC: Deloitte Center for Health Solutions.

Keen, J. D., and J. E. Keen. 2008. "How Does Age Affect Baseline Screening Mammography Performance Measures? A Decision Model." *BMC Medical Informatics and Decision Making* 8: 40.

Keenan, P. S., M. N. Elliott, P. D. Cleary, A. M. Zaslavsky, and B. E. Landon. 2009. "Quality Assessments by Sick and Healthy Beneficiaries in Traditional Medicare and Medicare Managed Care." *Medical Care* 47 (8): 882–88.

Kemper, A. R., and S. J. Clark. 2005. "Physician Barriers to Lead Testing of Medicaid-Enrolled Children." *Ambulatory Pediatrics* 5 (5): 290–93.

Kerlikowske, K., P. Salzmann, K. A. Phillips, J. A. Cauley, and S. R. Cummings. 1999. "Continuing Screening Mammography in Women Aged 70 to 79 Years: Impact on Life Expectancy and Cost-Effectiveness." *Journal of the American Medical Association* 282 (22): 2156–63.

Kessel, R. 1958. "Price Discrimination in Medicine." *Journal of Law and Economics* 1 (1): 20–53.

Khan, N., R. Kaestner, J. W. Salmon, and B. Gutierrez. 2010. "Does Supply Influence Mammography Screening?" *American Journal of Health Behavior* 34 (4): 465–75.

Khaw, K. T., N. Wareham, S. Bingham, A. Welch, R. Luben, and N. Day. 2008. "Combined Impact of Health Behaviours and Mortality in Men and Women: The EPIC-Norfolk Prospective Population Study." *PLoS Medicine* 5(1): e12.

Khoury, M. J., M. Gwinn, and J. P. Ioannidis. 2010. "The Emergence of Translational Epidemiology: From Scientific Discovery to Population Health Impact." *American Journal of Epidemiology* 172 (5): 517–24.

Kilo, C. M., and J. H. Wasson. 2010. "Practice Redesign and the Patient-Centered Medical Home: History, Promises, and Challenges." *Health Affairs (Millwood)* 29 (5): 773–78.

Kim, J., and S. N. Jang. 2008. "Socioeconomic Disparities in Breast Cancer Screening Among US Women: Trends from 2000 to 2005." *Journal of Preventive Medicine and Public Health* 41 (3): 186–94.

Kindig, D. A. 1998. "Purchasing Population Health: Aligning Financial Incentives to Improve Health Outcomes." *Health Services Research* 33 (2 Pt. 1): 223–42.

———. 1997. *Purchasing Population Health: Paying for Results.* Ann Arbor, MI: University of Michigan Press.

———. 1996. "Strategic Issues for Managing the Future Physician Workforce." In *Strategic Choices for a Changing Health Care System*, edited by S. H. Altman and U. E. Reinhardt, 149–82. Chicago: Health Administration Press.

Kindig, D., and G. Stoddart. 2003. "What Is Population Health?" *American Journal of Public Health* 93 (3): 380–83.

Kingdon, J. W. 2010. *Agendas, Alternatives, and Public Policies*, second edition. New York: Longman.

Kissick, W. L. 1970. "Health-Policy Directions for the 1970s." *New England Journal of Medicine* 282 (24): 1343–54.

Kitzhaber, J. 2003. "The Road to Meaningful Reform: A Conversation with Oregon's John Kitzhaber. Interview by Jeff Goldsmith." *Health Affairs (Millwood)* 22 (1): 114–24.

Klein, R. 2006. "The Troubled Transformation of Britain's National Health Service." *New England Journal of Medicine* 355 (4): 409–15.

Klein, R. J., E. B. Reidy, S. P. Hallquist, and A. Ryskulova. 2006. "Healthy People 2010 Mid-Decade Assessment of Progress: Methods and Results." Presentation at the National Center for Health Statistics Data Users Conference, Washington, DC, July 12.

Koh, H. K., J. J. Piotrowski, S. Kumanyika, and J. E. Fielding. 2011. "*Healthy People*: A 2020 Vision for the Social Determinants Approach." *Health Education & Behavior* 38 (6): 551–57.

Kohler, H. 1990. *Intermediate Microeconomics: Theory and Applications*, third edition. Glenview, IL: Scott, Foresman and Co.

Kolm, S. C. 1996. *Modern Theories of Justice*. Cambridge, MA: MIT Press.

Komen Foundation. 2012. "Susan G. Komen for the Cure." ww5.komen.org.

Komaroff, A. L. 1971. "Regional Medical Programs in Search of a Mission." *New England Journal of Medicine* 284 (14): 758–64.

Kono, S. 2010. "Host and Environmental Factors Predisposing to Cancer Development." *Gan To Kagaku Ryoho* 37 (4): 571–76.

Kretzmann, J. P., and J. L. McKnight. 1993. *Building Communities from the Inside Out: A Path Toward Finding and Mobilizing a Community's Assets*. Chicago: ACTA Publications.

Krieger, N. 2002. "A Glossary for Social Epidemiology." *Epidemiological Bulletin* 23 (1): 7–11.

Kuder, J. M., and G. S. Levitz. 1985. "Visits to the Physician: An Evaluation of the Usual-Source Effect." *Health Services Research* 20 (5): 579–96.

Kullgren, J. T., A. A. Galbraith, V. L. Hinrichsen, I. Miroshnik, R. B. Penfold, M. B. Rosenthal, B. E. Landon, and T. A. Lieu. 2010. "Health Care Use and Decision Making Among Lower-Income Families in High-Deductible Health Plans." *Archives of Internal Medicine* 170 (21): 1918–25.

Kuper, D. E. 1998. "Newborns' and Mothers' Health Protection Act: Putting the Brakes on Drive-Through Deliveries." *Specialty Law Digest. Health Care Law* 227: 9–31.

Labonte, R. 1994. "Health Promotion and Empowerment: Reflections on Professional Practice." *Health Education Quarterly* 21 (2): 253–68.

Lairson, D. R., M. DiCarlo, R. E. Myers, T. Wolf, J. Cocroft, R. Sifri, M. Rosenthal, S. W. Vernon, and R. Wender. 2008. "Cost-Effectiveness of Targeted and Tailored Interventions on Colorectal Cancer Screening Use." *Cancer* 112 (4): 779–88.

Lalonde, M. 1975. *A New Perspective on the Health of Canadians: A Working Document*. Ottawa, Canada: Information Canada.

Lamb, H. R., and L. E. Weinberger. 2005. "One-Year Follow-Up of Persons Discharged from a Locked Intermediate Care Facility." *Psychiatric Services* 56 (2): 198–201.

Lamb, S. E., C. Becker, L. D. Gillespie, J. L. Smith, S. Finnegan, R. Potter, and K. Pfeiffer. 2011. "Reporting of Complex Interventions in Clinical Trials: Development of a Taxonomy to Classify and Describe Fall-Prevention Interventions." *Trials* 12 (1): 125.

Lambrew, J. M. 2001. "Diagnosing Disparities in Health Insurance for Women: A Prescription for Change." Published August 1. New York: The Commonwealth Fund.

Lambrew, J. M., G. H. DeFriese, T. S. Carey, T. C. Ricketts III, and A. K. Biddle. 1996. "The Effects of Having a Regular Doctor on Access to Primary Care." *Medical Care* 34 (2): 138–51.

Lamphere, J. A., P. Neuman, K. Langwell, and D. Sherman. 1997. "The Surge in Medicare Managed Care: An Update." *Health Affairs (Millwood)* 16 (3): 127–33.

Landon, B. E., A. M. Zaslavsky, S. L. Bernard, M. J. Cioffi, and P. D. Cleary. 2004. "Comparison of Performance of Traditional Medicare vs Medicare Managed Care." *Journal of the American Medical Association* 291 (14): 1744–52.

Lantz, P. M., M. Mujahid, K. Schwartz, N. K. Janz, A. Fagerlin, B. Salem, L. Liu, D. Deapen, and S. J. Katz. 2006. "The Influence of Race, Ethnicity, and Individual Socioeconomic Factors on Breast Cancer Stage at Diagnosis." *American Journal of Public Health* 96 (12): 2173–78.

Lantz, P. M., and S. Soliman. 2009. "An Evaluation of a Medicaid Expansion for Cancer Care: The Breast and Cervical Cancer Prevention and Treatment Act of 2000." *Women's Health Issues* 19 (4): 221–31.

Lantz, P. M., C. S. Weisman, and Z. Itani. 2003. "A Disease-Specific Medicaid Expansion for Women. The Breast and Cervical Cancer Prevention and Treatment Act of 2000." *Women's Health Issues* 13 (3): 79–92.

Lasker, R. D., E. S. Weiss, and R. Miller. 2001. "Partnership Synergy: A Practical Framework for Studying and Strengthening the Collaborative Advantage." *Milbank Quarterly* 79 (2): 179–205, III–IV.

Lasswell, H. D. 1951. "The Policy Orientation." In *The Policy Sciences: Recent Developments in Scope and Methods*, edited by D. Lerner and H. D. Lasswell, 3–15. Stanford, CA: Stanford University Press.

Lauer, M. S., and F. S. Collins. 2010. "Using Science to Improve the Nation's Health System: NIH's Commitment to Comparative Effectiveness Research." *Journal of the American Medical Association* 303 (21): 2182–83.

LaVeist, T. A. 1994. "Beyond Dummy Variables and Sample Selection: What Health Services Researchers Ought to Know About Race as a Variable." *Health Services Research* 29 (1): 1–16.

Lavis, J. N., S. E. Ross, J. E. Hurley, J. M. Hohenadel, G. L. Stoddart, C. A. Woodward, and J. Abelson. 2002. "Examining the Role of Health Services Research in Public Policymaking." *Milbank Quarterly* 80 (1): 125–54.

Lee-Feldstein, A., P. J. Feldstein, T. Buchmueller, and G. Katterhagen. 2000. "The Relationship of HMOs, Health Insurance, and Delivery Systems to Breast Cancer Outcomes." *Medical Care* 38 (7): 705–18.

Legler, J., H. I. Meissner, C. Coyne, N. Breen, V. Chollette, and B. K. Rimer. 2002. "The Effectiveness of Interventions to Promote Mammography Among Women with Historically Lower Rates of Screening." *Cancer Epidemiology, Biomarkers & Prevention* 11 (1): 59–71.

Le Grand, J. 2002. "Further Tales from the British National Health Service." *Health Affairs (Millwood)* 21 (3): 116–28.

Lehrer, J. 2010. "The Truth Wears Off—Is There Something Wrong with the Scientific Method?" *New Yorker* (December 13).

Leibenstein, H. 1966. "Allocative Efficiency vs. 'X-Efficiency.'" *American Economic Review* 56 (3): 392–415.

Leibowitz, A. A. 2004. "The Demand for Health and Health Concerns After 30 Years." *Journal of Health Economics* 23 (4): 663–71.

Lesser, C. S., P. B. Ginsburg, and K. J. Devers. 2003. "The End of an Era: What Became of the 'Managed Care Revolution' in 2001?" *Health Services Research* 38 (1 Pt. 2): 337–55.

Levit, K. R., H. C. Lazenby, and L. Sivarajan. 1996. "Health Care Spending in 1994: Slowest in Decades." *Health Affairs (Millwood)* 15 (2): 130–44.

Levit, K., C. Smith, C. Cowan, H. Lazenby, A. Sensenig, and A. Catlin. 2003. "Trends in U.S. Health Care Spending, 2001." *Health Affairs (Project Hope)* 22 (1): 154–64.

Levy, A. R., C. Mitton, K. M. Johnston, B. Harrigan, and A. H. Briggs. 2010. "International Comparison of Comparative Effectiveness Research in Five Jurisdictions: Insights for the US." *PharmacoEconomics* 28 (10): 813–30.

Lewin, L. S., and R. A. Derzon. 1982. "Health Professions Education: State of Responsibilities Under the New Federalism." *Health Affairs (Millwood)* 1 (2): 69–85.

Lewis, C. E. 1969. "Variations in the Incidence of Surgery." *New England Journal of Medicine* 281 (16): 880–84.

Li, C. I. 2005. "Racial and Ethnic Disparities in Breast Cancer Stage, Treatment, and Survival in the United States." *Ethnicity & Disease* 15 (2 Suppl. 2): S5–9.

Lian, O. S. 2003. "Convergence or Divergence? Reforming Primary Care in Norway and Britain." *Milbank Quarterly* 81 (2): 305–30.

Liberati, A., D. G. Altman, J. Tetzlaff, C. Mulrow, P. C. Gotzsche, J. P. Ioannidis, M. Clarke, P. J. Devereaux, J. Kleijnen, and D. Moher. 2009. "The PRISMA Statement for Reporting Systematic Reviews and Meta-Analyses of Studies That Evaluate Healthcare Interventions: Explanation and Elaboration." *BMJ* 339: b2700.

Liebhaber, A., and J. M. Grossman. 2007. "Physicians Moving to Mid-Sized, Single-Specialty Practices." *Tracking Report/Center for Studying Health System Change* 18: 1–5.

Lillie-Blanton, M., and T. A. LaVeist. 1996. "Race/Ethnicity, the Social Environment, and Health." *Social Science & Medicine* 43 (1): 83–91.

Lin, C. J., D. Musa, M. Silverman, and H. B. Degenholtz. 2005. "Do Managed Care Plans Reduce Racial Disparities in Preventive Care?" *Journal of Health Care for the Poor and Underserved* 16 (1): 139–51.

Lindblom, C. 1959. "The Science of Muddling Through." *Public Administration Review* 19 (2): 79–88.

Link, B. G., and J. Phelan. 1995. "Social Conditions as Fundamental Causes of Disease." *Journal of Health and Social Behavior* 35 (Extra Issue): 80–94.

Lipscomb, C. E. 2002. "Lister Hill and His Influence." *Journal of the Medical Library Association* 90 (1): 109–10.

Lleras-Muney, A. 2002. *The Relationship Between Education and Adult Mortality in the United States.* Cambridge, MA: National Bureau of Economic Research.

Lo, K. M., and K. G. Fulda. 2008. "Impact of Predisposing, Enabling, and Need Factors in Accessing Preventive Medical Care Among U.S. Children: Results of the National Survey of Children's Health." *Osteopathic Medicine and Primary Care* 2: 12.

Loh, A., R. Leonhart, C. E. Wills, D. Simon, and M. Härter. 2007. "The Impact of Patient Participation on Adherence and Clinical Outcome in Primary Care of Depression." *Patient Education and Counseling* 65 (1): 69–78.

Lohr, K. N., K. Eleazer, and J. Mauskopf. 1998. "Health Policy Issues and Applications for Evidence-Based Medicine and Clinical Practice Guidelines." *Health Policy* 46 (1): 1–19.

Lohr, K. N., and D. M. Steinwachs. 2002. "Health Services Research: An Evolving Definition of the Field." *Health Services Research* 37 (1): 7–9.

Longest, B. B. Jr. 2009. *Health Policymaking in the United States,* fifth edition. Chicago: Health Administration Press.

———. 2005. *Health Policymaking in the United States,* fourth edition. Chicago: Health Administration Press.

Lorant, V., B. Boland, P. Humblet, and D. Deliège. 2002. "Equity in Prevention and Health Care." *Journal of Epidemiology & Community Health* 56 (7): 510–16.

Love, D., W. Custer, and P. Miller. 2010. *All-Payer Claims Databases: State Initiatives to Improve Health Care Transparency.* Issue Brief, Commonwealth Fund Pub. 1439, Vol. 99. http://apcdcouncil.org/sites/apcdcouncil.org/files/All-Payer%20Claims%20Databases%20State%20Initiatives%20to%20Improve%20Health%20Care%20Transparency.pdf.

Luft, H. S. 1978. "How Do Health-Maintenance Organizations Achieve Their 'Savings'?" *New England Journal of Medicine* 298 (24): 1336–43.

Luft, H. S., J. P. Bunker, and A. C. Enthoven. 1979. "Should Operations Be Regionalized? The Empirical Relation Between Surgical Volume and Mortality." *New England Journal of Medicine* 301 (25): 1364–69.

Lugtenberg, M., J. S. Burgers, and G. P. Westert. 2009. "Effects of Evidence-Based Clinical Practice Guidelines on Quality of Care: A Systematic Review." *Quality & Safety in Health Care* 18 (5): 385–92.

Luke, R. D., J. W. Begun, and D. D. Pointer. 1989. "Quasi Firms: Strategic Interorganizational Forms in the Health-Care Industry." *Academy of Management Review* 14 (1): 9–19.

Lurie, N. 2002. "Measuring Disparities in Access to Care." In *Guidance for the National Healthcare Disparities Report,* edited by Institute of Medicine, 99–147. Washington, DC: National Academies Press.

Ma, J., M. Lu, and H. Quan. 2008. "From a National, Centrally Planned Health System to a System Based on the Market: Lessons from China." *Health Affairs (Millwood)* 27 (4): 937–48.

Macdonald, S. M., B. A. Reeder, Y. Chen, and J. P. Després. 1997. "Obesity in Canada: A Descriptive Analysis. Canadian Heart Health Surveys Research Group." *Canadian Medical Association Journal* 157 (Suppl. 1): S3–9.

MacDowell, M., M. Glasser, M. Fitts, K. Nielsen, and M. Hunsaker. 2010. "A National View of Rural Health Workforce Issues in the USA." *Rural Remote Health* 10 (3): 1531.

Maciosek, M. V., A. B. Coffield, T. J. Flottemesch, N. M. Edwards, and L. I. Solberg. 2010. "Greater Use of Preventive Services in U.S. Health Care Could Save Lives at Little or No Cost." *Health Affairs (Millwood)* 29 (9): 1656–60.

MacRae, D., and D. Whittington. 1997. *Expert Advice for Policy Choice: Analysis and Discourse*. Washington, DC: Georgetown University Press.

Manning, W. G., J. P. Newhouse, N. Duan, E. B. Keeler, A. Leibowitz, and M. S. Marquis. 1987. "Health Insurance and the Demand for Medical Care: Evidence from a Randomized Experiment." *American Economic Review* 77 (3): 251–77.

Mansyur, C. L., B. C. Amick III, L. Franzini, and R. E. Roberts. 2009. "Culture and the Social Context of Health Inequalities." *International Journal of Health Services* 39 (1): 85–106.

Mansyur, C., B. C. Amick, R. B. Harrist, and L. Franzini L. 2008. "Social Capital, Income Inequality, and Self-Rated Health in 45 Countries." *Social Science & Medicine* 66 (1): 43–56.

Marchessault, G. 2010. "The Story of the Manitoba Centre for Health Policy." Winnipeg, Manitoba: Manitoba Centre for Health Policy, Department of Community Health Sciences, Faculty of Medicine, University of Manitoba. http://umanitoba.ca/faculties/medicine/units/mchp/media/Story_of _MCHP.pdf.

Marder, W. D., and S. Zuckerman. 1985. "Competition and Medical Groups: A Survivor Analysis." *Journal of Health Economics* 4 (2): 167–76.

Marincowitz, G. J. O. 2004. "Mutual Participation in the Health Worker-Patient Relationship." *South African Family Practice* 46 (3): 30–33.

Marmot, M., S. Friel, R. Bell, T. A. Houweling, and S. Taylor. 2008. "Closing the Gap in a Generation: Health Equity Through Action on the Social Determinants of Health." *Lancet* 372 (9650): 1661–69.

Marquis, M. S., and S. H. Long. 2001. "To Offer or Not to Offer: The Role of Price in Employers' Health Insurance Decisions." *Health Services Research* 36 (5): 935–58.

Marseille, E., J. G. Kahn, and J. Saba. 1998. "Cost-Effectiveness of Antiviral Drug Therapy to Reduce Mother-to-Child HIV Transmission in Sub-Saharan Africa." *AIDS* 12 (8): 939–48.

Marsh, D. R., D. G. Schroeder, K. A. Dearden, J. Sternin, and M. Sternin. 2004. "The Power of Positive Deviance." *BMJ* 329 (7475): 1177–79.

Marshall, M. N., P. G. Shekelle, S. Leatherman, and R. H. Brook. 2000. "The Public Release of Performance Data: What Do We Expect to Gain? A Review of the Evidence." *Journal of the American Medical Association* 283 (14): 1866–74.

Marsteller, J. A., R. R. Bovbjerg, and L. M. Nichols. 1998. "Nonprofit Conversion: Theory, Evidence, and State Policy Options." *Health Services Research* 33 (5 Pt. 2): 1495–535.

Martin, A., D. Lassman, L. Whittle, A. Catlin, J. Benson, C. Cowan, B. Dickensheets, M. Hartman, P. McDonnell, O. Nuccio, and B. Washington. 2011. "Recession Contributes to Slowest Annual Rate of Increase in Health Spending in Five Decades." *Health Affairs (Millwood)* 30 (1): 11–22.

Martin, L. 2011. "Eight Key Lessons for Managing Care in Medicaid in 2011 and Beyond." Center for Health Care Strategies policy brief, published in May. www.chcs.org/usr_doc/Eight_Key_Lessons_FINAL.pdf.

Martin-Moreno, J. M., J. L. Alfonso-Sanchez, M. Harris., and B. G. Lopez-Valcarcel. 2010. "The Effects of the Financial Crisis on Primary Prevention of Cancer." *European Journal of Cancer* 46 (14): 2525–33.

Mason, J. O., and J. M. McGinnis. 1990. "'Healthy People 2000': An Overview of the National Health Promotion and Disease Prevention Objectives." *Public Health Reports* 105 (5): 441–46.

Masten, A. S. 2001. "Ordinary Magic. Resilience Processes in Development." *American Psychologist* 56 (3): 227–38.

Mayberry, R. M., F. Mili, and E. Ofili. 2000. "Racial and Ethnic Differences in Access to Medical Care." *Medical Care Research & Review* 57 (Suppl. 1): 108–45.

Mayes, R. 2007. "The Origins, Development, and Passage of Medicare's Revolutionary Prospective Payment System." *Journal of the History of Medicine Allied Sciences* 62 (1): 21–55.

Mayes, R., and R. A. Berenson. 2006. *Medicare Prospective Payment and the Shaping of U.S. Health Care.* Baltimore, MD: The Johns Hopkins University Press.

McAlearney, A. S., K. W. Reeves, C. Tatum, and E. D. Paskett. 2007. "Cost as a Barrier to Screening Mammography Among Underserved Women." *Ethnicity & Health* 12 (2): 189–203.

McAlearney, J. S. 2002. "The Financial Performance of Community Health Centers, 1996–1999." *Health Affairs (Project Hope)* 21 (2): 219–25.

McCall, N., J. Korb, A. Petersons, and S. Moore. 2003. "Reforming Medicare Payment: Early Effects of the 1997 Balanced Budget Act on Postacute Care." *Milbank Quarterly* 81 (2): 277–303, 172–73.

McCarthy, T., and K. L. White. 2000. "Origins of Health Services Research." *Health Services Research* 35 (2): 375–87.

McClellan, M. 1997. "Hospital Reimbursement Incentives: An Empirical Analysis." *Journal of Economics & Management Strategy* 6 (1): 91–128.

McClellan, M. B., J. S. Benner, A. M. Garber, D. O. Meltzer, S. R. Tunis, and S. Pearson. 2009. *Implementing Comparative Effectiveness Research: Priorities, Methods, and Impact.* Washington, DC: The Brookings Institution.

McClellan, M., A. N. McKethan, J. L. Lewis, J. Roski, and E. S. Fisher. 2010. "A National Strategy to Put Accountable Care into Practice." *Health Affairs (Millwood)* 29 (5): 982–90.

McGinnis, J. M., and W. H. Foege. 1993. "Actual Causes of Death in the United States." *Journal of the American Medical Association* 270 (18): 2207–12.

McGinnis, J. M., and P. R. Lee. 1995. "Healthy People 2000 at Mid Decade." *Journal of the American Medical Association* 273 (14): 1123–29.

McGlynn, E. A., S. M. Asch, J. Adams, J. Keesey, J. Hicks, A. DeCristofaro, and E. A. Kerr. 2003. "The Quality of Health Care Delivered to Adults in the United States." *New England Journal of Medicine* 348 (26): 2635–45.

McKeown, T. 1990. "Determinants of Health." In *The Nation's Health*, edited by P. R. Lee and C. L. Estes, 6–13. Boston: Jones and Bartlett.

McKinlay, J. B., S. M. McKinlay, and R. Beaglehole. 1989. "A Review of the Evidence Concerning the Impact of Medical Measures on Recent Mortality and Morbidity in the United States." *International Journal of Health Services* 19 (2): 181–208.

McKinney, M. 2010. "Where You Live = How You Die: 'Geography Is Destiny' for End-of-Life Care, Which Often Is Costly, Aggressive." *Modern Healthcare* 40 (47): 6–7, 16, 1.

McLeroy, K. R., and C. E. Crump. 1994. "Health Promotion and Disease Prevention: A Historical Perspective." *Generations* 18 (1): 9–17.

MCOL Research. 2013. "Managed Care Fact Sheets from National Statistics." www .mcareol.com/factshts/factnati.htm.

McPherson, K., P. M. Strong, A. Epstein, and L. Jones. 1981. "Regional Variations in the Use of Common Surgical Procedures: Within and Between England and Wales, Canada and the United States of America." *Social Science & Medicine. Part A, Medical Sociology* 15 (3 Pt. 1): 273–88.

McPherson, K., J. E. Wennberg, O. B. Hovind, and P. Clifford. 1982. "Small-Area Variations in the Use of Common Surgical Procedures: An International Comparison of New England, England, and Norway." *New England Journal of Medicine* 307 (21): 1310–14.

McWilliams, J. M., E. Meara, A. M. Zaslavsky, and J. Z. Ayanian. 2009. "Medicare Spending for Previously Uninsured Adults." *Annals of Internal Medicine* 151 (11): 757–66.

———. 2007. "Use of Health Services by Previously Uninsured Medicare Beneficiaries." *New England Journal of Medicine* 357 (2): 143–53.

Mead, H., L. Cartwright-Smith, K. Jones, C. Ramos, K. Woods, and B. Siegel. 2008. "Racial and Ethnic Disparities in U.S. Health Care: A Chartbook." Published March 13. New York: The Commonwealth Fund.

Mechanic, D. 1996. "Changing Medical Organization and the Erosion of Trust." *Milbank Quarterly* 74 (2): 171–89.

Medicare Payment Advisory Commission (MedPAC). 2010a. *A Data Book: Healthcare Spending and the Medicare Program.* Published in June. www.medpac .gov/documents/jun10databookentirereport.pdf.

———. 2010b. "Payment Basics: Physician Services Payment System." Published in October. www.medpac.gov/documents/MedPAC_Payment_Basics_10 _Physician.pdf.

Mennemeyer, S. T., M. A. Morrisey, and L. Z. Howard. 1997. "Death and Reputation: How Consumers Acted Upon HCFA Mortality Information." *Inquiry* 34 (2): 117–28.

Merzel, C., and J. Moon-Howard. 2002. "Access to Health Services in an Urban Community: Does Source of Care Make a Difference?" *Journal of Urban Health* 79 (2): 186–99.

Metzler, M., N. Kanarek, K. Highsmith, R. Straw, R. Bialek, J. Stanley, I. Auston, and R. Klein. 2008. "Community Health Status Indicators Project: The Development of a National Approach to Community Health." *Preventing Chronic Disease* 5 (3): A94.

Mhatre, S. L., and R. B. Deber. 1992. "From Equal Access to Health Care to Equitable Access to Health: A Review of Canadian Provincial Health Commissions and Reports." *International Journal of Health Services* 22 (4): 645–68.

Miller, A. M., and V. L. Champion. 1997. "Attitudes About Breast Cancer and Mammography: Racial, Income, and Educational Differences." *Women & Health* 26 (1): 41–63.

Miller, R. H., and H. S. Luft. 2002. "HMO Plan Performance Update: An Analysis of the Literature, 1997–2001." *Health Affairs (Millwood)* 21 (4): 63–86.

———. 1997. "Does Managed Care Lead to Better or Worse Quality of Care?" *Health Affairs (Millwood)* 16 (5): 7–25.

———. 1994. "Managed Care Plan Performance Since 1980: A Literature Analysis." *Journal of the American Medical Association* 271 (19): 1512–19.

Milstein, B. 2008. "Hygeia's Constellation—Navigating Health Futures in a Dynamic and Democratic World." Atlanta, GA: Centers for Disease Control and Prevention.

Minkler, M. 2010. "Linking Science and Policy Through Community-Based Participatory Research to Study and Address Health Disparities." *American Journal of Public Health* 100 (Suppl. 1): S81–87.

———. 1997. *Community Organizing and Community Building for Health.* Piscataway, NJ: Rutgers University Press.

Minkler, M., and N. Wallerstein, eds. 2003. *Community-Based Participatory Research for Health.* San Francisco: Jossey-Bass.

Misch, A., and L. Starke. 1994. "Assessing Environmental Health Risks." In *State of the World 1994*, edited by L. R. Brown, 117–36. New York: Norton & Co.

Mitchell, J. M. 2005. "Effects of Physician-Owned Limited-Service Hospitals: Evidence from Arizona." *Health Affairs (Millwood)* (Suppl. Web Exclusives): W5-481–90.

Mitchell, P. H., S. Ferketich, and B. M. Jennings. 1998. "Quality Health Outcomes Model. American Academy of Nursing Expert Panel on Quality Health Care." *Image—The Journal of Nursing Scholarship* 30 (1): 43–46.

Mohai, P., P. M. Lantz, J. Morenoff, J. S. House, and R. P. Mero. 2009. "Racial and Socioeconomic Disparities in Residential Proximity to Polluting Industrial

Facilities: Evidence from the Americans' Changing Lives Study." *American Journal of Public Health* 99 (Suppl. 3): S649–56.

Moher, D., K. F. Schulz, and D. G. Altman. 2001. "The CONSORT Statement: Revised Recommendations for Improving the Quality of Reports of Parallel-Group Randomised Trials." *Lancet* 357 (9263): 1191–94.

Mokdad, A. H., J. S. Marks, D. F. Stroup, and J. L. Gerberding. 2004. "Actual Causes of Death in the United States, 2000." *Journal of the American Medical Association* 291 (10): 1238–45.

Montazeri, A. 2008. "Health-Related Quality of Life in Breast Cancer Patients: A Bibliographic Review of the Literature from 1974 to 2007." *Journal of Experimental & Clinical Cancer Research* 27 (1): 32.

Montori, V. M., M. Bhandari, P. J. Devereaux, B. J. Manns, W. A. Ghali, and G. H. Guyatt. 2002. "In the Dark: The Reporting of Blinding Status in Randomized Controlled Trials." *Journal of Clinical Epidemiology* 55 (8): 787–90.

Mooney, G. 1998. "'Communitarian Claims' as an Ethical Basis for Allocating Health Care Resources." *Social Science & Medicine* 47 (9): 1171–80.

Morgan, A., and E. Ziglio. 2007. "Revitalising the Evidence Base for Public Health: An Assets Model." *Promotion & Education* Suppl. 2: 17–22.

Morgan, L. M. 2001. "Community Participation in Health: Perpetual Allure, Persistent Challenge." *Health Policy & Planning* 16 (3): 221–30.

Morgan, R. O., L. A. Petersen, J. C. Hasche, J. A. Davila, M. M. Byrne, N. I. Osemene, I. I. Wei, and M. L. Johnson. 2009. "VHA Pharmacy Use in Veterans with Medicare Drug Coverage." *American Journal of Managed Care* 15 (3): 1–8.

Morgan, R. O., and K. R. Sail. 2012. "Patient-Reported Outcome Data." In *Clinical Research Informatics*, edited by J. E. Andrews and R. L. Richesson, 203–20. London: Springer-Verlag.

Moss, S. M., H. Cuckle, A. Evans, L. Johns, M. Waller, and L. Bobrow. 2006. "Effect of Mammographic Screening from Age 40 Years on Breast Cancer Mortality at 10 Years' Follow-Up: A Randomised Controlled Trial." *Lancet* 368 (9552): 2053–60.

Moy, E., M. Barrett, and K. Ho. 2011. "Potentially Preventable Hospitalizations—United States, 2004–2007." *Morbidity and Mortality Weekly Report. Surveillance Summaries* 60 (Suppl.): 80–83.

Moy, E., E. Dayton, and C. M. Clancy. 2005. "Compiling the Evidence: The National Healthcare Disparities Reports." *Health Affairs (Millwood)* 24 (2): 376–87.

Mueller, K. J., S. T. Ortega, K. Parker, K. Patil, and A. Askenazi. 1999. "Health Status and Access to Care Among Rural Minorities." *Journal of Health Care for the Poor and Underserved* 10 (2): 230–49.

Muennig, P. 2008. *Cost-Effectiveness Analysis in Health: A Practical Approach*, second edition. San Francisco: Jossey-Bass.

Mukamel, D. B., and A. I. Mushlin. 1998. "Quality of Care Information Makes a Difference: An Analysis of Market Share and Price Changes After Publication of the New York State Cardiac Surgery Mortality Reports." *Medical Care* 36 (7): 945–54.

Mulhall, S., and A. Swift. 1996. *Liberals and Communitarians.* Cambridge, MA: Blackwell.

Mullan, F. 2002. "Time-Capsule Thinking: The Health Care Workforce, Past and Future." *Health Affairs (Millwood)* 21 (5): 112–22.

Munger, M. C. 2000. *Analyzing Policy: Choices, Conflicts, and Practices.* New York: W. W. Norton & Company.

Murray, C. J. L., and D. B. Evans, eds. 2003. *Health Systems Performance Assessment: Debates, Methods and Empiricism.* Geneva, Switzerland: World Health Organization.

Murray, C. J. L., J. A. Salomon, C. D. Mathers, and A. D. Lopez. 2002. *Summary Measures of Population Health: Concepts, Ethics, Measurement and Applications.* Geneva, Switzerland: World Health Organization.

National Association of County & City Health Officials (NACCHO). 2009. "2008 National Profile of Local Health Departments." Washington, DC: National Association of County & City Health Officials.

National Cancer Institute. 2011a. "Breast Cancer Screening: Mammogram." www.cancer.gov/cancertopics/pdq/screening/breast/Patient/page3#Key point6.

———. 2011b. "Overview of the Seer Program." http://seer.cancer.gov/about /overview.html.

———. 2010. *Cancer Trends Progress Report—2009/2010 Update: Breast Cancer Screening.* Bethesda, MD: National Institutes of Health, US Department of Health & Human Services.

National Center for Health Statistics (NCHS). 2012. "Health, United States, 2011: With Special Feature on Socioeconomic Status and Health." Washington, DC: US Government Printing Office.

———. 2011. "Health, United States, 2010: With Special Feature on Death and Dying." Washington, DC: US Government Printing Office.

———. 2010. "Health, United States, 2009: With Special Feature on Medical Technology." Washington, DC: US Government Printing Office.

———. 2005. "Health, United States, 2005: With Chartbook on Trends in the Health of Americans." Washington, DC: US Government Printing Office.

———. 1997. "Health, United States, 1996–97 and Injury Chartbook." Washington, DC: US Government Printing Office.

National Committee for Quality Assurance (NCQA). 2012. "Public Policy." www .ncqa.org/tabid/61/Default.aspx.

———. 2011. "HEDIS & Performance Measurement." www.ncqa.org/tabid/59 /Default.aspx.

————. 2010. "The State of Health Care Quality: Reform, the Quality Agenda and Resource Use." www.ncqa.org/portals/0/state%20of%20health%20 care/2010/sohc%202010%20-%20full2.pdf.

————. 2006. "Guidelines for Advertising." www.ncqa.org/Portals/0/Marketing /AdGuidelines/SoftCert.pdf.

National Information Center on Health Services Research and Health Care Technology (NICHSR). 2007. "Introduction to Health Services Research: A Self-Study Course." Bethesda, MD: US National Library of Medicine. www.nlm .nih.gov/nichsr/ihcm/hsrctoc.html.

National Opinion Research Center. 2009. "NORC Final Report: *Healthy People* User Study." Bethesda, MD: US Department of Health & Human Services.

National Research Council. 2001. *Mammography and Beyond: Developing Technologies for the Early Detection of Breast Cancer.* Washington, DC: National Academies Press.

National Science Foundation. 2011. *Grants.Gov Application Guide: A Guide for Preparation and Submission of NSF Applications via Grants.gov.* www.nsf .gov/pubs/policydocs/grantsgovguide0111.pdf?WT.mc_id=USNSF_179.

Nelson, W. A., and J. Campfield. 2006. "Ethical Implications of Transparency. Valid Justification Is Required When Withholding Information." *Healthcare Executive* 21 (6): 33–34.

Newhouse, J. P. 2004. "Consumer-Directed Health Plans and the RAND Health Insurance Experiment." *Health Affairs (Millwood)* 23 (6): 107–13.

————. 2002. *Pricing the Priceless: A Health Care Conundrum.* Cambridge, MA: MIT Press.

Newhouse, J. P., W. G. Manning, N. Duan, C. N. Morris, E. B. Keeler, A. Leibowitz, M. S. Marquis, W. H. Rogers, A. R. Davies, and K. N. Lohr. 1987. "The Findings of the RAND Health Insurance Experiment: A Response to Welch et al." *Medical Care* 25 (2): 157–79.

Nowell, B., and P. Foster-Fishman. 2010. "Examining Multi-Sector Community Collaboratives as Vehicles for Building Organizational Capacity." *American Journal of Community Psychology* (November 9).

Nowicki, M. 2004. *The Financial Management of Hospitals and Healthcare Organizations*, third edition. Chicago: Health Administration Press.

Nozick, R. 1993. *The Nature of Rationality.* Princeton, NJ: Princeton University Press.

————. 1990. *The Normative Theory of Individual Choice.* New York: Garland Publishing, Inc.

————. 1974. *Anarchy, State and Utopia.* New York: Basic Books.

Nutrition Committee of the Canadian Paediatric Society. 1976. "The Nutrition Canada Survey: A Review." *Canadian Medical Association Journal* 115 (8): 775–77.

O'Brien, E. 2005. "Medicaid's Coverage of Nursing Home Costs: Asset Shelter for the Wealthy or Essential Safety Net?" Georgetown University Long-Term

Care Financing Project. Issue brief, published in May. http://ltc.georgetown.edu/pdfs/nursinghomecosts.pdf.

O'Cathain, A. 2009. "Mixed Methods Research in the Health Sciences: A Quiet Revolution." *Journal of Mixed Methods Research* 3 (1): 3–6.

Office of Air and Radiation. 2011. *Summary Report: The Benefits and Costs of the Clean Air Act from 1990 to 2020.* Washington, DC: US Environmental Protection Agency.

Office of Disease Prevention and Health Promotion. 2012. "Healthy People 2020: About Healthy People." US Department of Health & Human Services. www.healthypeople.gov/2020/about/default.aspx.

Office of the Deputy Prime Minister. 2004. "The Social Exclusion Unit." http://webarchive.nationalarchives.gov.uk/+/http://www.cabinetoffice.gov.uk/media/cabinetoffice/social_exclusion_task_force/assets/publications_1997_to_2006/seu_leaflet.pdf.

Office of the Federal Register. *Federal Register, Volume 75, Number 8, January 13, 2010, Pages 1697–2052.* Washington, DC: UNT Digital Library. http://digital.library.unt.edu/ark:/67531/metadc52591.

Office of the Legislative Counsel. 2010. "Compilation of Patient Protection and Affordable Care Act." Published in May. http://housedocs.house.gov/energycommerce/ppacacon.pdf.

O'Malley, A. S., C. B. Forrest, and J. Mandelblatt. 2002. "Adherence of Low-Income Women to Cancer Screening Recommendations." *Journal of General Internal Medicine* 17 (2): 144–54.

110th Congress. 2008. "Medicare Improvements for Patients and Providers Act of 2008." Public Law 110–275, enacted July 15. www.gpo.gov/fdsys/pkg/PLAW-110publ275/pdf/PLAW-110publ275.pdf.

Ong, K. L., B. M. Cheung, Y. B. Man, C. P. Lau, and K. S. Lam. 2007. "Prevalence, Awareness, Treatment, and Control of Hypertension Among United States Adults 1999–2004." *Hypertension* 49 (1): 69–75.

Oreopoulos, P. 2006. "Estimating Average and Local Average Treatment Effects of Education When Compulsory Schooling Laws Really Matter." *American Economic Review* 96 (1): 152–75.

Organisation for Economic Co-operation and Development (OECD). 2012. "StatExtracts: Health." http://stats.oecd.org/Index.aspx?DatasetCode=HEALTH_STAT.

———. 2010a. "OECD Health Data 2010." Paris, France: OECD Publishing.

———. 2010b. "OECD Health Data 2009." Paris, France: OECD Publishing.

———. 2009. *Achieving Better Value for Money in Health Care.* Paris, France: OECD Publishing.

———. 2002. *Measuring Up: Improving Health System Performance in OECD Countries.* Paris, France: OECD Publishing.

Orszag, P. R. 2008. *The Overuse, Underuse, and Misuse of Health Care.* Washington, DC: Congressional Budget Office. www.cbo.gov/sites/default/files/cbofiles /ftpdocs/95xx/doc9567/07-17-healthcare_testimony.pdf.

Orszag, P. R., and E. J. Emanuel. 2010. "Health Care Reform and Cost Control." *New England Journal of Medicine* 363 (7): 601–603.

Pande, A. H., D. Ross-Degnan, A. M. Zaslavsky, and J. A. Salomon. 2011. "Effects of Healthcare Reforms on Coverage, Access, and Disparities: Quasi-Experimental Analysis of Evidence from Massachusetts." *American Journal of Preventive Medicine* 41 (1): 1–8.

Parchman, M. L., and S. K. Burge. 2004. "The Patient–Physician Relationship, Primary Care Attributes, and Preventive Services." *Family Medicine* 36 (1): 22–27.

Parker, E., L. H. Margolis, E. Eng, and C. Henríquez-Roldan. 2003. "Assessing the Capacity of Health Departments to Engage in Community-Based Participatory Public Health." *American Journal of Public Health* 93 (3): 472–76.

Patel, N., S. Bae, and K. P. Singh. 2010. "Association Between Utilization of Preventive Services and Health Insurance Status: Findings from the 2008 Behavioral Risk Factor Surveillance System." *Ethnicity & Disease* 20 (2): 142–47.

Patient-Centered Primary Care Collaborative. 2007. "Joint Principles of the Patient-Centered Medical Home." www.pcpcc.net/content/joint-principles-patient-centered-medical-home.

Patton, C. V., and D. S. Sawicki. 1993. *Basic Methods of Policy Analysis and Planning.* Englewood Cliffs, NJ: Prentice Hall.

Pear, R. 2010a. "Health Plans Must Provide Some Tests at No Cost." *New York Times* (July 14).

———. 2010b. "Medicare Advantage Premiums to Fall in 2011." *New York Times* (September 21).

———. 1997. "New Options Include Shift into Preventive Benefits, and Slightly Higher Costs." *New York Times* (July 30).

Peelen, L., N. de Keizer, N. Peek, G. Scheffer, P. van der Voort, and E. de Jonge. 2007. "The Influence of Volume and Intensive Care Unit Organization on Hospital Mortality in Patients Admitted with Severe Sepsis: A Retrospective Multicentre Cohort Study." *Critical Care* 11 (2): R40.

Penrod, J. D., R. L. Kane, M. D. Finch, and R. A. Kane. 1998. "Effects of Post-Hospital Medicare Home Health and Informal Care on Patient Functional Status." *Health Services Research* 33 (3 Pt. 1): 513–29.

Perez, L. M., and J. Martinez. 2008. "Community Health Workers: Social Justice and Policy Advocates for Community Health and Well-Being." *American Journal of Public Health* 98 (1): 11–14.

Perkins, C. I., W. E. Wright, M. Allen, S. J. Samuels, and P. S. Romano. 2001. "Breast Cancer Stage at Diagnosis in Relation to Duration of Medicaid Enrollment." *Medical Care* 39 (11): 1224–33.

Perloff, J. D., P. R. Kletke, J. W. Fossett, and S. Banks. 1997. "Medicaid Participation Among Urban Primary Care Physicians." *Medical Care* 35 (2): 142–57.

Phillips, C. E., J. D. Rothstein, K. Beaver, B. J. Sherman, K. M. Freund, and T. A. Battaglia. 2010. "Patient Navigation to Increase Mammography Screening Among Inner City Women." *Journal of General Internal Medicine* 26 (2): 123–29.

Phillips, K. A., K. Kerlikowske, L. C. Baker, S. W. Chang, and M. L. Brown. 1998. "Factors Associated with Women's Adherence to Mammography Screening Guidelines." *Health Services Research* 33 (1): 29–53.

Phillips, K. A., M. L. Mayer, and L. A. Aday. 2000. "Barriers to Care Among Racial /Ethnic Groups Under Managed Care." *Health Affairs (Millwood)* 19 (4): 65–75.

Phillips, K. A., K. R. Morrison, R. Andersen, and L. A. Aday. 1998. "Understanding the Context of Healthcare Utilization: Assessing Environmental and Provider-Related Variables in the Behavioral Model of Utilization." *Health Services Research* 33 (3 Pt. 1): 571–96.

Physician Payment Review Commission (PPRC). 1991. *Annual Report to Congress, 1991*. Washington, DC: PPRC.

Pindyck, R. S., and D. L. Rubinfeld. 2008. *Microeconomics*, seventh edition. Upper Saddle River, NJ: Pearson Prentice Hall.

Pittman, P. 2010. "Health Services Research in 2020: Data and Methods Needs for the Future." *Health Services Research* 45 (5 Pt. 2): 1431–41.

Platner, J. H., L. M. Bennett, R. Millikan, and M. D. Barker. 2002. "The Partnership Between Breast Cancer Advocates and Scientists." *Environmental & Molecular Mutagenesis* 39 (2–3): 102–107.

Plowden, K. O., and A. E. Young. 2003. "Sociostructural Factors Influencing Health Behaviors of Urban African-American Men." *Journal of National Black Nurses' Association* 14 (1): 45–51.

Politzer, R. M., S. R. Gamliel, J. M. Cultice, C. M. Bazell, M. L. Rivo, and F. Mullan. 1996. "Matching Physician Supply and Requirements: Testing Policy Recommendations." *Inquiry* 33 (2): 181–94.

Portnoy, B., J. Miller, K. Brown-Huamani, and E. DeVoto. 2007. "Impact of the National Institutes of Health Consensus Development Program on Stimulating National Institutes of Health–Funded Research, 1998 to 2001." *International Journal of Technology Assessment in Health Care* 23 (3): 343–48.

Pourat, N., M. Kagawa-Singer, and S. P. Wallace. 2006. "Are Managed Care Medicare Beneficiaries with Chronic Conditions Satisfied with Their Care?" *Journal of Aging and Health* 18 (1): 70–90.

Powers, M., and R. Faden. 2006. *Social Justice: The Moral Foundation of Public Health and Health Policy*. New York: Oxford University Press, Inc.

Prasad, V., A. Cifu, and J. P. Ioannidis. 2012. "Reversals of Established Medical Practices: Evidence to Abandon Ship." *Journal of the American Medical Association* 307 (1): 37–38.

Press Ganey. 2013. "Gain the Advantage with Press Ganey HHCAHPS Expertise." www.pressganey.com/researchResources/governmentInitiatives/HHCAHPS .aspx.

Preyra, C., and G. Pink. 2006. "Scale and Scope Efficiencies Through Hospital Consolidations." *Journal of Health Economics* 25 (6): 1049–68.

Proenca, E. J., M. D. Rosko, and J. S. Zinn. 2000. "Community Orientation in Hospitals: An Institutional and Resource Dependence Perspective." *Health Services Research* 35 (5 Pt. 1): 1011–35.

Pronovost, P. J., and C. A. Goeschel. 2011. "Time to Take Health Delivery Research Seriously." *Journal of the American Medical Association* 306 (3): 310–11.

Public Health Accreditation Board (PHAB). 2011. "Standards & Measures, Version 1.0." www.phaboard.org/wp-content/uploads/PHAB-Standards-and -Measures-Version-1.0.pdf.

Quast, T., D. E. Sappington, and E. Shenkman. 2008. "Does the Quality of Care in Medicaid MCOs Vary with the Form of Physician Compensation?" *Health Economics* 17 (4): 545–50.

Qureshi, M., H. L. Thacker, D. G. Litaker, and C. Kippes. 2000. "Differences in Breast Cancer Screening Rates: An Issue of Ethnicity or Socioeconomics?" *Journal of Women's Health & Gender-Based Medicine* 9 (9): 1025–31.

Rabinowitz, H. K., J. J. Diamond, F. W. Markham, and A. J. Santana. 2010. "Increasing the Supply of Rural Family Physicians: Recent Outcomes from Jefferson Medical College's Physician Shortage Area Program (PSAP)." *Academic Medicine* 86 (2): 264–69.

Racine, A. D., R. Kaestner, T. J. Joyce, and G. J. Colman. 2001. "Differential Impact of Recent Medicaid Expansions by Race and Ethnicity." *Pediatrics* 108 (5): 1135–42.

Radin, B. 2000. *Beyond Machiavelli: Policy Analysis Comes of Age.* Washington, DC: Georgetown University Press.

Ramirez, A. G., L. Suarez, L. Laufman, C. Barroso, and P. Chalela. 2000. "Hispanic Women's Breast and Cervical Cancer Knowledge, Attitudes, and Screening Behaviors." *American Journal of Health Promotion* 14 (5): 292–300.

Ramsey, S., E. Whitley, V. W. Mears, J. M. McKoy, R. M. Everhart, R. J. Caswell, K. Fiscella, T. C. Hurd, T. Battaglia, and J. Mandelblatt; Patient Navigation Research Program Group. 2009. "Evaluating the Cost-Effectiveness of Cancer Patient Navigation Programs: Conceptual and Practical Issues." *Cancer* 115 (23): 5394–403.

Ramsey, S. D., S. B. Zeliadt, L. C. Richardson, L. Pollack, H. Linden, D. K. Blough, and N. Anderson. 2008. "Disenrollment from Medicaid After Recent Cancer Diagnosis." *Medical Care* 46 (1): 49–57.

Raphael, D., and T. Bryant. 2002. "The Limitations of Population Health as a Model for a New Public Health." *Health Promotion International* 17 (2): 189–99.

Rawls, J. 2001. *The Law of Peoples with "The Idea of Public Reason Revisited."* Cambridge, MA: Harvard University Press.

———. 1971. *A Theory of Justice.* Cambridge, MA: Harvard University Press.

Rawls, J., and E. Kelly. 2001. *Justice as Fairness: A Restatement.* Cambridge, MA: Harvard University Press.

Rayburn, J. M. 1992. "History and Process of the Medicare Reimbursement Programs." *Health Marketing Quarterly* 9 (3–4): 115–31.

Rea, D. M. 2004. "Changing Practice: Involving Mental Health Service Users in Planning Service Provision." *Social Work in Health Care* 39 (3–4): 325–42.

Reinhardt, U. E. 2010. "The Little-Known Decision-Makers for Medicare Physicians Fees." *New York Times* (December 10). http://economix.blogs.nytimes.com/2010/12/10/the-little-known-decision-makers-for-medicare-physicans-fees.

———. 1998. *Accountable Health Care: Is It Compatible with Social Solidarity?* London: Office of Health Economics.

———. 1991. "Health Manpower Forecasting: The Case of Physician Supply." In *Health Services Research: Key to Health Policy*, edited by E. Ginzberg, 234–83. Cambridge, MA: Harvard University Press.

———. 1990. "What Can Americans Learn from Europeans? Respondent." In *Health Care Systems in Transition: The Search for Efficiency.* Paris, France: Organisation for Economic Co-operation and Development.

———. 1987. "A Clarification of Theories and Evidence on Supplier-Induced Demand for Physicians' Services." *Journal of Human Resources* 22 (4): 621–23.

———. 1975. *Physician Productivity and the Demand for Health Manpower: An Economic Analysis.* Cambridge, MA: Ballinger Publishing Company.

———. 1972. "A Production Function for Physician Services." *Review of Economics and Statistics* 54 (1): 55–66.

Reinhardt, U. E., P. S. Hussey, and G. F. Anderson. 2002. "Cross-National Comparisons of Health Systems Using OECD Data, 1999." *Health Affairs (Millwood)* 21 (3): 169–81.

Relman, A. S. 1980. "The New Medical-Industrial Complex." *New England Journal of Medicine* 303 (17): 963–70.

Resnicow, K., and S. E. Page. 2008. "Embracing Chaos and Complexity: A Quantum Change for Public Health." *American Journal of Public Health* 98 (8): 1382–89.

Reynolds, P. P. 1997. "Hospitals and Civil Rights, 1945–1963: The Case of Simkins v Moses H. Cone Memorial Hospital." *Annals of Internal Medicine* 126 (11): 898–906.

Rice, T., B. Biles, E. R. Brown, F. Diderichsen, and H. Kuehn. 2000. "Reconsidering the Role of Competition in Health Care Markets: Introduction." *Journal of Health Politics Policy and Law* 25 (5): 863–73.

Rice, T. H., and L. Unruh. 2009. *The Economics of Health Reconsidered*, third edition. Chicago: Health Administration Press.

Richardson, E. A., R. Mitchell, N. K. Shortt, J. Pearce, and T. P. Dawson. 2010. "Developing Summary Measures of Health-Related Multiple Physical Environmental Deprivation for Epidemiological Research." *Environment and Planning A* 42 (7): 1650–68.

Richardson, L. C., L. Tian, L. Voti, A. G. Hartzema, I. Reis, L. E. Fleming, and J. Mackinnon. 2006. "The Roles of Teaching Hospitals, Insurance Status, and Race/Ethnicity in Receipt of Adjuvant Therapy for Regional-Stage Breast Cancer in Florida." *American Journal of Public Health* 96 (1): 160–66.

Ricketts, T. C. III. 2002. "Geography and Disparities in Health Care." In *Guidance for the National Healthcare Disparities Report*, edited by E. K. Swift, 149–80. Washington, DC: National Academies Press.

Ricketts, T. C. III, L. A. Savitz, W. M. Gesler, and D. N. Osbourne. 1994. *Geographic Methods for Health Services Research: A Focus on the Rural–Urban Continuum*. Lanham, MD: University Press of America, Inc.

Rijnsburger, A. J., I. M. Obdeijn, R. Kaas, M. M. Tilanus-Linthorst, C. Boetes, C. E. Loo, M. N. Wasser, E. Bergers, T. Kok, S. H. Muller, H. Peterse, R. A. Tollenaar, N. Hoogerbrugge, S. Meijer, C. C. Bartels, C. Seynaeve, M. J. Hooning, M. Kriege, P. I. Schmitz, J. C. Oosterwijk, H. J. de Koning, E. J. Rutgers, and J. G. Klijn. 2009. "BRCA1-Associated Breast Cancers Present Differently from BRCA2-Associated and Familial Cases: Long-Term Follow-Up of the Dutch MRISC Screening Study." *Journal of Clinical Oncology* 28 (36): 5265–73.

Riley, G. F., and J. D. Lubitz. 2010. "Long-Term Trends in Medicare Payments in the Last Year of Life." *Health Services Research* 45 (2): 565–76.

Riley, G. F., J. L. Warren, A. L. Potosky, C. N. Klabunde, L. C. Harlan, and M. B. Osswald. 2008. "Comparison of Cancer Diagnosis and Treatment in Medicare Fee-for-Service and Managed Care Plans." *Medical Care* 46 (10): 1108–15.

Ringwalt, C., A. A. Vincus, S. Hanley, S. T. Ennett, J. M. Bowling, and L. A. Rohrbach. 2009. "The Prevalence of Evidence-Based Drug Use Prevention Curricula in U.S. Middle Schools in 2005." *Prevention Science* 10 (1): 33–40.

Robert Graham Center. 2005. "The Family Physician Workforce: The Special Case of Rural Populations." *American Family Physician* 72 (1): 147.

Robertson, A. 1998. "Critical Reflections on the Politics of Need: Implications for Public Health." *Social Science & Medicine* 47 (10): 1419–30.

Robertson, A., and M. Minkler. 1994. "New Health Promotion Movement: A Critical Examination." *Health Education Quarterly* 21 (3): 295–312.

Robert Wood Johnson Foundation. 2010. "The Robert Wood Johnson Foundation Health Care Consumer Confidence Index: A Monthly Survey of Americans' Attitudes About Health Care—October Findings." Analysis provided by State Health Access Data Assistance Center. Published in November. www.rwjf.org/content/dam/web-assets/2010/11/robert-wood-johnson-foundation-health-care-consumer-confidence-i.

Robertson, R., A. Dixon, and J. Le Grand. 2008. "Patient Choice in General Practice: The Implications of Patient Satisfaction Surveys." *Journal of Health Services Research & Policy* 13 (2): 67–72.

Robinowitz, D. L., and R. A. Dudley. 2006. "Public Reporting of Provider Performance: Can Its Impact Be Made Greater?" *Annual Review of Public Health* 27: 517–36.

Robinson, J. C. 2002. "Renewed Emphasis on Consumer Cost Sharing in Health Insurance Benefit Design." *Health Affairs (Millwood)* (Suppl. Web Exclusives): W139–54.

———. 2001. "The End of Managed Care." *Journal of the American Medical Association* 285 (20): 2622–28.

Roland, M., and R. Rosen. 2011. "English NHS Embarks on Controversial and Risky Market-Style Reforms in Health Care." *New England Journal of Medicine* 364 (14): 1360–66.

Romano, P. S., J. A. Rainwater, and D. Antonius. 1999. "Grading the Graders: How Hospitals in California and New York Perceive and Interpret Their Report Cards." *Medical Care* 37 (3): 295–305.

Romano, P. S., and H. Zhou. 2004. "Do Well-Publicized Risk-Adjusted Outcomes Reports Affect Hospital Volume?" *Medical Care* 42 (4): 367–77.

Roos, N. P. 1984. "Hysterectomy: Variations in Rates Across Small Areas and Across Physicians' Practices." *American Journal of Public Health* 74 (4): 327–35.

Roos, N. P., C. Black, N. Frohlich, C. DeCoster, M. Cohen, D. J. Tataryn, C. A. Mustard, L. L. Roos, F. Toll, K. C. Carriere, C. A. Burchill, L. MacWilliam, and B. Bogdanovic. 1996. "Population Health and Health Care Use: An Information System for Policy Makers." *Milbank Quarterly* 74 (1): 3–31.

Roos, N. P., C. D. Black, N. Frohlich, C. DeCoster, M. M. Cohen, D. J. Tataryn, C. A. Mustard, F. Toll, K. C. Carriere, and C. A. Burchill. 1995. "A Population-Based Health Information System." *Medical Care* 33 (12 Suppl.): DS13–20.

Roos, N. P., C. Black, L. L. Roos, N. Frohlich, C. DeCoster, C. Mustard, M. D. Brownell, M. Shanahan, P. Fergusson, F. Toll, K. C. Carriere, C. Burchill, R. Fransoo, L. MacWilliam, B. Bogdanovic, and D. Friesen. 1999. "Managing Health Services: How the Population Health Information System (POPULIS) Works for Policymakers." *Medical Care* 37 (6 Suppl.): JS27–41.

Rose, D., J. Evans, A. Sweeney, and T. Wykes. 2011. "A Model for Developing Outcome Measures from the Perspectives of Mental Health Service Users." *International Review of Psychiatry* 23 (1): 41–46.

Rosenbaum, S., K. Johnson, C. Sonosky, A. Markus, and C. DeGraw. 1998. "The Children's Hour: The State Children's Health Insurance Program." *Health Affairs (Millwood)* 17 (1): 75–89.

Rosenthal, M. B. 2007. "P4P: Rumors of Its Demise May Be Exaggerated." *American Journal of Managed Care* 13 (5): 238–39.

Rosenthal, M. B., and J. P. Newhouse. 2002. "Managed Care and Efficient Rationing." *Journal of Health Care Finance* 28 (4): 1–10.

Ross, D. C., and C. Marks. 2009. "Challenges of Providing Health Coverage for Children and Parents in a Recession: A 50 State Update on Eligibility Rules, Enrollment and Renewal Procedures, and Cost-Sharing Practices in Medicaid and SCHIP in 2009." Kaiser Commission on Medicaid and the Uninsured; published January 23. www.kff.org/medicaid/upload/7855.pdf.

Rossi, P. H., M. W. Lipsey, and H. E. Freeman. 2003. *Evaluation: A Systematic Approach*, seventh edition. Thousand Oaks, CA: Sage Publications, Inc.

Roussos, S. T., and S. B. Fawcett. 2000. "A Review of Collaborative Partnerships as a Strategy for Improving Community Health." *Annual Review of Public Health* 21: 369–402.

Rowland, D., C. Hoffman, and M. McGinn-Shapiro. 2009. "Focus on Health Reform—Health Care and the Middle Class: More Costs and Less Coverage." Kaiser Family Foundation; published in July. www.kff.org/health reform/upload/7951.pdf.

Rowland, D., and B. Lyons. 1996. "Medicare, Medicaid, and the Elderly Poor." *Health Care Financing Review* 18 (2): 61–85.

Rush, A. J. 2007. "STAR*D: What Have We Learned?" *American Journal of Psychiatry* 164 (2): 201–204.

Russell, L. B. 1989. *Medicare's New Hospital Payment System: Is It Working?* Washington, DC: Brookings Institution Press.

Ryerson, A. B., J. W. Miller, C. R. Eheman, S. Leadbetter, and M. C. White. 2008. "Recent Trends in U.S. Mammography Use from 2000–2006: A Population-Based Analysis." *Preventive Medicine* 47 (5): 477–82.

Sabatino, S. A., R. J. Coates, R. J. Uhler, N. Breen, F. Tangka, and K. M. Shaw. 2008. "Disparities in Mammography Use Among US Women Aged 40–64 Years, by Race, Ethnicity, Income, and Health Insurance Status, 1993 and 2005." *Medical Care* 46 (7): 692–700.

Sackett, D. L. 1980. "Evaluation of Health Services." In *Maxcy-Rosenau Public Health and Preventive Medicine*, edited by J. Last, 1800–23. Norwalk, CN: Appleton-Century-Crofts.

Sackett, D. L., W. M. Rosenberg, J. A. Gray, R. B. Haynes, and W. S. Richardson. 1996. "Evidence Based Medicine: What It Is and What It Isn't." *BMJ* 312 (7023): 71–72.

Saha, S., D. D. Coffman, and A. K. Smits. 2010. "Giving Teeth to Comparative-Effectiveness Research—The Oregon Experience." *New England Journal of Medicine* 362 (7): e18.

Salganicoff, A., J. A. Beckerman, R. Wyn, and V. D. Ojeda. 2002. "Women's Health in the United States: Health Coverage and Access to Care." Washington, DC: Henry J. Kaiser Family Foundation.

Salsberg, E. S., and G. J. Forte. 2002. "Trends in the Physician Workforce, 1980–2000." *Health Affairs (Millwood)* 21 (5): 165–73.

Sandy, L. G., T. Bodenheimer, L. G. Pawlson, and B. Starfield. 2009. "The Political Economy of U.S. Primary Care." *Health Affairs (Millwood)* 28 (4): 1136–45.

Saywell, R. M. Jr., V. L. Champion, C. S. Skinner, D. McQuillen, D. Martin, and M. Maraj. 1999. "Cost-Effectiveness Comparison of Five Interventions to Increase Mammography Screening." *Preventive Medicine* 29 (5): 374–82.

Scheuplein, R. J. 1992. "Perspectives on Toxicological Risk: An Example—Food-borne Carcinogenic Risk." *Critical Reviews in Food Science & Nutrition* 32 (2): 105–21.

Schiff, G. D., and T. D. Rucker. 2001. "Beyond Structure-Process-Outcome: Donabedian's Seven Pillars and Eleven Buttresses of Quality." *Joint Commission Journal on Quality Improvement* 27 (3): 169–74.

Schiller, J. S., J. W. Lucas, B. W. Ward, and J. A. Peregoy. 2012. "Summary Health Statistics for U.S. Adults: National Health Interview Survey, 2010." National Center for Health Statistics. *Vital and Health Statistics* 10 (252).

Schneider, E. C., P. S. Hussey, and C. Schnyer. 2011. "Payment Reform: Analysis of Models and Performance Measurement Implications." Santa Monica, CA: RAND Corporation.

Schoen, C., and C. DesRoches. 2000. "Uninsured and Unstably Insured: The Importance of Continuous Insurance Coverage." *Health Services Research* 35 (1 Pt. 2): 187–206.

Schoen, C., R. Osborn, D. Squires, M. M. Doty, R. Pierson, and S. Applebaum. 2010. "How Health Insurance Design Affects Access to Care and Costs, by Income, in Eleven Countries." *Health Affairs (Millwood)* 29 (12): 2323–34.

Schoenbaum, S. C. 2006. "Keys to a High-Performance Health System for the United States." *Healthcare Financial Management* 60 (7): 60–64.

Schold, J. D. 2008. "Evaluation Criteria for Report Cards of Healthcare Providers." *Advances in Health Economics and Health Services Research* 19: 173–89.

Schuster, M. A., E. A. McGlynn, and R. H. Brook. 2005. "How Good Is the Quality of Health Care in the United States? 1998." *Milbank Quarterly* 83 (4): 843–95.

Schwartz, W. B., and D. N. Mendelson. 1991. "Hospital Cost Containment in the 1980s: Hard Lessons Learned and Prospects for the 1990s." *New England Journal of Medicine* 324 (15): 1037–42.

Segal, L., and J. Richardson. 1994. "Efficiency in Resource Allocation." In *Economics and Health: Proceedings of the 16th Australian Conference of Health Economists*, edited by A H. Harris, 231–55. Sydney, Australia: University of New South Wales.

Selvin, E., and K. M. Brett. 2003. "Breast and Cervical Cancer Screening: Sociodemographic Predictors Among White, Black, and Hispanic Women." *American Journal of Public Health* 93 (4): 618–23.

Sequist, T. D. 2011. "Ensuring Equal Access to Specialty Care." *New England Journal of Medicine* 364 (23): 2258–59.

Shadish, W. R., T. D. Cook, and D. T. Campbell. 2002. *Experimental and Quasi-Experimental Designs for Generalized Causal Inference*. Belmont, CA: Wadsworth Publishing.

Shaw, J. W., J. A. Johnson, and S. J. Coons. 2005. "US Valuation of the EQ-5D Health States: Development and Testing of the D1 Valuation Model." *Medical Care* 43 (3): 203–20.

Shen, Y. C., and S. K. Long. 2006. "What's Driving the Downward Trend in Employer-Sponsored Health Insurance?" *Health Services Research* 41 (6): 2074–96.

Sheppard, V. B., J. Wang, B. Yi, T. M. Harrison, S. Feng, E. E. Huerta, and J. S. Mandelblatt. 2008. "Are Health-Care Relationships Important for Mammography Adherence in Latinas?" *Journal of General Internal Medicine* 23 (12): 2024–30.

Shi, L. 1997. *Health Services Research Methods.* Albany, NY: Delmar Publishers Inc.

Shi, L., and G. D. Stevens. 2005. *Vulnerable Populations in the United States.* San Francisco: Jossey-Bass.

Shields, A. E., M. McGinn-Shapiro, and P. Fronstin. 2008. "Trends in Private Insurance, Medicaid/State Children's Health Insurance Program, and the Healthcare Safety Net: Implications for Vulnerable Populations and Health Disparities." *Annals of the New York Academy of Science* 1136: 137–48.

Shimada, S. L., A. M. Zaslavsky, L. B. Zaborski, A. J. O'Malley, A. Heller, and P. D. Cleary. 2009. "Market and Beneficiary Characteristics Associated with Enrollment in Medicare Managed Care Plans and Fee-for-Service." *Medical Care* 47 (5): 517–23.

Short, P. F., and V. A. Freedman. 1998. "Single Women and the Dynamics of Medicaid." *Health Services Research* 33 (5 Pt. 1): 1309–36.

Shortell, S. M., J. A. Alexander, P. P. Budetti, L. R. Burns, R. R. Gillies, T. M. Waters, and H. S. Zuckerman. 2001. "Physician-System Alignment: Introductory Overview." *Medical Care* 39 (7 Suppl. 1): I1–8.

Shortell, S. M., L. P. Casalino, and E. S. Fisher. 2010. "How the Center for Medicare and Medicaid Innovation Should Test Accountable Care Organizations." *Health Affairs (Millwood)* 29 (7): 1293–98.

Shortell, S. M., R. R. Gillies, and D. A. Anderson. 1994. "The New World of Managed Care: Creating Organized Delivery Systems." *Health Affairs (Millwood)* 13 (5): 46–64.

Shortell, S. M., R. R. Gillies, D. A. Anderson, K. M. Erickson, and J. B. Mitchell. 2000a. "Integrating Health Care Delivery." *Health Forum Journal* 43 (6): 35–39.

———. 2000b. *Remaking Health Care in America: The Evolution of Organized Delivery Systems,* second edition. San Francisco: Jossey-Bass.

Shortell, S. M., R. R. Gillies, D. A. Anderson, J. B. Mitchell, and K. L. Morgan. 1993. "Creating Organized Delivery Systems: The Barriers and Facilitators." *Hospital & Health Services Administration* 38 (4): 447–66.

Shortell, S. M., R. R. Gillies, and K. J. Devers. 1995. "Reinventing the American Hospital." *Milbank Quarterly* 73 (2): 131–60.

Shortell, S. M., and K. E. Hull. 1996. "The New Organization of the Health Care Delivery System." In *Strategic Choices for a Changing Health Care System,* edited by S. H. Altman and U. E. Reinhardt, 101–48. Chicago: Health Administration Press.

Shortell, S. M., and U. E. Reinhardt. 1992. *Improving Health Policy and Management: Nine Critical Research Issues for the 1990s.* Chicago: Health Administration Press.

Showstack, J. A., K. E. Rosenfeld, D. W. Garnick, H. S. Luft, R. W. Schaffarzick, and J. Fowles. 1987. "Association of Volume with Outcome of Coronary Artery Bypass Graft Surgery. Scheduled vs Nonscheduled Operations." *Journal of the American Medical Association* 257 (6): 785–89.

Shugarman, L. R., S. L. Decker, and A. Bercovitz. 2009. "Demographic and Social Characteristics and Spending at the End of Life." *Journal of Pain and Symptom Management* 38 (1): 15–26.

Sidani, S., D. M. Doran, and P. H. Mitchell. 2004. "A Theory-Driven Approach to Evaluating Quality of Nursing Care." *Journal of Nursing Scholarship* 36 (1): 60–65.

Silverstein, G., and B. Kirkman-Liff. 1995. "Physician Participation in Medicaid Managed Care." *Social Science & Medicine* 41 (3): 355–63.

Simera, I., D. Moher, A. Hirst, J. Hoey, K. F. Schulz, and D. G. Altman. 2010. "Transparent and Accurate Reporting Increases Reliability, Utility, and Impact of Your Research: Reporting Guidelines and the EQUATOR Network." *BMC Medicine* 8: 24.

Simera, I., D. Moher, J. Hoey, K. F. Schulz, and D. G. Altman. 2009. "The EQUATOR Network and Reporting Guidelines: Helping to Achieve High Standards in Reporting Health Research Studies." *Maturitas* 63 (1): 4–6.

Simon, C. J., and P. H. Born. 1996. "Physician Earnings in a Changing Managed Care Environment." *Health Affairs (Millwood)* 15 (3): 124–33.

Simon, C. J., D. Dranove, and W. D. White. 1998. "The Effect of Managed Care on the Incomes of Primary Care and Specialty Physicians." *Health Services Research* 33 (3 Pt. 1): 549–69.

Singh-Manoux, A., N. E. Adler, and M. G. Marmot. 2003. "Subjective Social Status: Its Determinants and Its Association with Measures of Ill-Health in the Whitehall II Study." *Social Science & Medicine* 56 (6): 1321–33.

Sinyor, M., A. Schaffer, and A. Levitt. 2010. "The Sequenced Treatment Alternatives to Relieve Depression (STAR*D) Trial: A Review." *Canadian Journal of Psychiatry* 55 (3): 126–35.

Sipkoff, M. 2010. "Higher Copayments and Deductibles Delay Medical Care, a Common Problem for Americans." *Managed Care* 19 (1): 46–49.

Siu, A. L., F. A. Sonnenberg, W. G. Manning, G. A. Goldberg, E. S. Bloomfield, J. P. Newhouse, and R. H. Brook. 1986. "Inappropriate Use of Hospitals in a Randomized Trial of Health Insurance Plans." *New England Journal of Medicine* 315 (20): 1259–66.

Skinner, J., and D. Staiger. 2009. "Technology Diffusion and Productivity Growth in Health Care." NBER Working Paper No. 14865. Cambridge, MA: National Bureau of Economic Research.

Skinner, J., D. Staiger, and E. S. Fisher. 2010. "Looking Back, Moving Forward." *New England Journal of Medicine* 362 (7): 569–74.

———. 2006. "Is Technological Change In Medicine Always Worth It? The Case of Acute Myocardial Infarction." *Health Affairs (Millwood)* 25 (2): w34–47.

Skocpol, T. 1996. *Boomerang: Clinton's Health Security Effort and the Turn Against Government in U.S. Politics.* New York: W. W. Norton & Company.

Smaldone, A., and M. Cullen-Drill. 2010. "Mental Health Parity Legislation: Understanding the Pros and Cons." *Journal of Psychosocial Nursing & Mental Health Services* 48 (9): 26–34.

Smart, D. R. 2010. *Physician Characteristics and Distribution in the US, 2011.* Chicago: American Medical Association.

Smigal, C., A. Jemal, E. Ward, V. Cokkinides, R. Smith, H. L. Howe, and M. Thun. 2006. "Trends in Breast Cancer by Race and Ethnicity: Update 2006." *CA: A Cancer Journal for Clinicians* 56 (3): 168–83.

Smith, A. D. 2008. "Managing the Quality of Health Information Using Electronic Medical Records: An Exploratory Study Among Clinical Physicians." *International Journal of Electronic Healthcare* 4 (3–4): 267–89.

Smith, K. R., M. Miller, and F. L. Golladay. 1972. "An Analysis of the Optimal Use of Inputs in the Production of Medical Services." *Journal of Human Resources* 7 (2): 208–55.

Smith, R. A., V. Cokkinides, D. Brooks, D. Saslow, and O. W. Brawley. 2010. "Cancer Screening in the United States, 2010: A Review of Current American Cancer Society Guidelines and Issues in Cancer Screening." *CA: A Cancer Journal for Clinicians* 60 (2): 99–119.

Sochalski, J. 2002. "Nursing Shortage Redux: Turning the Corner on an Enduring Problem." *Health Affairs (Millwood)* 21 (5): 157–64.

Solucient LLC. 2004. "Solucient 100 Top Hospitals: National Benchmarks for Success." Evanston, IL: Solucient LLC.

Sondik, E. J., J. H. Madans, and J. F. Gentleman. 2011. "Summary Health Statistics for the U.S. Population, 2011." National Center for Health Statistics. *Vital and Health Statistics* 10 (255).

Sox, H. C. 2010. "Comparative Effectiveness Research: A Progress Report." *Annals of Internal Medicine* 153 (7): 469–72.

Sox, H. C., and S. Greenfield. 2009. "Comparative Effectiveness Research: A Report from the Institute of Medicine." *Annals of Internal Medicine* 151 (3): 203–205.

Spitler, H. D. 2001. "Medical Sociology and Public Health: Problems and Prospects for Collaboration in the New Millennium." *Sociological Spectrum* 21 (3): 247–63.

Sprecher Institute for Comparative Cancer Research. 2013. "Breast Cancer and Environmental Risk Factors." http://ecommons.library.cornell.edu/handle/1813/14300.

Squiers, L. B., D. J. Holden, S. E. Dolina, A. E. Kim, C. M. Bann, and J. M. Renaud. 2011. "The Public's Response to the U.S. Preventive Services Task Force's

2009 Recommendations on Mammography Screening." *American Journal of Preventive Medicine* 40 (5): 497–504.

Staff of *The Washington Post*. 2010. *Landmark: The Inside Story of America's New Health-Care Law and What It Means for Us All.* New York: PublicAffairs.

Staiger, D. O., D. I. Auerbach, and P. I. Buerhaus. 2010. "Trends in the Work Hours of Physicians in the United States." *Journal of the American Medical Association* 303 (8): 747–53.

Statistics Canada. 2008. "Overview of the Canadian Health Measures Survey." www .library.carleton.ca/sites/default/files/find/data/surveys/pdf_files/chms -c1-07-09-ovr.pdf.

Steiner, E., D. Klubert, and D. Knutson. 2008. "Assessing Breast Cancer Risk in Women." *American Family Physician* 78 (12): 1361–66.

Stenger, J., S. B. Cashman, and J. A. Savageau. 2008. "The Primary Care Physician Workforce in Massachusetts: Implications for the Workforce in Rural, Small Town America." *Journal of Rural Health* 24 (4): 375–83.

Stephens, T. 1986. "Health Practices and Health Status: Evidence from the Canada Health Survey." *American Journal of Preventive Medicine* 2 (4): 209–15.

Stokey, E., and R. Zeckhauser. 1978. *A Primer for Policy Analysis.* New York: W.W. Norton & Co.

Stolpe, M. 2011. "Reforming Health Care—The German Experience." IMF Conference: Public Health Care Reforms: Challenges and Lessons for Advanced and Emerging Europe. Paris, France, June 21. www.imf.org/external/np /seminars/eng/2011/paris/pdf/stolpe.pdf.

Stone, D. 2001. *Policy Paradox: The Art of Political Decision Making*, revised edition. New York: W.W. Norton & Co.

Stone, J. 2002. "Race and Healthcare Disparities: Overcoming Vulnerability." *Theoretical Medicine & Bioethics* 23 (6): 499–518.

Street, A. 1994. "Purchaser/Provider Separation and Managed Competition: Reform Options for Australia's Health System." *Australian Journal of Public Health* 18 (4): 369–79.

Strunk, B. C., P. B. Ginsburg, and J. R. Gabel. 2002. "Tracking Health Care Costs: Growth Accelerates Again in 2001." *Health Affairs (Millwood)* (Suppl. Web Exclusives): W299–310.

Strunk, B. C., and J. D. Reschovsky. 2002. "Kinder and Gentler: Physicians and Managed Care, 1997–2001." *Tracking Report/Center for Studying Health System Change* 5: 1–4.

Stuart, A. L., S. Mudhasakul, and W. Sriwatanapongse. 2009. "The Social Distribution of Neighborhood-Scale Air Pollution and Monitoring Protection." *Journal of the Air & Waste Management Association* 59 (5): 591–602.

Sullivan, S. D., J. Watkins, B. Sweet, and S. D. Ramsey. 2009. "Health Technology Assessment in Health-Care Decisions in the United States." *Value in Health* 12 (Suppl. 2): S39–44.

Sultz, H. A., and K. M. Young. 2011. *Health Care USA: Understanding Its Organization and Delivery*, seventh edition. Sudbury, MA: Jones & Bartlett Learning.

Sunshine, J. H., D. R. Hughes, C. Meghea, and M. Bhargavan. 2010. "What Factors Affect the Productivity and Efficiency of Physician Practices?" *Medical Care* 48 (2): 110–17.

Swinehart, K. D., and A. E. Smith. 2004. "Customer Focused Health-Care Performance Instruments: Making a Case for Local Measures." *International Journal of Health Care Quality Assurance Incorporating Leadership in Health Services* 17 (1): 9–16.

Taira, D. A., D. G. Safran, T. B. Seto, W. H. Rogers, T. S. Inui, J. Montgomery, and A. R. Tarlov. 2001. "Do Patient Assessments of Primary Care Differ by Patient Ethnicity?" *Health Services Research* 36 (6 Pt. 1): 1059–71.

Talbott, J. A. 2004. "Deinstitutionalization: Avoiding the Disasters of the Past. 1979." *Psychiatric Services* 55 (10): 1112–15.

Taleb, N. N. 2007. "Black Swans and the Domains of Statistics." *American Statistician* 61 (3): 1–3.

Tanenbaum, S. J. 2009. "Comparative Effectiveness Research: Evidence-Based Medicine Meets Health Care Reform in the USA." *Journal of Evaluation in Clinical Practice* 15 (6): 976–84.

Tang, P. C., M. Ralston, M. F. Arrigotti, L. Qureshi, and J. Graham. 2007. "Comparison of Methodologies for Calculating Quality Measures Based on Administrative Data Versus Clinical Data from an Electronic Health Record System: Implications for Performance Measures." *Journal of the American Medical Informatics Association* 14 (1): 10–15.

Tarlov, A. R., and R. F. St. Peter. 2000. *The Society and Population Health Reader, Volume II: A State and Community Perspective*. New York: The New Press.

Tengs, T. O. 1996. "An Evaluation of Oregon's Medicaid Rationing Algorithms." *Health Economics* 5 (3): 171–81.

Tengs, T. O., M. E. Adams, J. S. Pliskin, D. G. Safran, J. E. Siegel, M. C. Weinstein, and J. D. Graham. 1995. "Five-Hundred Life-Saving Interventions and Their Cost-Effectiveness." *Risk Analysis* 15 (3): 369–90.

Tenopir, C., S. Allard, K. Douglass, A. U. Aydinoglu, L. Wu, E. Read, M. Manoff, and M. Frame. 2011. "Data Sharing by Scientists: Practices and Perceptions." *PLoS One* 6 (6): e21101.

Teutsch, S. M., and J. E. Fielding. 2011. "Applying Comparative Effectiveness Research to Public and Population Health Initiatives." *Health Affairs (Millwood)* 30 (2): 349–55.

Texas Department of State Health Services. 2013. "Breast and Cervical Cancer Services (BCCS) Program." www.dshs.state.tx.us/bccs/default.shtm.

———. 2012. "FY13 Policy Manual for BCCS." www.dshs.state.tx.us/bccs/contract only.shtm#manual.

———. 2010. "DSHS Community Health Services Forum—FY 10 Clinical Cost Worksheet." www.dshs.state.tx.us/chscontracts/all_forms.shtm#Clinical.

Thacker, S. B., J. P. Koplan, W. R. Taylor, A. R. Hinman, M. F. Katz, and W. L. Roper. 1994. "Assessing Prevention Effectiveness Using Data to Drive Program Decisions." *Public Health Reports* 109 (2): 187–94.

Thielen, L. 2004. "Exploring Public Health Experience with Standards and Accreditation: Is It Time to Stop Talking About How Every Health Department Is Unique?" Prepared for The Robert Wood Johnson Foundation; published in October. www.phaboard.org/wp-content/uploads/ExploringPublicHealth ExperiencewithStandardsandAccreditation.pdf.

Thorlby, R., and J. Maybin. 2010. *A High-Performing NHS? A Review of Progress 1997–2010.* London: The King's Fund.

Thorpe, K. E. 2005. "The Rise in Health Care Spending and What to Do About It." *Health Affairs (Millwood)* 24 (6): 1436–45.

Thorpe, K. E., and A. Atherly. 2002. "Medicare+Choice: Current Role and Near-Term Prospects." *Health Affairs (Millwood)* (Suppl. Web Exclusives): W242–52.

Thurston, W. E., G. MacKean, A. Vollman, A. Casebeer, M. Weber, B. Maloff, and J. Bader. 2005. "Public Participation in Regional Health Policy: A Theoretical Framework." *Health Policy (Amsterdam, Netherlands)* 73 (3): 237–52.

Timmermans, S., and A. Mauck. 2005. "The Promises and Pitfalls of Evidence-Based Medicine." *Health Affairs (Millwood)* 24 (1): 18–28.

Tomatis, L., J. Huff, I. Hertz-Picciotto, D. P. Sandler, J. Bucher, P. Boffetta, O. Axelson, A. Blair, J. Taylor, L. Stayner, and J. C. Barrett. 1997. "Avoided and Avoidable Risks of Cancer." *Carcinogenesis* 18 (1): 97–105.

Tomes, N. 2006. "The Patient as a Policy Factor: A Historical Case Study of the Consumer/Survivor Movement in Mental Health." *Health Affairs (Millwood)* 25 (3): 720–29.

Torrance, G. W., and D. Feeny. 1989. "Utilities and Quality-Adjusted Life Years." *International Journal of Technology Assessment in Health Care* 5 (4): 559–75.

Torrance, G. W., D. H. Feeny, W. J. Furlong, R. D. Barr, Y. Zhang, and Q. Wang. 1996. "Multiattribute Utility Function for a Comprehensive Health Status Classification System: Health Utilities Index Mark 2." *Medical Care* 34 (7): 702–22.

Trivedi, A. N., W. Rakowski, and J. Z. Ayanian. 2008. "Effect of Cost Sharing on Screening Mammography in Medicare Health Plans." *New England Journal of Medicine* 358 (4): 375–83.

Trivedi, A. N., A. M. Zaslavsky, E. C. Schneider, and J. Z. Ayanian. 2005. "Trends in the Quality of Care and Racial Disparities in Medicare Managed Care." *New England Journal of Medicine* 353 (7): 692–700.

Truffer, C. J., S. Keehan, S. Smith, J. Cylus, A. Sisko, J. A. Poisal, J. Lizonitz, and M. K. Clemens. 2010. "Health Spending Projections Through 2019: The Recession's Impact Continues." *Health Affairs (Millwood)* 29 (3): 522–29.

Tu, H. T. 2004. "Rising Health Costs, Medical Debt and Chronic Conditions." *Issue Brief (Center for Studying Health System Change)* 88: 1–5.

Tunis, S. R., D. B. Stryer, and C. M. Clancy. 2003. "Practical Clinical Trials: Increasing the Value of Clinical Research for Decision Making in Clinical and Health Policy." *Journal of the American Medical Association* 290 (12): 1624–32.

Tuohy, C. H. 2002. "The Costs of Constraint and Prospects for Health Care Reform in Canada." *Health Affairs (Millwood)* 21 (3): 32–46.

Turner, E. H. 2004. "A Taxpayer-Funded Clinical Trials Registry and Results Database." *PLoS Medicine* 1 (3): e60.

Turner, E. H., A. M. Matthews, E. Linardatos, R. A. Tell, and R. Rosenthal. 2008. "Selective Publication of Antidepressant Trials and Its Influence on Apparent Efficacy." *New England Journal of Medicine* 358 (3): 252–60.

Umscheid, C. A. 2010. "Maximizing the Clinical Utility of Comparative Effectiveness Research." *Clinical Pharmacology and Therapeutics* 88 (6): 876–79.

US Census Bureau. 2011. "Statistical Abstract of the United States: 2012." US Department of Commerce. www.census.gov/prod/www/abs/statab.html.

———. 2001. "Statistical Abstract of the United States: 2002." US Department of Commerce. www.census.gov/prod/www/abs/statab.html.

US Department of Health, Education, and Welfare (DHEW). 1979. *Healthy People: The Surgeon General's Report on Health Promotion and Disease Promotion.* DHEW (PHS) Publication No. 79-55071. Public Health Service, Office of the Assistant Secretary for Health and Surgeon General. Washington, DC: US Government Printing Office.

US Department of Health and Human Services (HHS). 2012. "HHS Announces 89 New Accountable Care Organizations." Press release, July 9. www.hhs.gov/news/press/2012pres/07/20120709a.html.

———. 2010. *Healthy People 2020.* Office of Health Promotion and Disease Prevention, Publication No. B0132. Published in November. www.healthypeople.gov/2020/TopicsObjectives2020/pdfs/HP2020_brochure_with_LHI_508.pdf.

———. 2000. *Healthy People 2010: Understanding and Improving Health*, second edition. Published in November. Washington, DC: US Government Printing Office. www.healthypeople.gov/2010/Document/pdf/uih/2010uih.pdf.

———. 1980. *Promoting Health/Preventing Disease: Objectives for the Nation.* Public Health Service, Office of the Assistant Secretary for Health; published in November. http://stacks.cdc.gov/view/cdc/5293.

US Department of Veterans Affairs (VA). 2001. "2001 National Survey of Veterans (NSV): Final Report." www.va.gov/VETDATA/docs/SurveysAndStudies/NSV_Final_Report.pdf.

US Food and Drug Administration (FDA). 2006. "Guidance for Clinical Trial Sponsors: Establishment and Operation of Clinical Trial Data Monitoring Committees." www.fda.gov/downloads/Regulatoryinformation/Guidances/ucm127073.pdf.

US Preventive Services Task Force. 2009. "Screening for Breast Cancer." Released in November, updated in December. www.uspreventiveservicestaskforce.org /uspstf/uspsbrca.htm.

————. 1989. *Guide to Clinical Preventive Services: An Assessment of the Effectiveness of 169 Interventions: Report of the U.S. Preventive Services Task Force.* Baltimore, MD: Williams & Wilkins.

Valdez, A., K. Banerjee, L. Ackerson, M. Fernandez, R. Otero-Sabogal, and C. P. Somkin. 2001. "Correlates of Breast Cancer Screening Among Low-Income, Low-Education Latinas." *Preventive Medicine* 33 (5): 495–502.

Valdmanis, V. G., M. D. Rosko, and R. L. Mutter. 2008. "Hospital Quality, Efficiency, and Input Slack Differentials." *Health Services Research* 43 (5 Pt. 2): 1830–48.

Vandenbroucke, J. P., E. von Elm, D. G. Altman, P. C. Gotzsche, C. D. Mulrow, S. J. Pocock, C. Poole, J. J. Schlesselman, and M. Egger. 2007. "Strengthening the Reporting of Observational Studies in Epidemiology (STROBE): Explanation and Elaboration." *PLoS Medicine* 4 (10): e297.

van Merode, F. 2010. "Judith D. de Jong: 'Explaining Medical Practice Variation—Social Organization and Institutional Mechanisms,' Utrecht, 2007." *Journal of Public Health* 18 (2): 205–206.

Vayda, E. 1973. "A Comparison of Surgical Rates in Canada and in England and Wales." *New England Journal of Medicine* 289 (23): 1224–29.

Veatch, R. M. 1989. *Death, Dying, and the Biological Revolution: Our Last Quest for Responsibility.* New Haven, CT: Yale University Press.

————. 1981. *A Theory of Medical Ethics.* New York: Basic Books.

Vernon, S. W., A. McQueen, J. A. Tiro, and D. J. del Junco. 2010. "Interventions to Promote Repeat Breast Cancer Screening with Mammography: A Systematic Review and Meta-Analysis." *Journal of the National Cancer Institute* 102 (14): 1023–39.

Vistnes, J., and T. Selden. 2011. "Premium Growth and Its Effect on Employer-Sponsored Insurance." *International Journal of Health Care Finance and Economics* 11 (1): 55–81.

Vita, M. G. 1990. "Exploring Hospital Production Relationships with Flexible Functional Forms." *Journal of Health Economics* 9 (1): 1–21.

von dem Knesebeck, O., G. Luschen, W. C. Cockerham, and J. Siegrist. 2003. "Socioeconomic Status and Health Among the Aged in the United States and Germany: A Comparative Cross-Sectional Study." *Social Science & Medicine* 57 (9): 1643–52.

von Elm, E., D. G. Altman, M. Egger, S. J. Pocock, P. C. Gotzsche, and J. P. Vandenbroucke. 2007. "Strengthening the Reporting of Observational Studies in Epidemiology (STROBE) Statement: Guidelines for Reporting Observational Studies." *BMJ* 335 (7624): 806–808.

Voti, L., L. C. Richardson, I. M. Reis, L. E. Fleming, J. Mackinnon, and J. W. Coebergh. 2006. "Treatment of Local Breast Carcinoma in Florida: The Role of the Distance to Radiation Therapy Facilities." *Cancer* 106 (1): 201–207.

Wagemakers, A., M. A. Koelen, J. Lezwijn, and L. Vaandrager. 2010. "Coordinated Action Checklist: A Tool for Partnerships to Facilitate and Evaluate Community Health Promotion." *Global Health Promotion* 17 (3): 17.

Wagner, E. H., T. M. Wickizer, A. Cheadle, B. M. Psaty, T. D. Koepsell, P. Diehr, S. J. Curry, M. Von Korff, C. Anderman, W. L. Beery, D. C. Pearson, and E. B. Perrin. 2000. "The Kaiser Family Foundation Community Health Promotion Grants Program: Findings from an Outcome Evaluation." *Health Services Research* 35 (3): 561–89.

Waitzkin, H., T. Britt, and C. Williams. 1994. "Narratives of Aging and Social Problems in Medical Encounters with Older Persons." *Journal of Health & Social Behavior* 35 (4): 322–48.

Wang, C. J., K. N. Conroy, and B. Zuckerman. 2009. "Payment Reform for Safety-Net Institutions—Improving Quality and Outcomes." *New England Journal of Medicine* 361 (19): 1821–23.

Ward, P. R., S. B. Meyer, F. Verity, T. K. Gill, and T. C. Luong. 2011. "Complex Problems Require Complex Solutions: The Utility of Social Quality Theory for Addressing the Social Determinants of Health." *BMC Public Health* 11: 630.

Ware, J. E. Jr., M. Kosinski, and B. Gandek. 2002. *SF-36 Health Survey: Manual and Interpretation Guide*. Lincoln, RI: QualityMetric Inc.

Ware, J. E. Jr., J. Phillips, B. B. Yody, and J. Adamczyk. 1996. "Assessment Tools: Functional Health Status and Patient Satisfaction." *American Journal of Medical Quality* 11 (1): S50–53.

Wassenaar, J. D., and S. L. Thran, eds. 2003. *Physician Socioeconomic Statistics, 2003 Edition*. Chicago: AMA Press.

Weech-Maldonado, R., L. S. Morales, K. Spritzer, M. Elliott, and R. D. Hays. 2001. "Racial and Ethnic Differences in Parents' Assessments of Pediatric Care in Medicaid Managed Care." *Health Services Research* 36 (3): 575–94.

Weeks, W. B., D. J. Gottlieb, D. J. Nyweide, J. M. Sutherland, J. Bynum, L. P. Casalino, R. R. Gillies, S. M. Shortell, and E. S. Fisher. 2010. "Higher Health Care Quality and Bigger Savings Found at Large Multispecialty Medical Groups." *Health Affairs (Millwood)* 29 (5): 991–97.

Weimer, D. L., and A. R. Vining. 1999. *Policy Analysis: Concepts and Practice*. Upper Saddle River, NJ: Prentice Hall.

Weiner, J. P. 1994. "Forecasting the Effects of Health Reform on US Physician Workforce Requirement: Evidence from HMO Staffing Patterns." *Journal of the American Medical Association* 272 (3): 222–30.

Weissman, J. S., A. M. Zaslavsky, R. E. Wolf, and J. Z. Ayanian. 2008. "State Medicaid Coverage and Access to Care for Low-Income Adults." *Journal of Health Care for the Poor and Underserved* 19 (1): 307–19.

Wennberg, J. E. 2005. "Variation in Use of Medicare Services Among Regions and Selected Academic Medical Centers: Is More Better?" Published December 13. New York: The Commonwealth Fund.

———. 2004. "Practice Variations and Health Care Reform: Connecting the Dots." *Health Affairs (Millwood)* Suppl. Variation: VAR140–44.

———. 1990. "Small Area Analysis and the Medical Care Outcome Problem." In *Research Metholology: Strengthening Causal Interpretations of Nonexperimental Data*, edited by L. Sechrest, E. Perrin, and J. Bunker, 177–206. Rockville, MD: US Department of Health and Human Services.

———. 1984. "Dealing with Medical Practice Variations: A Proposal for Action." *Health Affairs (Millwood)* 3 (2): 6–32.

Wennberg, J. E., J. P. Bunker, and B. Barnes. 1980. "The Need for Assessing the Outcome of Common Medical Practices." *Annual Review of Public Health* 1: 277–95.

Wennberg, J. E., E. S. Fisher, D. C. Goodman, and J. S. Skinner. 2008. *Tracking the Care of Patients with Severe Chronic Illness: The Dartmouth Atlas of Health Care 2008.* Lebanon, NH: Dartmouth Institute for Health Policy and Clinical Practice, Center for Health Policy Research.

Wennberg, J. E., E. S. Fisher, J. S. Skinner, and K. K. Bronner. 2007. "Extending the P4P Agenda, Part 2: How Medicare Can Reduce Waste and Improve the Care of the Chronically Ill." *Health Affairs (Millwood)* 26 (6): 1575–85.

Wennberg, J. E., and A. Gittelsohn. 1973. "Small Area Variations in Health Care Delivery." *Science* 182 (4117): 1102–108.

White, K. L., ed. 1992. *Health Services Research: An Anthology.* PAHO Scientific Publication 534. Washington, DC: Pan American Health Organization.

Wholey, D., R. Feldman, J. B. Christianson, and J. Engberg. 1996. "Scale and Scope Economies Among Health Maintenance Organizations." *Journal of Health Economics* 15 (6): 657–84.

Wickizer, T. M., M. Von Korff, A. Cheadle, J. Maeser, E. H. Wagner, D. Pearson, W. Beery, and B. M. Psaty. 1993. "Activating Communities for Health Promotion: A Process Evaluation Method." *American Journal of Public Health* 83 (4): 561–67.

Williams, A. H. 1990. "Ethics, Clinical Freedom and the Doctor's Role." In *Competition in Health Care: Reforming the NHS*, edited by A. J. Culyer, A. K. Maynard, and J. W. Posnett, 178–91. Basingstoke, UK: Palgrave Macmillan.

———. 1974. "'Need' as a Demand Concept (with special reference to health)." In *Economic Policies and Social Goals: Aspects of Public Choice*, edited by A. J. Culyer, 60–76. London: Martin Robertson.

Williams, D. R. 1994. "The Concept of Race in Health Services Research: 1966 to 1990." *Health Services Research* 29 (3): 261–74.

Williams, D. R., and S. A. Mohammed. 2009. "Discrimination and Racial Disparities in Health: Evidence and Needed Research." *Journal of Behavioral Medicine* 32 (1): 20–47.

Williams, S., F. Potter, N. Diaz-Tena, and R. Strouse. 2006. "Community Tracking Study Physician Survey Methodology Report 2004–05 (Round Four)." Washington, DC: Center for Studying Health System Change. http://hschange.org/CONTENT/888/888text.pdf.

Williams-Piehota, P., J. Pizarro, T. R. Schneider, L. Mowad, and P. Salovey. 2005. "Matching Health Messages to Monitor-Blunter Coping Styles to Motivate Screening Mammography." *Health Psychology* 24 (1): 58–67.

Williamson, J. W. 1978. "The Estimation of Achievable Health Care Benefit." In *Assessing and Improving Health Care Outcomes: The Health Accounting Approach to Quality Assurance*, edited by J. W. Williamson and R. Wilson, 51–69. Cambridge. MA: Ballinger Publishers.

Wolfe, B. L., and J. R. Behrman. 1987. "Women's Schooling and Children's Health: Are the Effects Robust with Adult Sibling Control for the Women's Childhood Background?" *Journal of Health Economics* 6 (3): 239–54.

Wolinsky, F. D. 1980. "The Performance of Health Maintenance Organizations: An Analytic Review." *Milbank Memorial Fund Quarterly. Health and Society* 58 (4): 537–87.

Woolhandler, S., T. Campbell, and D. U. Himmelstein. 2004. "Health Care Administration in the United States and Canada: Micromanagement, Macro Costs." *International Journal of Health Services* 34 (1): 65–78.

———. 2003. "Costs of Health Care Administration in the United States and Canada." *New England Journal of Medicine* 349 (8): 768–75.

World Health Organization (WHO). 2010. "Building Healthy Communities and Populations." Published September 1. www.wpro.who.int/regional_director/regional_directors_report/2010/media/rd10_3_dhp.pdf.

———. 2008. "The World Health Report 2008: Primary Health Care (Now More than Ever)." Geneva, Switzerland: WHO Press. www.who.int/whr/2008/whr08_en.pdf.

———. 2002. "The World Health Report 2002: Reducing Risks, Promoting Healthy Life." Geneva, Switzerland: World Health Organization. www.who.int/whr/2002/en/whr02_en.pdf.

———. 1999. "Healthy Cities: Evaluation of Programs." www.who.int/hpr2/archive/cities/evaluation.html.

Worrall, G., P. Chaulk, and D. Freake. 1997. "The Effects of Clinical Practice Guidelines on Patient Outcomes in Primary Care: A Systematic Review." *Canadian Medical Association Journal* 156 (12): 1705–12.

Xu, K. T. 2002. "Usual Source of Care in Preventive Service Use: A Regular Doctor Versus a Regular Site." *Health Services Research* 37 (6): 1509–29.

Yabroff, K. R., N. Breen, S. W. Vernon, H. I. Meissner, A. N. Freedman, and R. Ballard-Barbash. 2004. "What Factors Are Associated with Diagnostic Follow-Up After Abnormal Mammograms? Findings from a U.S. National Survey." *Cancer Epidemiology, Biomarkers & Prevention* 13 (5): 723–32.

Yu, H., and A. W. Dick. 2009. "Recent Trends in State Children's Health Insurance Program Eligibility and Coverage for CSHCN." *Pediatrics* 124 (Suppl. 4): S337–42.

Zakus, J. D., and C. L. Lysack. 1998. "Revisiting Community Participation." *Health Policy & Planning* 13 (1): 1–12.

Zarabozo, C., and S. Harrison. 2009. "Payment Policy and the Growth of Medicare Advantage." *Health Affairs (Millwood)* 28 (1): w55–67.

Zerzan, J., T. Edlund, L. Krois, and J. Smith. 2007. "The Demise of Oregon's Medically Needy Program: Effects of Losing Prescription Drug Coverage." *Journal of General Internal Medicine* 22 (6): 847–51.

Zweifel, P., F. Breyer, and M. Kifmann. 2009. *Health Economics*, second edition. New York: Springer.

INDEX

A/B/A trial study design, 43
A/B trial study design, 42–43
ACA. *See* Patient Protection and Affordable Care Act of 2010
Academy for Health Services Research and Health Policy committee, 2
AcademyHealth, 2
Access to care: Andersen–Aday model of, 29, 33, 136, 140, 214; effective, efficient, and equitable, 182; as a goal of equity, 161; health policy role in, 13; indicators of equity of, 185; for minorities, 175; potential access, 167–69; realized access, 169; socio-behavioral model of, 211. *See also* Delivery system of health services
Accountable care organizations (ACOs): ACA encouragement of, 60; characteristics of, 121; defining of, 109–10; as new delivery model, 18; payment incentives of, 19, 60, 78, 107; Shortell's models similarities to, 78
Aday, LuAnn, 3, 141, 165
Adjusted models, 51
Administration and production efficiency, 119–20
African Americans: breast cancer in, 20, 182–83; health disparities of, 72, 163–64; physician visits relative to need by, 192; uninsured, 190; unmet need of, 194; utilization of services by, 191–92; volume of use by, 193
Agency for Health Care Policy and Research (AHCPR), 9
Agency for Healthcare Research and Quality (AHRQ): clinical guidelines for policy analysis, 206; data resources of, 156; evolution of, 9; Medical Expenditure Panel Survey, 55; Patient Outcomes Research Teams, 97; practice guidelines of, 61–62; Quality Indicators program, 66; "Quality Information & Improvement" effort, 48; reporting of hospital mortality rates by, 62–63
AHA Commission on Financing, 8
AIDS/HIV, 163–64
Alliance for Health Policy and Systems Research (of WHO), 26
Allocative efficiency: achieving, 126; in evidence of efficiency, 110–17; in market-minimized systems, 105; overview of, 81, 83–86; in policy analysis, 208, 209, 211, 217; production functions applied to, 94; used in programmatic investments, 98. *See also* Efficiency/efficacy
American Cancer Society, 220
American College of Physicians, 97
American Hospital Association (AHA), 8, 156
American Medical Association (AMA), 7, 91, 156
American Recovery and Reinvestment Act (ARRA) of 2009, 9, 63, 65
Analytical research, 158–59, 216
Andersen–Aday model of access to care, 29, 33, 136, 140, 214
Attitudinal scales, 176
Australia, 196–97

Balanced Budget Act of 1997, 106, 121
Behavioral Risk Factor Surveillance System, 55. *See also* CDC
Bias: in A/B/A trial designs, 43; controlling of by statistical design, 50–51, 159; in evaluation of evidence, 33; in generalizability, 35; types of, 42, 43, 45, 52, 54
Biomedical research, focus of, 3, 4
Blacks. *See* African Americans
Blind trials, 44–45
Breast cancer: equity promotion in screening and treatment of, 177–83, 178–80; Georgia MBCCP findings, 226; in Hispanics, 183, 240; Medicaid for Breast and Cervical Cancer Program (MBCCP), 221–22; National Breast and Cervical Cancer Early Detection Program (NBCCEDP), 183, 219–21; outcomes in African-Americans, 20; Texas Breast and Cervical Cancer Services (TBCCS), 181. *See also* Mammography screening
Breast cancer case study: analyzing results, 231–38; background, 219–22; BCCS eligibility process, 223; cases detected through BCCS/MBCCP, 233, 233, 238; conclusion and recommendations, 238–43; cost-effectiveness analysis, 236, 237; criteria and measures for evaluation, 224, 224–31; decision tree model of efficiency analysis, 227, 227–29; identifying objectives, 222–23; logic model of impact, 222–23, 223; mammography screening program extension data, 234; overview, 219; reimbursement rates for screening and diagnostic services, 235; Texas Breast and Cervical Cancer Services (TBCCS), 183, 221

California Relative Value Scale, 91
Canada: administrative costs in, 119; consumer satisfaction in, 109, 196–97; disease-specific comparisons of US and, 98; healthcare spending in, 117; health indicator monitoring in, 75–76; hospital payment methods in, 108–109; Lalonde report, 66, 68; pharmacoeconomics in, 96; physician payment methods in, 107–108; population-based surveys in, 68; service utilization in, 114, 116
Cancer, 20, 73–74, 112, 154–55. *See also* Breast cancer
Capital theory, 94
Case study designs, 39–41
Center for Studying Health System Change, 157
Centers for Disease Control and Prevention (CDC): data resources of, 156; health indicator data role, 70; Healthy Communities Program, 162; public health funding by, 22; role in breast cancer prevention, 220. *See also* Behavioral Risk Factor Surveillance System; National Center for Health Statistics
Centers for Medicare & Medicaid Services (CMS): data resources of, 156, 157; Hospital Compare